Disc	Root	MotorF	Sensory	Reflex
C5–6	C6	Biceps, wrist ext.	Med. arm and hand	Biceps
C6–7*	C7	Triceps, wrist flex.	Middle finger	Triceps
C7-T1	C8	Finger flex.	Lat. hand	Finger
L3–4	L4	Quadriceps	Med. calf	Knee
L4–5*	L5	Dorsiflexors	Med. foot	—
L5-S1	S1	Plantar flexors	Lat. foot	Ankle

* Most common.

Table 1. Symptoms of disc herniation.

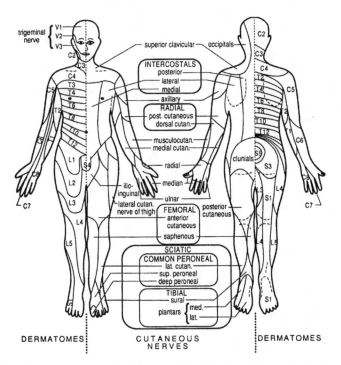

Figure 2. Dermatomes and peripheral nerve territories. (From Patton HD, et al. *Introduction to Basic Neurology.* Philadelphia: Saunders, 1976, with permission.)

EMERGENCIES

THE
MASSACHUSETTS GENERAL HOSPITAL
Handbook of Neurology

SECOND EDITION

Alice W. Flaherty
Natalia S. Rost

Contributors:
Beau Bruce, M.D.
Andrew Chi, M.D., Ph.D.
Tracey Cho, M.D.
Edward Gilmore, M.D.
Andrew Norden, M.D.
Kevin Sheth, M.D.

*Massachusetts General Hospital,
Harvard Medical School
Boston, Massachusetts*

Wolters Kluwer | Lippincott Williams & Wilkins
Health
Philadelphia · Baltimore · New York · London
Buenos Aires · Hong Kong · Sydney · Tokyo

Acquisitions Editor: Frances Destefano
Managing Editor: Leanne McMillan
Project Manager: Alicia Jackson
Manufacturing Manager: Kathleen Brown
Marketing Manager: Kimberly Schonberger
Creative Director: Doug Smock
Producti
Printer

© 200

530 W
Philad
LWW.

First E

All rig
form b
tem wi
ical ar
cial du

Printe
Libra
Flaher
  The
contri
  p
  Incl
  ISB
  ISB
  1. N
3. Me
Handt
  [DN
2007]
  RC
  616

Care l
accept
sions
expre
the p
respo
Mark

The a
forth
tion.
of inf
insert
This

Som
(FDA
provi

To pt
fax o

Visit
custo

CONTENTS

ABBREVIATIONS

Abbreviations used only locally are defined in that section.

A fib: atrial fibrillation
Ab: antibody
Abx: antibiotics
ABG: acute blood gas
ACA: anterior cerebral artery
ACD: anticonvulsant drug
ACE: angiotensin-converting enzyme
ACE-I: ACE inhibitor
ACh: acetylcholine
A-comm: anterior communicating artery
AFB: acid fast bacillus stain for TB
Ag: antigen
AICA: anterior inferior cerebellar artery
AKA: also known as
ALS: amyotrophic lateral sclerosis
ANA: antinuclear antibody
ANS: autonomic nervous system
ant.: anterior
AV: atrioventricular
AVM: arteriovenous malformation
bid: twice a day (Latin: *bis in die*)
BP: blood pressure
BUN: blood urea nitrogen
bx: biopsy
Ca: calcium
CAD: coronary artery disease
CBC: complete blood count
CHF: congestive heart failure
Cl: chloride
CMV: cytomegalovirus
CN: cranial nerve
CNS: central nervous system
COPD: chronic obstructive pulmonary
        disease
CPAP: continuous positive airway
        pressure
CPK: creatine phosphokinase
Cr: creatinine
CJD: Creutzfeldt-Jacob disease
CSF: cerebrospinal fluid
CT: computed tomography
CXR: chest x-ray
D5: 5% dextrose
DA: dopamine
DBP: diastolic blood pressure
d/c: discontinue

DDx: differential diagnosis
DIC: disseminated intravascular
        coagulation
DM: diabetes mellitus
DPH: phenytoin (diphenyl hydantoin)
DTR: deep tendon reflex
DVT: deep venous thrombosis
DWI: diffusion-weighted MRI
DWM: dead white male
dz: disease
EBV: Epstein-Barr virus
EEG: electroencephalogram
EKG: electrocardiogram
EMG: electromyography
EOM: extraocular movement
ER: emergency room
esp.: especially
ESR: erythrocyte sedimentation rate
ETT: exercise tolerance test
EVD: external ventricular drain
GABA: gamma-aminobutyric acid
GBM: glioblastoma multiforme
GBS: Guillain-Barré syndrome
GI: gastrointestinal
H&P: history and physical exam
h/o: history of
HA: headache
HCG: human chorionic gonadotropin
Hct: hematocrit
Hg: mercury
HLA: human leukocyte group A
HOB: head of bed
HR: heart rate
HSV: herpes simplex virus
5-HT: serotonin
HTN: hypertension
I/Os: inputs and outputs
ICA: internal carotid artery
ICH: intracranial hemorrhage
ICP: intracranial pressure
ICU: intensive care unit
Ig: immunoglobulin
IM: intramuscular
inf.: Inferior
INR: international normalized PTT ratio
IQ: intelligence quotient

IU: international units
IV: intravenous
IVDA: intravenous drug abuse
IVIg: intravenous immunoglobulins
K: potassium level
L: left
LFT: liver function test
LMN: lower motor neuron
LOC: loss of consciousness
LP: lumbar puncture
LV: left ventricle
MAOI: monoamine oxidase inhibitor
Max.: maximum
MCA: middle cerebral artery
MCV: mean corpuscular volume
MI: myocardial infarction
MLF: medial longitudinal fasciculus
MRA: magnetic resonance angiogram
MRI: magnetic resonance image
MS: multiple sclerosis
N/V: nausea and vomiting
NCS: nerve conduction studies
NE: norepinephrine
nl: normal
NMJ: neuromuscular junction
NPH: normal pressure hydrocephalus
NPO: nothing by mouth
NS: normal saline
NSAID: nonsteroidal anti-inflammatory drug
nu.: nucleus
OCD: obsessive-compulsive disorder
OR: operating room
PCA: posterior cerebral artery
P-comm: posterior communicating artery
PCR: polymerase chain reaction
PE: pulmonary embolus
PET: positron emission tomography
PICA: posterior inferior cerebellar artery
PMN: polymorphonuclear leukocyte
PNS: peripheral nervous system
PO: by mouth
post.: posterior
Post-op: postoperative
PPD: purified protein derivative test (TB)
Pre-op: preoperative
prn: as needed (Latin: *pro re nata*)
PSNS: parasympathetic nervous system
PSP: progressive supranuclear palsy
pt: patient
PT: prothrombin time

PTT: partial thromboplastin time
PTX: pneumothorax
q: every (Latin: *quaque*)
qd: daily
qhs: nightly
qid: four times a day
qod: every other day
R: right
r/o: rule out
RBC: red blood cell
REM: rapid eye movement sleep
RF: rheumatoid factor
RPR: rapid plasmin reagent test
RV: right ventricle
Rx: treatment
SAH: subarachnoid hemorrhage
SBP: systolic blood pressure
SC: subcutaneous
SCA: superior cerebellar artery
SDH: subdural hemorrhage
SE: side effect
SIADH: syndrome of inappropriate antid-iuretic hormone secretion
SIEP: serum immunoelectrophoresis
SL: sublingual
SLE: systemic lupus erythematosus
SNRI: serotonin-norepinephrine reuptake inhibitor
SPECT: single photon emission CT
SSRI: selective serotonin reuptake inhibitor
stat: immediate (Latin: *statim*)
sup.: superior
Sx: symptoms, signs
TB: tuberculosis
TCA: tricyclic antidepressant
TEE: transesophageal echocardiogram
TIA: transient ischemic attack
tid: three times a day (Latin: *ter in die*)
TSH: thyroid stimulating hormone
UA: urinalysis
UBJ: urine Bence-Jones protein
UMN: upper motor neuron
V fib: ventricular fibrillation
V/Q: ventilation-perfusion lung scan
VDRL: venereal disease research lab test
VP: ventriculoperitoneal
VS: vital signs
VZV: varicella zoster virus
WBC: white blood cell
XRT: radiation therapy

FOREWORD TO THE SECOND EDITION

As with the first edition, this handbook's goals are to quickly remind and update the reader. It therefore strives to be well cross-referenced, terse, and thin—a pocket book should really fit in the pocket. We have tried to keep in mind that the head is actually connected to the body, and include sections on medicine and other related disciplines. The book provides a clear framework for action, without neglecting the complexity that arises when protocols are applied to real patients. Its tendency towards algorithm makes it a practical tool for non-neurologists.

In the second edition we have added 20% more material, including revolutionary advances in fields like cerebrovascular disease and neuroimaging, without skimping on such common problems as migraine. We also tried to make the prose 10% less sedating than other leading neurology texts.

This second edition owes its existence to Natalia Rost, who first coaxed me into starting the revision, then donated more assistance than I ever expected, and finally changed the shape of many sections by—always tactfully—leading me out of conceptual errors. Drs. Beau Bruce, Andrew Chi, Tracey Cho, Edward Gilmore, Andrew Norden and Kevin Sheth at MGH made inestimable contributions in updating the book. Editors Fran Destefano, Leanne McMillan, and Angelique Amig helped greatly, as did (and does) my first editor Charley Mitchell.

Many other colleagues have influenced both the book and us, including William I. (not J.) Bennett, Robert Brown, Ferdinando Buonanno, Keith Chiappa, Andrew Cole, William Copen, Bradford Dickerson, Gregory Fricchione, Michael Greene, John Growdon, Timothy Hain, John Henson, John Herman, Daniel Hoch, David Hooper, Paymon Hosseini, Farish Jenkins, Barry Kosofsky, Robert LaZebnik, Beverly Mahfuz, Jerrold Rosenbaum, Jonathan Rosand, Lee Schwamm, Katherine Sims, Lisa Townsend, Katharina Trede, Marion Stein, Shirley Wray, and—always both last and first—Anne Young.

Natalia and I would love to thank our husbands, Abdul Traish and Andrew Hrycyna respectively, but want to neglect that acknowledgment ritual of calling spouses "long-suffering."

The book is dedicated to Walter Koroshetz, who departed this MGH life—for the NINDS—as galleys went to press. We wish we had more than words to offer in thanks for all that he has taught us by example.

Alice Flaherty, M.D., Ph.D.
Director, Movement Disorders Fellowship,
Massachusetts General Hospital
Harvard Medical School

ADMISSIONS

A. Note: Most important features are underlined, but these are guidelines only. It can be wasteful and, in emergencies, even dangerous to test everything.

GENERAL EXAM

A. VS: <u>BP, HR, temperature</u>, respirations, orthostatic BP.
B. Skin: Petechiae, rash, striae, telangiectasias, caput medusae.
C. Head: For trauma exam, see p. 119.
   1. Eye: <u>Papilledema</u>, retinopathy, icterus.
   2. Skull: Trauma, craniotomy.
   3. Other: Temporal wasting or tenderness, ears, nose, throat, thrush.
D. Neck: <u>Stiffness, carotids/bruits</u>, thyroid, jugular distension, nodes.
E. Back: <u>Lungs</u>, spine tenderness, pelvic stability.
F. Chest: <u>Heart</u>, breasts, nodes.
G. Abdomen: Bowel sounds, bruits, palpation, nodes, liver, hernias, scars.
H. Genitourinary: Hair, testis size/masses, lesions, pelvic exam.
I. Rectal: <u>Guaiac</u>, masses, tenderness, tone.
J. Limbs: <u>Pulses</u>, color, edema, splinters/clubbing, calf pain, Homan's sign, range of motion, straight leg raise.

NEUROLOGICAL EXAM

A. Mental status: For coma exam, see p. 30. For psychiatric mental status exam (including the Mini-Mental Status Exam), see p. 98
   1. Orientation: <u>Self, date, place</u>.
   2. Attention: <u>Say months backwards</u>; spell "world" backwards.
   3. Memory: <u>3 objects, presidents</u>.
   4. Speech: <u>Naming, fluency, comprehension, repetition,</u> read/writing.
      a. F test: Number of words beginning with F in 60 sec (>12 if high school education).
      b. Passive construction comprehension.
   5. Frontal:
      a. Perseveration: Go-no go task, copying Luria diagram.
      b. Disinhibition: Snout, grasp, imitation behavior.
      c. Abulia: Affect, response latency.
   6. Parietal:
      a. Neglect: Limb recognition, clock draw, bisect line.
      b. Calculations: Serial 7's, etc.
      c. Praxis: Blowing out a match, tying a shoe.
      d. Spatial orientation: Directions, commands across midline.
      e. Agnosia: Finger agnosia, anosognosia, alexia without agraphia, color naming.
   7. Cognition: Insight, judgment, logic, proverbs, subjunctives.

8. Thought content: Hallucinations, delusions, paranoia.
9. Mood: SIGECAPS criteria, suicidal or homicidal ideation, mania.

B. Cranial nerves:

CN I: Smell.

CN II: Pupils, fundi; fields, acuity, blink to threat, red desaturation. Pts with hysterical blindness (see p. 104) or cortical blindness have normal pupils, blink to threat.

CN III, IV, VI: Horner's, EOMs, saccades, pursuit, optokinetic reflex, cover-uncover test, red glass test, upper lid.

CN V: Sensation of forehead/cheek/chin, corneals, jaw.

CN VII: Symmetry, brow raise, eye close, nose wrinkle, grimace, cheek puff, anterior taste.

CN VIII: Tympani, hearing (see p. 54), balance Bárány's test.

CN IX-XII: Palate, gag, sternocleidomastoid, trapezius, tongue.

C. Motor:

1. **Strength:** <u>Drift, fine finger movements</u>, heel/toe walk, knee bends.
   a. **Individual muscles:** Include hip adductors, pronation/supination, inversion/eversion, abdominal muscles.
   b. **Subtle signs:** Wartenberg's (pull flexed fingers; thumb flexes), stress gait (walk on outside of feet, look for posturing), mirror movements with finger sequencing, testing multiple repeats.
2. **Bulk:** Atrophy, fasciculations.
3. **Tone:** Rigidity, spasticity, cogwheeling, dystonic posturing, myotonia. If pt. not cooperative, drop limb to test tone (malingering pts. may not let limb hit face).
4. **Extra movements:** Tremor, dysmetria, myoclonus, tics, dyskinesias, asterixis.
5. **Reflexes:** Biceps, triceps, brachioradialis, knee, ankle, Babinski.
   a. **If brisk:** Check clonus, spreading, palmomental, jaw jerk, Hoffman's sign (flick nail down, watch for thumb contraction).
   b. **If frontal damage:** Glabellar, grasp, snout, suck.
   c. **If spinal cord injury:** Abdominals, suprapubic, cremasteric, wink, bulbocavernosus.
6. **Tests for hysterical weakness:** See p. 103.

D. Cerebellar:

1. **Appendicular:** Finger-to-nose, rapid alternating movements, fine finger movements, finger following ("mirror test"), lack of check, toe tapping, heel-to-shin, decreased tone, arm swings after shaking shoulders (nl <3), pendular reflexes.
2. **Axial:** Gait, tandem, axial stability, stand on line, walk in circle, march with eyes closed (advancing more than a few feet or rotating more than 30 degrees in 30 sec is abnormal).
3. **Voice:** Dysarthria, holding a tone, la-la-la, say "Methodist-Episcopal," count to 20 fast.

E. Sensory:

1. **Pin:** All 4 limbs; trunk for level; nerve distributions, summation.
2. **Light touch:** Cotton wisp; 2-point discrimination.
3. **Proprioception:** Joint position, vibration, Romberg, nose touch.
4. **Cortical:** Dual simultaneous extinction, stereognosis, graphesthesia.

5. **Temperature:** Try side of tuning fork or alcohol swab.
6. **Anal:** If you suspect spinal cord lesion, check anal wink, tone, bulbocavernosus reflex.
7. **Tests for hysterical weakness:** See p. 103.

ADMISSION ORDERS

A. **Notifications:** Speak to family members; the senior resident; private neurologist; internist, floor or nurse accepting the pt.
B. **Orders:** ADCVAANDISCL.
   1. **Admit:** Service, admitting physician, resident to page.
   2. **Diagnosis:** Be specific.
   3. **Condition:** Good, fair, guarded, critical.
   4. **Vital signs:** Specify only if other than per routine.
   5. **Allergies:** List the reaction too, e.g., "contrast dye → anaphylaxis."
   6. **Activity:** Bedrest with head up 30 degrees? Up with assist? Ad lib?
   7. **Nursing:** Pneumo-boots? Guaiac all stools? Etc. Nurses get annoyed that MDs call this category "nursing"—it is all nursing.
   8. **Diet:** NPO? Aspiration precautions? Low salt or cholesterol? DM? Renal? Dysphagia?
   9. **Ins/Outs:** Done automatically in most ICUs; harder to do on general wards. If it is important, consider a bladder catheter. Daily weights may need a special request outside the ICU.
   10. **Special:**
       a. **Oxygen or ventilator settings.**
       b. **Bleed risk?** Blood bank sample, guaiac stools, orthostatic BP, large-bore IV.
       c. **CHF?** Strict I/Os, daily weights.
       d. **Chest pain?** Oxygen, cardiac monitor, bedside commode, CPK/isoenzymes/troponins q8h × 3.
       e. **Mental status change?** (see p. 42) Restraint × 72 h prn safety, aspiration precautions.
       f. **Clot risk?** Pneumo-boots, SC or low MW heparin (if DVT, full anticoagulation, elevate foot, bedrest), neurovascular checks.
       g. **Hyper- or hypotension:** BP parameters and drugs.
       h. **Skin care.**
   11. **Consults:** Consider social service, physical therapy, occupational therapy, speech/swallow. . .
   12. **Tests (Labs):** bid PTT? Daily PT/INR? qod electrolytes/BUN/Cr?
C. **Drugs:** Consider
   1. **Rehydration?** D5NS at 60 cc/h if concern for brain edema.
   2. **Sleeping pill?** (Avoid if pt confused). See p. 112. Zolpidem 5-10 mg, diphenhydramine 25-50 mg, or lorazepam 0.5-1.0 mg.
   3. **Pain?** Acetaminophen 650 mg q4h prn, opiate + constipation rx, etc.
   4. **GI?** E.g., senna tablets, omeprazole 20 mg qd, bisacodyl (Dulcolax) + PR qd prn, milk of magnesia 30 cc q8h prn.

    5. Diabetes? NPH insulin + regular (CZI) sliding scale: for BG <200: 0U; 200-249: 2U; 250-299: 4U; 300-349: 6U; 350-399: 8U; >400: 10U. Alternatively, substitute aspart or lispro at night.

      a. Hypertension? E.g., captopril 25 mg PO, or metoprolol 50 mg PO bid prn SBP >180. For IV drugs, see p. 172.

      b. Hypotension? IV fluids; consider midodrine 10 mg PO tid or IV drugs (see p. 172).

    6. Chest pain? Avoid hypotension in stroke or carotid dz.

      a. SL nitroglycerine: 0.3 mg q5min prn × 3 while SBP >120.

      b. NTP SS: q4h for SBP <120: wipe, 120-134: 0.5 in.; 135-149: 1 in.; 150-164: 1.5 in.; >165: 2 in.

D. Admission note: Age, handedness, chief complaint, history of present illness, past medical history, allergies, medicines, family and social history (always include education), review of systems, physical exam, labs, assessment, plan.

    1. Assessment by issues: Neuro, cardiovascular (pump, rate, rhythm, valves, etc.), pulmonary, renal, fluids/electrolytes/nutrition, infectious dz, GI, GU, hematologic, endocrine, dermatologic, oncologic, orthopedic, psychiatric, rheumatologic, code status, discharge plan.

    2. Etiologies: Traumatic, vascular, high ICP, toxic, metabolic, psychiatric, infectious, inflammatory, neoplastic, epileptic, degenerative.

ADULT NEUROLOGY
APHASIA, AGNOSIA, APRAXIA, AND AMNESIA

A. **Aphasia:** Language disorder—versus the motor disorder of dysarthria.
   1. **Three questions:** Is the pt.'s speech fluent? Does pt. comprehend speech? Can pt. repeat it? See endpapers at back of book for picture naming and reading samples.

Type of Aphasia	Speech Fluent?	Compre-hends?	Repeats Phrases?	Lesion Location
Global	No	No	No	Does not localize
Expressive (Broca's)	No	Yes	No	Inf. frontal gyrus
Receptive (Wernicke's)	Yes	No	No	Sup. temporal gyrus
Transcortical motor	No	Yes	Yes	Premotor cortex
Transcortical sensory	Yes	No	Yes	Occipitotemporal cx.
Conductive	Yes	Yes	No	Subcortical MCA territ.
Amnestic (anomia)	Yes	Yes	Yes	Alzheimer's, etc.

Table 2. Major aphasia categories.

   2. **Jargon-based aphasia of the physician (JBAP):** Onset between the third year of medical school and internship. Speech fluent but incomprehensible in severe cases. JBAP lowers pt compliance (see p. 105). Pathognomonic signs include saying "lower extremity" instead of "leg" to a pt., or saying "micturition" to anyone at all.

B. **Evolution of aphasia:** Expressive or receptive aphasia from strokes commonly starts as global aphasia acutely; only later becomes clearly productive or receptive aphasia. The amnestic aphasia of Alzheimer's dz may evolve into a full-blown receptive aphasia.

C. **Alexia, agraphia, and acalculia:** Respectively, inability to read, write, or do arithmetic. Usually from lesions of the left angular gyrus. For alexia without agraphia, see Eyes and Vision, p. 44.

D. **Amnesia:** Poor memory storage (anterograde amnesia) or recall (retrograde amnesia). Often a hippocampal or paramedian thalamic lesion.

E. **Agnosia:** Impairment of recognition in a single modality, as opposed to amnesia, in which impairment includes all modalities.
   1. **Anosognosia:** Unawareness of neurological deficit. Usually from right parietotemporal lesion.
   2. **Neglect:** Disregard of stimuli arising from one side of the body, usually the left, from right parietal lesion.
   3. **Object agnosia:** Usually from bilateral posterior temporal lobe lesion.
   4. **Visual agnosias:** See p. 45.

F. Apraxia: Inability to do a task for cognitive rather than motor reasons.
   1. **Ideomotor apraxia:** Disordered complex movement sequencing, e.g., perseveration or distortion. Often L premotor or parietal lesion.
   2. **Constructional apraxia:** Disorder of spatial design, drawing. Usually R parietal lesion.

BRAINSTEM ANATOMY

A. See also: Figure 6, Cranial nerve nuclei, p. 34.

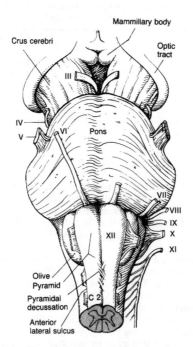

Figure 3. The ventral surface of the brainstem. (From Duus P. *Topical Diagnosis in Neurology*. New York: Thieme, 1983:101, with permission.)

B. Slice anatomy: For easier comparison with MRIs, the five images in Figure 4 are in radiologic convention, as if looking up from the feet, upside down and backwards from neuropathologic convention. In order, they show the upper medulla, lower pons, midpons, upper pons, and midbrain.

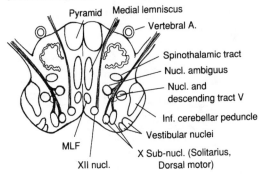

UPPER MEDULLA

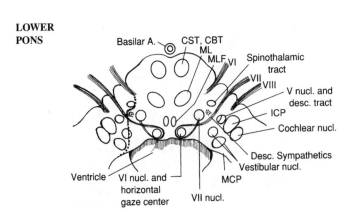

LOWER PONS

Figure 4. Brainstem cross-sections drawn in radiologic convention. (From Schwamm L. In Batjer HH, ed. *Cerebrovascular Disease*. Philadelphia: Lippincott, 1996, with permission.) Continued on next page.

MID-PONS

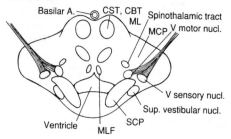

UPPER PONS

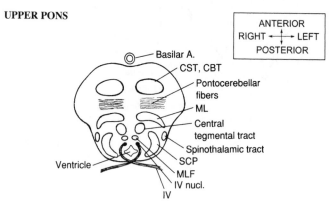

MID-BRAIN

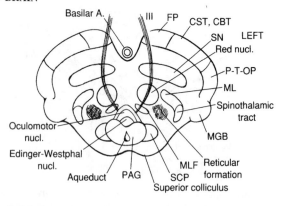

Figure 4. (Continued)

Condition	OP (cm H$_2$O)	Color	Cells/mm^3	Protein (mg%)	Glucose (CSF ÷ serum)	Miscellaneous
Normal adult	6-20	Clear	0 PMN, 0 RBC, <5 mono	15-45	0.5	Lymph/PMN ratio = 100/0
Normal child	6-20	Clear	<5 WBCs	5-40	~0.5	
Normal term	8-10	Clear	<8 WBCs	90	~0.5	Lymph/PMN = 40/60
Normal preemie		Clear	<9 WBCs	115	~0.5	Lymph/PMN = 40/60
Acute bacterial meningitis	~Up	Turbid	>100 WBCs, mostly PMNs	100-1,000	<0.2	Do rapid antigen tests
Viral meningoen-cephalitis	nl	Clear	10-350 WBCs, mostly monos	40-100	nl	PMNs early
Toxoplasmosis	~Up	Clear	nl or up	Usually high	~Up	CSF often nl
Tuberculous meningitis	~Up	Pearly, clumps	50-500 lymphs and monos	60-700	0.2-0.4	Do AFB culture and stain
Fungal meningitis	~Up	Pearly monos (PMNs early)	30-300	100-700	<0.3	Do India ink prep for crypto
HSV encephalitis	~Up	Pink	High monos and RBCs	High (nl early)	~Down	WBCs nl in 3%; PCR for antigen
Parameningeal infection	Up if block	Clear	0-800 WBCs	High	nl	E.g., epidural abscess
Neurosyphilis	nl	Clear	0-300	High (nl late)	nl	Oligoclonal band, antitreponema Ab
Leptome-ningeal metastasis	~Up	~Clear	0-500	nl or up	~Down	Cytology shows tumor in 50%
Multiple sclerosis	nl	Clear	5-50 monos	nl-800	nl	Oligoclonal bands
Guillain-Barré syndrome	nl	Clear	nl to 100 monos	50-1,000	nl	Protein nl early
Bloody tap (traumatic)	nl	Pink → yellow	RBC/WBC ratio like blood	Slightly up	nl	Less blood in following tubes
Subarachnoid hemorrhage	Up	Pink → yellow	RBC/WBC < blood (nl early)	50-800	nl	RBCs last 2 wks; xantho longer
Pseudotumor cerebri	25-50	Clear	nl	nl	nl	Do large-volume therapeutic tap

Table 3. CSF findings by disease.

CEREBROSPINAL FLUID

A. Lumbar puncture technique: See p. 224.
B. CSF findings by dz:
C. Dz by CSF profile:
1. **Many PMNs, low sugar, high protein:**
    a. **Infectious:** Bacterial meningitis, early viral or TB meningitis, parameningeal infections, septic emboli.
    b. **Noninfectious:** Chemical meningitis, Behçet's dz, Mollaret's recurrent meningitis.
2. **Many lymphocytes, low sugar, high protein:** TB, fungal, or partially treated/resolving bacterial meningitis, viral meningitis, carcinomatous meningitis, meningeal sarcoidosis.
3. **Many lymphocytes, normal sugar, high protein:** Viral meningitis or encephalitis, partially treated/resolving bacterial meningitis, para-meningeal infections, early fungal or TB meningitis, parasitic infections, postinfectious encephalomyelitis, active demyelinating dz.
D. Skull CSF leak: May be a sign of CSF obstruction.
1. **H&P:** Skull trauma, transsphenoidal surgery, clear watery nasal or ear drainage when leaning forward or sneezing. Have pt. lean forward for several min to elicit nasal discharge.
2. **Tests:** To tell CSF from nasal secretions.
    a. **Handkerchief test:** When CSF dries on tissue (e.g., Kleenex), it is still flexible. Snot is stiff.
    b. **Vodka test:** Nasal mucin precipitates in alcohol; CSF does not.
    c. **Dip stick:** Glucose is positive in CSF, not in snot.
    d. **Labs:** CSF glucose >20, chloride > serum Cl. Tau/transferrin.
3. **Rx:** Elevate the HOB. If there is a transsphenoidal incision, reinforce it with more sutures or several coats of colloidon. Lumbar drain; pro-phylactic nafcillin × 3 days. Hang drain bag as low as possible with-out causing headache (usually level of heart).
E. LP headache/spinal CSF leak: See Headache, p. 52.

CEREBROVASCULAR ISCHEMIA

A. Acute stroke evaluation: Always an emergency because aggressive emergent rx is available (see below).
1. **The ABBA of acute stroke:** Determines whether pt is eligible for intervention. Emergent CT/CTA helps with the last two.
    a. **Acuity?** When did symptoms start?
    b. **Badness?** How severe are they?
    c. **Bleeding?** Intracranial blood is an absolute contraindication for tPA
    d. **Anterior vs. posterior?** I.e., carotid vs. vertebrobasilar territory.
2. **Acuity:** If pt. awoke with sx, count time from when last seen normal. Time of onset cutoffs for acute stroke rx vary with vascular source.
    a. **Anterior circulation:** Acute usually defined as sx beginning <3 h ago, but rx now available for anterior circulation strokes up to 9 h (or more if sx fluctuate, esp. with BP).
    b. **Posterior circulation:** Up to 24 h for posterior circulation strokes.

3. **NIH Stroke Scale:** This standardized exam will answer the first two questions of ABBA. Add scores for total. Higher score is worse.
   a. **Level of consciousness:** 0 = alert and responsive; 1 = arousable to minor stimuli; 2 = arousable only to pain; 3 = reflex responses or unarousable.
   b. **Orientation:** Ask pt.'s name and month. Must be exact. 0 = both correct; 1 = one correct (or dysarthria, intubated, foreign language); 2 = neither correct.
   c. **Commands:** Open/close eyes, grip and release nonparetic hand (mimicry or another 1-step command okay). 0 = both correct (okay if impaired by weakness); 1 = one correct; 2 = neither correct.
   d. **Best gaze:** Horizontal EOM by voluntary or Doll's test. 0 = normal; 1 = partial palsy (abnormal in one or both eyes); 2 = forced eye deviation or total paresis that cannot be overcome by Doll's.
   e. **Visual field:** Use visual threat if necessary. If monocular, score field of good eye. 0 = normal; 1 = quadrantanopia, partial hemianopia, or extinction; 2 = complete hemianopia; 3 = blindness.
   f. **Facial palsy:** If stuporous, check grimace to pain. 0 = normal; 1 = minor paralysis (flat nasolabial fold, asymmetric smile); 2 = partial paralysis (lower face); 3 = complete paralysis (lower and upper face).
   g. **Motor arms:** Arms outstretched 90 degrees (sitting) or 45 degrees (supine) for 10 sec. Encourage best effort. 0 = no drift × 10 sec; 1 = drift but does not hit bed; 2 = some antigravity effort, but cannot sustain; 3 = no antigravity effort, but even minimal movement counts; 4 = no movement at all; X = cannot assess due to amputation, fracture, etc.
   h. **Motor legs:** Score like motor arms (see above).
   i. **Limb ataxia:** Check finger-nose and heel-shin; score only if out of proportion to paresis. 0 = no ataxia (or aphasia, hemiplegic); 1 = ataxia in arm or leg; 2 = ataxia in arm AND leg; X = unable to assess, as above.
   j. **Sensory:** Use pin. Check grimace or withdrawal if stuporous. Score only stroke-related losses. 0 = normal; 1 = mild-moderate unilateral loss but pt. aware of touch (or aphasic or confused); 2 = total unilateral loss, pt. unaware of touch; 3 = bilateral loss or coma.
   k. **Best language:** Describe cookie jar or picture; name objects; read sentences. May use repeating, writing, stereognosis. 0 = normal; 1 = mild-mod aphasia (but comprehensible); 2 = severe aphasia (almost no info exchanged); 3 = mute, no one-step commands, coma.
   l. **Dysarthria:** Read list of words. 0 = normal; 1 = mild-mod slurring; 2 = severe, unintelligible, or mute; X = intubation or mechanical barrier.
   m. **Extinction/neglect:** Simultaneously touch pt on both hands, show fingers in both visual fields, ask about deficit, left hand. 0 = normal; 1 = neglects or extinguishes to double stimulation in any modality; 2 = profound neglect in more than one modality.
4. **Bleed risk:** Ask about anticoagulant use, HA, neck/eye pain, recent trauma, rectal bleeding. Visible stroke on CT increases bleed risk.

5. **Anterior vs. posterior circulation stroke:** Save more precise localization for later. The following sx are a <u>rough</u> guide.
   a. **Anterior:** Preserved alertness, aphasia; neglect; both weak and numb in face + arm without leg OR in leg without face + arm; horizontal gaze palsy in which pt. looks away from paretic side.
   b. **Posterior:** Ataxia; vertigo, N/V; cranial nerve deficits; altered consciousness; bilateral or crossed sensory and motor deficits; crossed dissociation of proprioception from pain sensation, horizontal gaze palsy in which pt looks towards paretic side.
6. **The rest of the H&P:** Do this only after the NIH Stroke Scale and getting pt at top of queue for emergent CT.
   a. **Other causes and complications:** LOC, seizure-like activity, previous strokes and their deficits, etc.
   b. **Vascular risk factors:** HTN, smoking, obesity, DM, hyperlipidemia, male sex, age, angina, MIs, PVD, pregnancy, oral contraceptive use, family history of early MIs or strokes.
   c. **Detailed exam:** See sx of specific stroke syndromes, p. 26.

B. **See also:** venous sinus thrombosis, p. 126; transient monocular blindness, p. 45; hemorrhagic strokes, p. 61.

C. **Tests:**
1. **Blood:**
   a. **General:** Glucose, BUN/Cr, CBC, PTT (q6h on heparin until in range), PT, INR, ESR, Hgb A1c, RPR, homocysteine.
      1) **False positives:** Glucose, WBC, ESR, and CRP are all mildly high post stroke. Check Hgb A1c if glucose >130. CPK rises 4-7 d post stroke.
   b. **Lipids:** Total cholesterol, LDL, HDL, triglycerides.
   c. **Hypercoagulability panel** for pts <60 (lupus anticoagulant and anticardiolipin Ab, D-dimer, fibrinogen, Lp(a), protein C&S, factor V Leiden, prothrombin gene mutation, antithrombin III Ab).
2. **Imaging:** (See imaging, p. 179.)
   a. **Emergent head CT:** To rule out bleed. Best to do head and neck CTA at same time; it may detect persistent clot or arterial stenosis (contraindications: confirmed contrast allergy, Cr >1.7). Consider CT perfusion scan to assess area at risk for further ischemia.
   b. **Follow-up scan:** To assess stroke territory, e.g., MRI with diffusion-weighted image (DWI), or repeat CT in 6-12 h. Consider diffusion-perfusion MRI to look for territory at risk in pts whose exam fluctuates or iron-susceptibility sequence to rule out small bleeds from amyloid angiopathy.
   c. **Vascular studies:** Carotid ultrasound, anterior and posterior transcranial Doppler (TCD), MRA (time-of-flight or with gadolinium), or CT angiogram. Consider conventional angiogram [diagnostic or therapeutic (IA tPA)].
3. **Cardiac workup:** EKG; echocardiogram + bubble study, or TEE, to rule out LV clot, patent foramen ovale, atrial septal aneurysm. Consider bubble TCD. Holter to rule out A fib.

D. **DDx of stroke:** Cerebral bleed, TIA, postictal (Todd's) paralysis, spinal cord lesion, peripheral nerve injury (e.g., Bell's palsy, Saturday night palsy), MS flare, vasculitis, hemiplegic migraine, transient global amnesia, venous infarct, acute illness causing flare of an old stroke's sx, hypoglycemia. . . .

E. **Mechanisms of ischemic stroke:**
  1. **Thrombus:** ~40% of strokes
     a. **Large artery:** (~15% of strokes) Arterial dissection, atherosclerosis.
     b. **Penetrating artery:** (~25%) Lacunar, from hypertensive lipohyalinosis.
     c. **Venous thrombosis:** (See p. 126.)
  2. **Embolus:**
     a. **Cardiac:** About 20% of all ischemic strokes. Causes: A fib, sustained A flutter, rheumatic valve dz/mechanical valves, LV clot (recent MI, dilated cardiomyopathy), endocarditis, myxoma, hypercoagulable state (see p. 192).
     b. **Paradoxical embolus:** Via patent foramen ovale, atrial septal aneurysm, atrial or ventricular septal defect; or clot from lung.
     c. **Artery-to-artery embolus:** E.g., from carotid plaque.
     d. **Other:** Fat, air, or septic embolus.
  3. **Coagulopathy or platelet disorder:** <5%. See p. 192.
  4. **Low flow:** <5%; border-zone ischemia during systemic hypotension, often in the setting of pre-existing large-artery atherosclerosis.
  5. **Vasculopathy:** <5%; infectious (e.g., syphilis, TB, VZV), vasospasm (e.g., cocaine, migraine), collagen vascular dz, primary CNS vasculitis, moya-moya dz, fibromuscular dysplasia, homocystinuria, Fabry's dz.
  6. **Cryptogenic:** ~30% of all ischemic strokes. A dx of exclusion.
F. **Transient ischemic attack (TIA) vs. stroke:** TIA was originally defined as a deficit lasting <24 h; now defined as a brief deficit, typically lasting < 1 h, caused by a focal CNS ischemia without evidence of infarction. Treat TIA as an impending stroke (10% of TIA develop stroke within 90 d, of which 50% occur in the first 2 d).
  1. **Predictive factors for stroke after TIA:** Age >60, DM, sx duration >10 mins, weakness and/or speech impairment. Diagnostic workup for TIA is similar to stroke and warrants an admission to expedite. Management is guided by underlying etiology.
  2. **Embolic TIA:** Sx usually of vascular territory ischemia, last minutes to hours before embolus breaks up.
  3. **Lacunar TIA:** Sx often of white matter ischemia, often stuttering or stereotyped.
  4. **Low-flow TIA:** Sx usually of watershed ischemia, often blood pressure dependent, stereotyped, or crescendo, with evidence of large-artery atherosclerosis.
  5. **Amyloid angiopathy:** Sx usually of cortical ischemia, often spreading across to adjacent body parts over a few minutes.
G. **Rx of acute stroke:**
  1. **Emergent thrombolysis:** Use NIH tPA protocol for acute stroke in every pt. <3 hours of witnessed (confirmed) symptom onset. Can be given by *any* physician and does not require informed consent (standard of practice).
     a. **Contraindications:** Large stroke on noncontrast head CT (>1/3 arterial territory); blood on CT; minor (except aphasia) or

resolving deficit; history of ICH; recent stroke, head trauma, or intracranial procedure (<3 mo); seizure at symptom onset; suspicion of SAH; recent trauma or surgery (<14 d); active internal bleeding; history of GI/UT bleeding (<21 d); recent LP or non-compressible arterial puncture; bleeding diathesis (INR >1.2, abnormal PTT, plts <100); uncontrollable HTN; serum glucose <50 or >400.

   b. IV tissue plasminogen activator (tPA): Give <3 h after symptom onset. 0.9 mg/kg up to 90 mg, 10% of total dose as IV bolus (over 1 min), and remainder IV over 60 min.

   c. Intra-arterial tPA: Experimental, multiple agents and variations used. Informed consent required by family. IA tPA is given with angiographic guidance at site of clot, less than 6 h after symptom onset for anterior circulation clot; 12 h (and up to 24 h if no MR/CT evidence of infarct and/or hemorrhagic transformation) for posterior circulation clot.

     1) Pre-op and post-op angio orders: See p. 177.

     2) Blood pressure management after lysis: Keep SBP <180, DBP <105, with labetalol or nitroprusside if necessary.

2. Mechanical clot disruption or retrieval: up to 9 (ant)-24 (post) hrs.

3. Intracranial stents or bypass.

4. Anticoagulants: See also p. 160.

   a. Contraindications: Recent CNS bleed, surgery (relative).

   b. Aspirin: If no bleed on CT and pt is not a candidate for thrombolysis, have pt chew 325 mg.

   c. Other antiplatelet agents: If pt has had stroke on aspirin or cannot tolerate it.

     1) Clopidogrel: Indicated alone for secondary stroke prevention but showed higher risk of bleeding complications when combined with ASA.

     2) Aspirin-dipyridamole: Combination (25/200) is protective, but cost and HA may be problems.

   d. IV heparin:

     1) Indications: Symptomatic carotid stenosis, neck artery dissection, cerebral venous thrombosis, intracardiac clot. Less evidence for anticoagulation in acute new-onset A fib, intracranial atherosclerosis, lacunar infarcts, etc.

     2) Administration: Avoid loading boluses (e.g., 3,000-5,000 units) except if systemic indication (e.g., DVT with paradoxical embolism, unstable angina with MI and cardiac thrombus). In septic emboli, anticoagulation can be initiated after infection has been sufficiently treated with antibiotics.

   e. Heparin alternatives: If h/o heparin-induced thrombocytopenia.

   f. Consider warfarin: INR goal usually 2-3, but 3-4.5 for metal heart valves.

     1) Short-term warfarin: For cerebral venous thrombosis, carotid or vertebral dissection. Warfarin for 3-6 months; then may discontinue if cause no longer present and vessel reconstitution is confirmed by imaging.

    2) Long-term warfarin:

      a) Indication: Atrial fibrillation (including paroxysmal), mechanical heart valve, hypercoagulable disorder.

      b) <u>No</u> evidence for warfarin in these: Prevention of stroke recurrence, embolus of unknown origin, intracranial stenosis, and inoperable extracranial stenosis is <u>not</u> currently supported by evidence.

5. Maintain blood pressure: Allow or even assist HTN in acute strokes—the brain needs a higher perfusion pressure.

    a. Exceptions: Evidence of end-organ damage—MI, CHF, aortic dissection, h/o severe CAD, large stroke, hemorrhagic transformation of stroke.

      1) In non-tPA pts.: Avoid sustained (2 readings 5 min apart) SBP >185 or DBP >110

      2) In pts. with a procedure (tPA, thromborrhexis, CEA): Avoid SBP >140 to prevent reperfusion syndrome.

    b. Hold routine BP meds: As long as the above exceptions are not present.

    c. Avoid dehydration: When giving IV fluids to avoid dehydration, use D5NS to avoid cerebral edema.

    d. Hypertensive therapy: Consider IV pressors in pts with diffusion-perfusion mismatch and variation of sx with SBP.

      1) Pressor trial: Use peripheral neosynephrine to see if HTN helps stroke sx. If sx improve at SBP ≤180, pt. will require ICU monitoring for the duration of treatment.

      2) Contraindications: Active or history of severe coronary dz; SBP >180 required to show benefit; large infarct or evidence of hemorrhagic transformation.

    e. Antihypertensives: Short acting is better, so use IV drugs if possible

      1) Order of use: β-blocker first, then add calcium channel blockers, then ACEI, then nitrates, then hydralazine, then α_1-blockers.

      a) IV: Labetalol → nicardipine → enalapril → nitroprusside → hydralazine.

      b) PO: Lopressor → diltiazem → captopril → isosorbide → hydralazine.

      2) Avoid: Drugs that can make BP plummet (nifedipine) or directly dilate arteries (hydralazine, nitrates). The latter could hinder autoregulation of cerebral vasculature. Clonidine can be too sedating (sometimes useful for agitation).

6. Prevent cerebral edema: IVF of choice is D5NS to aim for hypertonic isovolemia. If there is progressive mass effect or signs of brainstem herniation, treat high ICP aggressively; see p. 68. See also Herniation, p. 181.

7. Oxygen:

    a. Hyperbaric oxygen: For ischemia related to carbon monoxide poisoning, air emboli, etc.

    b. O_2 via nasal cannula in the EW.

8. Treat fever: If temperature >100.4°F, treat with acetaminophen, ice packs, cooling blankets.

9. **Treat hyperglycemia:** Keep glucose <130, with insulin drip if needed, to decrease oxidative metabolism.
10. **Drugs to avoid:** haloperidol, benzodiazepines, opiates, α-antagonists, nifedipine.
11. **Aspiration precautions:** Keep NPO until bedside swallow or official S&S evaluation is done; may need NGT early on for meds.
12. **Monitor coagulation factors:** If on heparin, PTT q6h until therapeutic. If on warfarin, PT/INR qd.
13. **Physical, occupational, and speech/swallow therapy evaluation:** Wait until pt is hemodynamically stable and can cooperate with therapist.

H. **Surgical interventions for secondary stroke prevention:**
1. **Carotid endarterectomy (CEA):** Indications are:
   a. **Carotid stenosis:** Greater than 70% (from NASCET study); debatable between 50%-70%.
   b. **Deficit:** TIA or infarct in vascular territory distal to lesion ("symptomatic stenosis").
   c. **No severe distal stenoses:** Downstream from lesion.
   d. **Good surgical candidate:** Age <75, no serious cardiac disorders. (See preoperative cardiac evaluation, p. 210.)
   e. **Stable CNS:** No intracerebral hemorrhage or extensive fresh infarct (may postpone operation 2+ weeks to prevent "reperfusion injury").
2. **Carotid stenting:** An option for those who cannot get CEA. Higher risk of reocclusion but fewer intraoperative complications.
3. **Patent foramen ovale closure:**
   a. **Indications:** Young patients with PFO-associated stroke (large PFO/atrial septal aneurysm; temporal evidence of clot by DVT/MRV of pelvic veins, etc.).
   b. **Alternatives:** ASA vs. warfarin for PFO with associated atrial septal aneurysm in young patients.

I. **Vascular territories and stroke syndromes:**
1. **See also:** Angiographic anatomy, p. 175.
2. **Anterior vs. posterior circulation:** The latter are more dangerous. See p. 22.
3. **Middle cerebral artery (MCA):**
   a. **Superior division:** Weak face/arm > leg, expressive aphasia.
   b. **Inferior division:** Mild or transient motor/sensory deficit, fluent aphasia, neglect, sometimes field cut (Meyer's loop infarct causes superior quadrantanopia, not hemianopsia), Gerstmann's syndrome (dominant inferior parietal lobule, with acalculia, L-R dissociation, finger agnosia, agraphia).
4. **Anterior cerebral artery (ACA):** Contralateral leg weak, grasp reflex, gegenhalten, abulia, gait disorder, perseveration, urinary incontinence. Sometimes bilateral if both ACAs have common origin.
5. **ACA-MCA watershed:** Contralateral trunk > weakness. Bilateral watershed gives man-in-the-barrel syndrome, with proximal > distal weakness.
6. **MCA-PCA watershed:** Parietal lobe dysfunction, Balint syndrome (if bilateral).

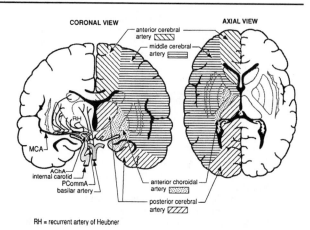

Figure 5. Cerebrovascular territories. (From Greenberg MS. *Handbook of Neurosurgery*. 3rd ed. Lakeland, FL: Greenberg Graphics; 1994, with permission.)

7. **Posterior cerebral artery (PCA):** Contralateral field cut. Sometimes memory loss, color anomia, alexia without agraphia, hemisensory loss, mild hemiparesis. Spatial disorientation is nondominant superior parietal lobule. Complications of PCA stroke include:
   a. **Brainstem ischemia:** PCA stroke can be the beginning of a top-of-the-basilar syndrome.
   b. **Uncal herniation** can pinch off PCAs.
   c. **Hemorrhagic transformations** are common after PCA infarcts.
8. **Subcortical arteries:**
   a. **Heubner and other medial striates:** AKA recurrent artery of Heubner. See expressive aphasia, mild hemiparesis arm > leg, proximal > distal. Comes off ACA or A-comm to anterior hypothalamus, globus pallidus, putamen, head of caudate nucleus.
   b. **Anterior choroidal and other lenticulostriates:** Contralateral sensorimotor loss, homonymous hemianopsia. The anterior choroidal comes off ICA to posterior limb of int. capsule, cerebral peduncle, and medial globus pallidus.
9. **Basilar artery:** Infarct causes pontine and cerebellar signs.
   a. **Occlusion:** Frequently bilateral signs, e.g., quadriplegia, conjugate horizontal gaze palsies, coma, "locked-in" syndrome.
   b. **Top of the basilar embolus:**
      1) **Sx:** Usually see oculomotor problems, altered mental status, dorsal midbrain syndrome, bilateral thalamic stroke.

      2) **Embolic complications:** Emboli from basilar clot can cause occipital, thalamic, cerebellar, and brainstem infarcts with contralateral hemiplegia but ipsilateral horizontal gaze palsy (opposite of cerebral lesion), INO, palatal myoclonus, etc.

  c. **Basilar scrape syndrome:**

      1) **Sx:** Progressive brainstem and cerebellar sx as basilar thrombosis sequentially occludes PICA, AICA, paramedian basilar aa., perforators, SCA, etc. Often bilateral or alternating sides.

      2) **Prognosis:** Usually ends with complete occlusion, top-of-the-basilar syndrome, and infarct.

10. **Midbrain strokes:** From occlusion of basilar branches. Damage to oculomotor, Edinger-Westphal, red, trochlear, or lateral geniculate nuclei; reticular activating system.

  a. **Dorsal midbrain syndrome:** (Parinaud's syndrome) See p. 48.

  b. **Rostral interstitial nucleus:** From branch of PCA. Infarct of single side can give a bilateral upgaze palsy because the infarct catches crossing fibers en passant.

  c. **Ventral midbrain syndrome:** Bilateral down gaze paralysis, paralysis of convergence, obtundation.

  d. **Named midbrain syndromes:** Varying degree of CN III palsy and contralateral motor system dysfunction, namely Weber's, with contralateral weakness; Claude's, with contralateral rubral tremor; and Benedikt's, with both.

      1) **Eponym rant:** Why immortalize very dead guys when you could use descriptive names? That would spare the energy wasted on keeping similar eponyms straight (e.g., Bell's palsy, Bell's reflex, Bell's nerve, and Bell's law), the problem of diseases named after Nazis (e.g., Hallervorden-Spatz), etc.

      2) **Syndrome rant:** "But," you protest, "it's hard to find descriptive names that distinguish syndromes as similar as Benedikt's, Claude's, and Weber's." Why even bother? Simply describing the sx helps pt management more and makes your notes clearer to nonneurologists.

11. **Pontine strokes:** From occlusion of basilar branches. Damages nuclei of V, VII, and VIII, reticular activating system.

  a. **"Locked-in" syndrome:** From basis pontis lesion, sparing tegmentum. Frequently, the only motor function preserved is vertical gaze. Sx may be mistaken for coma or nonconvulsive status epilepticus.

  b. **Pontine rigors:** The jerking movements sometimes seen in bilateral pontine strokes.

12. **Cerebellar strokes:** Vertigo, N/V, nystagmus, ataxia, poor smooth pursuit, often headache; often with brainstem signs including ipsilateral hearing loss, ipsilateral Horner's, contralateral pain, and temperature loss. SCA and AICA are off basilar; PICA off vertebral.

  a. <u>**Large cerebellar strokes are an emergency**</u> because of the risk of herniation. Consider neurosurgical decompression if >3 cm or if edema/hemorrhagic transformation. Pt. can die within hours of first brainstem signs.

   b. Superior cerebellar artery (SCA): Ataxia. Usually embolic. Rarely causes hydrocephalus (7%).

   c. Posterior inferior cerebellar artery (PICA): Vertigo, N/V. Often with lateral medullary syndrome (see below). Embolus and stenosis are equally likely. If whole territory is infarcted, there is a 25% risk of hydrocephalus.

   d. Anterior inferior cerebellar artery (AICA): Hearing loss, weak/numb face, ataxia, vertigo. Rare; usually thrombotic; usually with brainstem infarct too.

13. Medullary stroke: From vertebral artery lesion. Signs of damage to VIII, IX-XII, spinal tract, and nucleus of V. Hemiparesis implies more medial involvement or higher lesion.

   a. Lateral medullary syndrome (Wallenberg's):

      1) Vestibular sx: Vertigo, N/V, nystagmus, diplopia.

      2) Crossed sensory loss: Sensory loss on <u>ipsilateral</u> face; poor pain and temperature sensation on <u>contralateral</u> body.

      3) Horner's syndrome: Ipsilateral.

      4) Poor speech and swallow: Dysphagia, hoarseness, hiccups, ipsilateral poor gag. From cranial nerve IX, X palsies.

      5) Ataxia: Ipsilateral.

   b. Medial medullary syndrome (Déjèrine's): Ipsilateral tongue weakness and deviation, contralateral hemiparesis and poor proprioception, but cutaneous sensation spared.

14. Lacunar syndromes: Thought to be from hypertensive lipohyalinosis; probably not helped by heparin.

   a. Typical locations: In order of decreasing frequency: putamen, caudate, thalamus, pons, internal capsule, corona radiata.

   b. Pure sensory: Ventral posterolateral or posteromedial nucleus of the thalamus.

   c. Pure motor: Posterior limb of internal capsule, corona radiata, basis pontis, or cerebral peduncle.

   d. Sensorimotor: Contralateral face, arm, and leg involvement due to a lesion in the thalamus and adjacent posterior limb of internal capsule.

   e. Ataxic hemiparesis: Ataxia >>> weakness on same side. Often leg > arm > face. From basis pontis (upper third, midline), or ventral anterior thalamus + adjacent internal capsule, or superior cerebellar peduncle.

   f. Dysarthria-clumsy hand: Weak face, dysphagia, and ipsilateral clumsy hand. From lesion of basis pontis, genu of internal capsule, or immediately subcortical white matter.

COMA AND BRAIN DEATH

A. See also Trauma, p. 119.

B. Levels of decreased consciousness:

   1. Confusion: Decreased attention but relatively normal alertness.

2. **Drowsiness:** (~lethargy, somnolence). Arouses to voice and can respond verbally.
3. **Stupor:** (~obtundation). No response to voice, no spontaneous speech. Incomplete but purposeful response to pain.
4. **Coma:** Nonpurposeful or no response to pain ("unarousable unresponsiveness").

C. **Other alterations in consciousness:** See p. 42.

D. **Initial coma evaluation:** CPR if needed → IV access → draw labs (include tox screen, ?carbon monoxide level) → give dextrose, thiamine, naloxone → do coma exam (see below) → treat suspected high ICP, meningitis, or seizures → get head CT → treat metabolic problems.

E. **Coma exam:** VS (and note pattern of breathing), cardiac rhythm, response to voice, lids (spontaneously closed?), pupils, eye movements (spontaneous, doll's, calorics), corneals, grimace to nasal tickle, gag, cough, motor response to pain, tone (lift and drop arm), reflexes.
  1. **Decorticate posturing** (lesion is above midbrain):
     a. **Arm:** Flexed elbow, wrist, fingers.
     b. **Leg:** Extended and internally rotated leg, with plantar flexion.
  2. **Decerebrate posturing** (lesion is above medulla):
     a. **Head:** Clenched jaw, extended neck.
     b. **Arm:** Adducted and internally rotated shoulder, extended elbow, pronated wrist, flexed fingers.
     c. **Leg:** Extended and internally rotated leg, plantar flexion.

F. **Glasgow Coma Scale (GCS):** Range 3-15 (pt. gets 3 points for just being there). GCS <8 is indication for intubation and poor prognosis.

Points	Eye Opening	Verbal	Motor
6			Obeys
5		Oriented	Localizes pain
4	Spontaneous	Confused	Withdraws to pain
3	To speech	Inappropriate	Flexion (decort.)
2	To pain	Unintelligible	Extensor (decereb.)
1	None	None	None

Table 4. Glasgow Coma Scale.

G. **Causes of coma with normal head CT:**
  1. **Drug overdose or reaction:** Especially sedatives, anticholinergics, and poisons, but also including neuroleptic malignant syndrome.
  2. **Anoxia or ischemia:** Cardiac arrest, brainstem stroke, fat or cholesterol emboli, DIC, thrombotic thrombocytopenic purpura, vasculitis.
  3. **Trauma:** Diffuse axonal injury, bilateral isodense SDH, high ICP.
  4. **Metabolic encephalopathy:** Low or high glucose, low or high Na, high Ca, alkalosis or acidosis, hypercapnia, adrenal crisis, low or high thyroid, uremia, high ammonia, thiamine deficiency, hyperthermia or hypothermia.

5. **Infection or inflammation:** Meningitis, encephalitis, sepsis, cerebritis (SLE), sarcoidosis, Behçet's, etc.
6. **Seizure disorder:** Nonconvulsive status epilepticus, postictal state.
7. **Central pontine myelinolysis:** See p. 197. Usually presents as mutism, oculobulbar palsies, quadriparesis. After rapid Na correction.

H. **Prognosis in <u>non</u>traumatic coma:**
  1. **Confounding factors:** All drug effects, reversible metabolic factors, and hypothermia must be corrected first.
  2. **Prognosis by etiology:** Those with hepatic cause do best, hypoxic-ischemic intermediate, vascular worst.
  3. **Prognosis by neurological exam:**
    a. **Day of presentation:** Look for corneal, pupillary, and oculocephalic (doll's) or caloric test responses.
      1) **1 of 3 absent:** 95% of pts. → vegetative or badly disabled.
      2) **2 of 3 absent:** 99% of pts. → vegetative or badly disabled.
    b. **Day 1:**
      1) **Spontaneous eye movements:** 99% of pts. who do not have spontaneous conjugate roving eye movements or better will be vegetative or severely disabled.
      2) **Motor withdrawal:** Of pts. with spontaneous eye movements but no purposeful withdrawal to pain, 90% will be vegetative or severely disabled.
    c. **Day 3:**
      1) **Motor withdrawal:** Of pts. with no purposeful withdrawal to pain, 100% will be vegetative or severely disabled.
      2) **Spontaneous eye opening:** Of pts. who withdraw but keep eyes closed, 80% will be vegetative or severely disabled.
    d. **Day 7:**
      1) **Spontaneous eye opening:** Of pts. who withdraw but keep eyes closed, 100% will be vegetative.
      2) **Obeying commands:** Of pts. with spontaneous eye opening who do not follow commands, about 80% will be vegetative or severely disabled.
    e. **Day 14:**
      1) **Abnormal oculocephalic reflex:**
        a) **Not following commands or opening eyes spontaneously:** 100% vegetative.
        b) **Following commands or opening eyes spontaneously:** 80% vegetative or severely disabled.
      2) **Normal oculocephalic reflex:** Only 20% will be severely disabled or worse.

I. **Vegetative state:** Similar to coma but pt may have sleep-wake cycles and eye opening to auditory stimuli, with no awareness of environment or self, no ability to communicate, and no purposeful motor activity.

J. **Brain death:** An attending must see the pt before he is declared brain dead. If there may be litigation about the death, get legal counsel first. The following criteria should be met:
  1. **Known cause.**
  2. **No masking conditions:** No hypothermia (<32°C), CNS depressants, nl electrolytes.

3. **No evidence of brainstem function:**
   a. **Reflexes:** No pupillary, corneal, oculovestibular, gag, cough, or other brainstem reflexes.
   b. **No motor response to deep central pain:** There should be neither decerebrate nor decorticate posturing, but spinal reflexes including flexor withdrawal ("triple flexion") can be seen after brain death, as well as deep tendon reflexes. There should be no change in heart rate to pain.
4. **Apnea test:** Criteria are no spontaneous breaths and pCO_2 >60 (unreliable in pt with COPD and CO_2 retention).
   a. **Preoxygenate:** 15 min of ventilation with 100% O_2 beforehand. Need pCO_2 <45 and normal pH before further testing.
   b. **Disconnect ventilator;** give O_2 8-12 L/min by tracheal cannula; observe for spontaneous breaths.
   c. **Draw ABG** after about 8-10 min (depends on pt stability).
   d. **Terminate test if:**
      1) **pCO_2 >60:** Positive for brain death.
      2) **Pt breathes:** Negative.
      3) **Systemic instability:** Hypotension, cardiac arrhythmia, or O_2 saturation <80%: inconclusive test.
5. **Observation period:** Use clinical judgment. Recommendations:
   a. **24 h:** For anoxic brain injury and no confirmatory tests.
   b. **12 h:** For clearly irreversible condition, no confirmatory tests.
   c. **6 h:** For clearly irreversible condition, confirmatory tests.
6. **Optional confirmatory tests** (not necessary):
   a. **Flat EEG:** Isoelectric at high gain.
   b. **Absent cerebral blood flow:** e.g., an ICP > SBP for 1 hour or transcranial ultrasound showing reversible flow velocities.

K. **Organ and tissue donation:**
   1. **Eligibility criteria:** Candidates may be any age. Next of kin does not disapprove (this may hold even if pt. had an organ donor card). There are additional exclusion criteria not listed (e.g. HIV infection), but call the transplant coordinator and let them decide.
      a. **Organ donation:** Brain dead, intact circulation, ventilated.
      b. **Tissue donation:** Anyone with irreversible absence of respiration and circulation.
   2. **Transplant coordinator:** Call early, 1-800-446-6362, even if you have not yet asked the family. You can ask afterwards; the organ bank will not approach the family without your permission.
   3. **When and how to ask the family:** In some states, you ask all families of eligible donors about organ donation. Especially in ICUs, the nurses have had much experience with this. Ask their advice, if possible.
   4. **Management after brain death for organ donation:** The transplant team will help once the pt. is declared brain dead. Before that, of course, you should treat pts. with their best interest in mind only.

CRANIAL NERVES

A. **See also:** Brainstem Anatomy, p.16.

	CNS Nucleus	Function
I	Olfactory bulb	Smell
II	Retina; lat. geniculate	Vision
III	Oculomotor nu. (somatic motor)	EOM except sup. oblique and lat. rectus
	Edinger-Westphal (PSNS)	Pupillary constriction
IV	Trochlear nu.	Superior oblique muscle
V	Spinal nu.	Pain and temp from face, dura, tympani
	Main sensory nu.	Light touch from face
	Mesencephalic nu.	Mechanoreceptors of face, mouth
	Trigeminal motor nu.	Muscles of chewing, tensor tymp.
VI	Abducens nu	Lateral rectus muscle (p. 48)
VII	Facial motor nu.	Facial expression and stapedius
	Spinal trigeminal nu.	Ear and tympanic memb. sensation
	Solitary nu.	Taste from ant. 2/3 of tongue
	Sup. salivatory nu.	Salivation and lacrimation
VIII	Cochlear nu.	Hearing (p. 54)
I	Vestibular nu.	Balance (p. 127)
IX	Nu. ambiguus	Pharyngeal muscles
	Spinal trigeminal nu.	Sensation of ear, post. 1/3 of tongue
	Solitary nu.	Taste from post. 1/3 tongue
	Solitary and spinal trigem.	Carotid, oropharynx sensation
	Inf. salivatory nu.	Parotid gland secretion
X	Nu. ambiguus	Larynx/pharynx muscles
	Spinal trigeminal nu.	Sensory from external ear
	Solitary nu.	Taste buds of epiglottis
	Solitary and spinal trigeminal nu.	Larynx/pharynx sensation; PSNS from chest and abdomen
	Dorsal motor nu.	PSNS to chest and abdomen
XI	Nu. ambiguus	Larynx and pharynx muscles
	Accessory nu.	Sternocleidomastoid and trapezius
XII	Hypoglossal nu.	Intrinsic tongue muscles

Table 5. Cranial nerve nuclei and their function.

DEMYELINATING DISEASE

A. **Multiple sclerosis:** Multiple CNS demyelinating attacks, disseminated in time and space.
   1. **Definitions:**
      a. **Attack** (exacerbation, relapse): Inflammatory and demyelinating lesion lasting >24 h, objective clinical findings, separated by 30 d between onset of attacks.
      b. **Course:** Relapsing-remitting, secondary progressive, primary progressive.

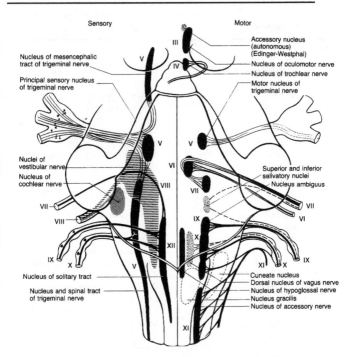

Sensory · Motor

III · Accessory nucleus (autonomous) (Edinger-Westphal) · Nucleus of oculomotor nerve · Nucleus of trochlear nerve · Motor nucleus of trigeminal nerve

Nucleus of mesencephalic tract of trigeminal nerve

Principal sensory nucleus of trigeminal nerve

Nuclei of vestibular nerve
Nucleus of cochlear nerve

Superior and inferior salivatory nuclei · Nucleus ambiguus

Nucleus of solitary tract
Nucleus and spinal tract of trigeminal nerve

Cuneate nucleus · Dorsal nucleus of vagus nerve · Nucleus of hypoglossal nerve · Nucleus gracilis · Nucleus of accessory nerve

Figure 6. Cranial nerve nuclei. (Reprinted with permission from Duus P. *Topical Diagnosis in Neurology.* New York: Thieme; 1983:105.)

   c. MRI Criteria: Three of the following: at least one gad+ lesion or nine T2 lesions, one infratentorial lesion, one juxtacortical lesion, at least three periventricular lesions. Spinal cord lesions considered equivalent to infratentorial lesion, enhancing brain lesion, and T2 lesion.

   d. % criteria: Diagnostic criteria for "MS," "possible MS," and "not MS."

2. H&P:

   a. Common presenting sx: Optic neuritis, weakness and numbness, diplopia, vertigo, myelitis, urinary retention. Sx worse with heat (Uthoff's phenomenon).

   b. Other MS sx: Urinary retention, pain, fatigue, Lhermitte's phenomenon (tingling on neck flexion), internuclear ophthalmoplegia, cognitive changes. Weakness frequently worst in hands and hips.

   c. MS flare: Usually subacute (>1 wk) deterioration. Acute (1-3 d) deterioration suggests an infection that is briefly exacerbating MS sx. Does the pt. use catheters?

MCDONALD CRITERIA FOR DIAGNOSIS OF MS	
Clinical Presentation	*Additional Data Needed for DX*
≥2 attacks, and ≥2 lesions with objective clinical evidence	None
≥2 attacks and 1 lesion with objective clinical evidence	Dissemination in space, by MRI *or* ≥2 MRI lesions plus + CSF *or* 2nd clinical attack at different site
1 attack, and ≥2 lesions with objective clinical evidence	Dissemination in time, by MRI *or* 2nd clinical attack
1 attack, and 1 lesion with objective clinical evidence (clinically isolated syndrome)	Dissemination in space, by MRI *or* ≥2 MRI lesions plus + CSF *and* dissemination in time (disseminated by MRI *or* second clinical attack)
Insidious neurological progression suggestive of MS	One year of progression *and* 2 of the following 3: (A) + Brain MRI (9 T2 lesions or 4+ T2 lesions with + VEP); (B) + spinal cord MRI (2 T2 lesions); (C) + CSF

Table 6. McDonald criteria for diagnosis of MS.

3. Tests:
   a. Initial workup:
      1) MRI brain + contrast: See p. 188. Pts. with a first MS-like neurological event and significant white matter lesions on MRI have a 5-year incidence of MS of about 80%. If no lesions, risk is about 5%.
      2) MRI spinal cord + contrast only if clinically suspicious.
      3) If unusual clinical picture or criteria not fulfilled: CSF for elevated IgG index or oligoclonal bands (WBC should be <50) and VEP (delayed but preserved wave form).
      4) Consider Lyme titer, RPR, B_{12} level, HIV, ESR, ANA, ACE, HTLV.
   b. MS attack: CBC, urinalysis, CXR and ESR to help r/o infection that could mimic an attack; consider tests to r/o disc herniation or entrapment neuropathy.
4. DDx:
   a. DDx of MS: Acute disseminated encephalomyelitis, antiphospholipid syndrome, carotid dissection, cervical cord compression, CNS lymphomas and gliomas, vasculitis, lupus, myelitis, infection (HIV, Lyme, HTLV, syphilis), neurosarcoid, Chiari malformations, B_{12} deficiency, arylsulfatase or hexosaminidase A deficiencies, CADASIL, paraneoplastic syndrome, mitochondrial dzs....
   b. Neuromyelitis optica (Devic's syndrome): Severe opticospinal recurrent demyelinating disease, either variant of MS or separate disease. Serum NMO antibody is sensitive and specific.

    c. **DDx of MS attack in pt. with known MS:** Infection
(*bladder* > teeth > URI), cervical or lumbar disc herniation,
entrapment neuropathy....

5. **Rx of MS:**
    a. **Immunomodulators:** Approved for relapsing-remitting MS.
Reduce clinical and MRI indicators of disease activity, possibly
may alter course.
       1) **Avonex** (β-IFN 1a): 30 μg IM q wk. May delay progression.
       2) **Rebif** (high-dose β-IFN 1a): 22 or 44 μg SC qod. Possible dose-
related benefit, much higher rate of neutralizing antibodies.
       3) **Betaseron** (β-IFN 1b): 8 MIU IU SC qod. May delay progres-
sion in active relapsing-remitting or secondary progressive MS.
       4) **Glatiramer** (Copaxone): Fragments of myelin basic protein.
20 μg SC qd.
       5) **Mitoxantrone:** FDA approved for active relapsing-remitting or
secondary progressive MS. Has a lifetime dose limit.
       6) **Cyclophosphamide** (Cytoxan): Controversial. For aggressively
progressive MS.
    b. **MS attack:** High-dose steroids (methylprednisolone IV
1,000 mg $\times$ 3 d, $\pm$ prednisone taper) speed clinical recovery but
no long-term benefit. For prevention of steroid side effects,
see p. 173.
    c. **Rx of secondary sx:** See rx for spasticity, p. 176; pain, p. 155;
tremor, p. 79; and spastic bladder or bladder-sphincter dyssynergia, p. 126. Fatigue: modafinil 100-200 mg in AM and at noon.
Brief, painful, focal seizures sometimes resolve after a few weeks
of low-dose ACD.

B. **Other CNS demyelinating conditions:**
1. **Transverse myelitis:** Isolated spinal cord inflammation without com-
pressive lesion.
    a. **H&P:** Back pain, sudden paresthesias, myelopathy (see Spinal
Cord Disorders, p. 113) over hours to weeks.
    b. **Tests:** CSF, MRI spine with gado, consider MRA or CTA spine,
CT myelogram more sensitive for dural AVF, infectious workup,
ANA, ESR, ANCA, SSA/SSB, ACE, B$_{12}$ and Vit E levels.
    c. **Causes:** Idiopathic, postinfectious (*M. pneumonia*, otitis media,
skin infections, Lyme, VZV, HSV, CMV, TB, HTLV, HIV, syphilis,
influenza, echovirus, hepatitis A, rubella, schistosomiasis), post-
vaccine. Associated with SLE, Sjögren's, sarcoid. Can be first
attack of MS, may be secondary to ischemia.
    d. **DDx:** Some infections, e.g., TB. Structural myelopathy, infarct,
hemorrhage, AVM, dural AV fistula, cord contusion, vasculitis,
vitamin B$_{12}$ and E deficiency.
    e. **Rx:** Steroids (1 g methylprednisolone IV or 100 mg dexametha-
sone IV for at least 3 days), consider IVIg.
    f. **Prognosis:** Rarely recurs. Recovery starts in 2-12 wk, up to 2 years.
1/3 good recovery, 1/3 can walk but have deficits, 1/3 paraplegic.
2. **Acute disseminated encephalomyelitis (ADEM):** Multifocal
demyelination similar to MS but acute, monophasic, sometimes
postinfectious.

      a. H&P: Recent viral infection or vaccination.

      b. DDx: Infectious encephalomyelitis.

      c. Rx: Consider steroids, plasmapheresis.

  3. Acute hemorrhagic leukoencephalitis: A hyperacute ADEM, often with fever, seizures, obtundation.

  4. Cerebellitis: See p. 145.

  5. Brainstem (Bickerstaff) encephalitis: Adolescents and young adults.

C. Guillain-Barré syndrome: AKA acute idiopathic demyelinating polyradiculoneuritis (AIDP, as opposed to CIDP).

  1. <u>GBS is an emergency:</u> There is danger of sudden respiratory collapse, even in pts without severe limb weakness. 25% of pts. need intubation.

  2. H&P: Infection (1/4 have prior *Campylobacter jejuni*), vaccination, or surgery in previous 1-3 wk; pregnancy. Rapid (days to 1 mo) symmetric weakness, weak or absent DTRs, facial diplegia, poor swallowing or breathing, stocking/glove numbness in hands and feet. Sometimes proximal > distal (vs. other peripheral neuropathies), ANS instability, diffuse back pain.

  3. Variants:

      a. Miller Fisher variant: Areflexia, sensory ataxia, ophthalmoparesis. GQ1b Ab is sensitive and specific.

      b. Axonal variants: Can be pure motor or motor + sensory. EMG shows the axon damage. Ganglioside antibodies, e.g., GM1, are common.

      c. Polyneuritis cranialis: A variant that often presents with bifacial weakness.

      d. Acute pandysautonomia: ANS dysfunction, papilledema, upgoing toes. No meningeal signs.

  4. Tests:

      a. Respiratory: Vital capacity tid. Remember that O_2 saturation is not sensitive; pt will become hypercarbic before becoming hypoxic.

      b. Blood: β-HCG, heterophile Ab and EBV titers, *Campylobacter*, HIV, CMV, RF, ANA, hepatitis titers, serum GM1 and GQ1b antibodies.

      c. NCS: Conduction block, usually low velocity, high latency, decreased F-wave conduction (poor correlation with sx, can be nl early in dz).

      d. Biopsy: Focal demyelination. Biopsy only if dx unclear.

      e. CSF: Protein usually up after first few days. Cell count usually normal; sometimes 10-100 monocytes.

  5. DDx of GBS: CIDP, other neuropathies (see p. 93); neuromuscular problem, e.g., myasthenia or botulism, Lyme, MS, foramen magnum or other spine tumor, polio, hypophosphatemia (during long TPN course), tick paralysis. . . .

  6. Rx: Intubate if vital capacity <15 cc/kg or 0.6 L, or higher if falling fast. Plasmapheresis (ANS instability is a relative contraindication) and IVIg are equally effective, limit severity and hasten recovery. No role for steroids (although help CIDP). Protect eyes from drying. Back pain may require narcotics. Watch for SIADH.

      a. Prognosis: Fatal in 4-15%, 20% disabled, and 35% have permanent deficit. 10% relapse. 50% nadir in 1 wk; 90% in 1 mo. Poorer outcomes with axonal variants, elderly, bed-bound or intubated, more rapid onset, prior diarrheal illness, motor amplitude <250.

D. Chronic inflammatory demyelinating polyradiculoneuropathy (CIDP):

   1. CIDP vs. GBS: CIDP progresses or relapses for 2 months or more; usually legs > arms; incidence peaks at age 50-60. Like GBS, it is probably autoimmune.

   2. Tests: NCS show demyelination, CSF protein >45 mg/dL, cell count <10/μL, sural nerve biopsy shows de- and remyelination with perivascular inflammation.

   3. DDx: Other neuropathies, e.g., DM, metabolic, toxic, infectious (HIV, HCV), paraneoplastic, paraproteinemias, lymphoma, vasculitis.

   4. Rx: Steroids, plasma exchange, and IVIg are equally effective; 60% respond. Second line = combinations of these or immunosuppressants (cyclosporine, mycophenolate, etc.).

   5. Multifocal motor neuropathy (MMN): Purely motor variant of CIDP.

      a. H&P: Age 20-50 at onset, progressive, asymmetric weakness in distribution of individual nerves, upper > lower limbs, multifocal conduction block, GM1 Ab.

      b. Rx of MMN: Long-term IVIg; 80% respond but dose lasts only few weeks. Plasma exchange and steroids do not work. Immunosuppressants for refractory dz.

DYSARTHRIA AND DYSPHAGIA

A. Dysarthria: Abnormal articulation, as opposed to aphasia.

   1. H&P: Abnormal articulation, rhythm, or volume. Ask about diurnal fluctuations (suggests myasthenia), improvement with alcohol (suggests essential tremor). Assess palatal elevation when pt says a long "a" or "coca-cola." Assess ability to hold a tone or sing. Look especially for other cranial nerve signs, dysmetria, tremor, dystonia, or spasticity.

   2. Tests: MRI, laryngoscopy, consider EMG of orofacial muscles (hurts).

   3. Causes: See also bulbar vs. pseudobulbar palsy, p. 129.

      a. Peripheral: Flaccid. Myasthenia, polyneuritis, myopathy, cranial nerve lesions, maxillofacial lesions.

      b. Central: Spastic (corticospinal tract damage), ataxic (cerebellar lesion), bradykinetic (parkinsonism), hyperkinetic (chorea, dystonia).

      c. Mixed: Spastic-flaccid (ALS), spastic-ataxic (MS, Wilson's dz, encephalitis).

   4. DDx:

      a. Spasmodic dysphonia: Often associated with face or neck dystonia. Not present when whispering or singing.

         1) Abductor dysphonia: Choppy and strained; words drop out.

      2) **Adductor dysphonia:** Breathy, whispery.
      3) **Rx:** Botulinum toxin.
    b. **Dysfluency:** E.g., stuttering, palilalia. In frontal lesion, Parkinson's.
    c. **Other:** Aphasia, stuttering, intoxication or delirium.
  5. **Rx:** Treat underlying dz.
B. **Dysphagia:** Abnormal swallowing.
  1. **H&P:** Choking, coughing after swallowing, weight loss, recurrent pneumonias. Is it worse with liquids or solids? Watch pt. swallow water, assess gag, other cranial nerves, motor exam.
  2. **Tests:** "Swallowing study" (cine-esophogram). Brain scan. CXR if you suspect aspiration pneumonia.
  3. **Causes:**
    a. **Neurological:** Upper or lower motor neuron lesion (stroke, brainstem mass, etc.), ALS, neuropathy, MS, myasthenia, Chiari malformation, syringobulbia, myopathy, Parkinson's dz, spinocerebellar degeneration, tardive dyskinesia, cerebral palsy.
    b. **Nonneurological:** Esophageal mass, scleroderma, achalasia, esophageal spasm, Sjögren's syndrome.
  4. **Rx:** "Aspiration precautions," swallowing therapy, dysphagia diets (e.g., purees), thickened liquids, nasogastric or gastric tube.

EEG (ELECTROENCEPHALOGRAPHY)

A. **Indications:** Confirming, localizing, or classifying seizures—but a normal EEG does not rule out the possibility of seizures. EEGs aid dx of CJD and encephalopathy.
B. **Montages:**
  1. **Bipolar:** Good for localization; bad because distort widely distributed potentials, e.g., vertex waves. Location of spike = at phase reversal.
  2. **Referential:** Good for sleep studies. More EKG artifact. Location of spike = at max. amplitude.
C. **Studies:**
  1. **Routine**
  2. **Sleep-deprived:** More sensitive for epileptiform activity, which is seen especially in sleep-wake transitions.
  3. **Continuous:** Indications include ACD coma in status epilepticus, nonconvulsive status, capturing seizures to determine the hemisphere in which the seizure began (for epilepsy surgery), and distinguishing electrographic seizures from nonepileptic spells (see p. 104).
D. **Normal rhythms:**
  1. **Alpha:** 8-12 Hz, posterior. Resting rhythm of thalamocortical network. Disappears when eyes open or when drowsy.
  2. **Beta:** Fast, 20-40 Hz, anterior. Cortical activity during alertness.
  3. **Theta:** 4-8 Hz. Normal during drowsiness or sleep; abnormal if alert.
  4. **Delta:** <4 Hz. Normal during drowsiness or sleep; abnormal if alert.
  5. **Gamma:** 40-80 Hz. Not analyzed in clinical EEG, but important for binding and coordinating the activity of different brain regions.

6. **Sleep:** Generalized slowing, vertex waves, K complexes, sleep spindles (14 Hz), drowsy hypersynchrony.
7. **Normal effects of stimulation:**
   a. **Hyperventilation:** Can cause generalized slowing in normals.
   b. **Photic stimulation:** Occipital driving; often more with eyes closed, can be normal.

E. **Abnormal rhythms:**
   1. **Slowing:** Theta or delta while alert. Nonspecific if generalized; may help localize lesion if focal.
   2. **Seizure:** High-voltage, chaotic or rhythmic, focal or generalized.
   3. **Spikes and sharp waves:** Interictal evidence for epilepsy.
   4. **FIRDA:** Frontal intermittent rhythmic delta activity. Nonspecific encephalopathy.
   5. **Diffuse periodic sharps:** DDx = CJD, lithium toxicity, baclofen toxicity, metabolic encephalopathy, subacute sclerosing panencephalitis (has complexes with longer periodicity).
   6. **PLEDS:** Periodic lateralized epileptiform discharges. Do not try to eradicate them; just aim for normal ACD levels. May have different meaning in different contexts.
   7. **Triphasic waves:** Usually from metabolic abnormality, although they look ictal.

EMG (ELECTROMYOGRAPHY) AND NERVE CONDUCTION STUDIES

	Conduction Velocity	Amplitude	F & H Latency	Distal Latency	Fibrillations
Axonal damage	>70%	↓	~↑	nl	↑
PNS demyelination	<50%	~↓	↑	~↑	Variable
LMN dz	>70%	↓ motor	~c	nl	↑
UMN dz	nl	nl	nl	nl	None
Radiculopathy	>80%	~↓	↑	nl	↑
NMJ dz	nl	nl/↓	nl	nl	None
Myopathy	nl	~↓	nl	nl	None

Table 7. EMG findings in neuromuscular diseases.

A. **Ordering tests:** Always give tentative dx; specify muscles, nerves of interest.
B. **Nerve conduction studies (NCS):** Measure electrical conduction along a nerve orthodromically (stimulate near cell bodies, record near terminals) or antidromically (vice versa).
   1. **Motor NCS:** Stimulate motor nerve and record muscle CMAP (compound muscle action potential), i.e., the sum of all axons directed to the muscle. CMAP depends on axon, NMJ, and muscle fibers.

       a. Amplitude: Reflects the number of conductive muscle fibers (therefore axons). It is decreased by damage to motor unit (axon + muscle fibers).

       b. Distal latency: Time between stimulus and recording, depends on conduction of axons (not NMJ or muscle). Slowed in demyelination.

       c. Conduction velocity: Divides the distal latency between two locations along the same nerve by the distance between them. Conduction block is the hallmark of demyelination.

2. Sensory NCS: Stimulate a nerve and record its sensory nerve action potential (SNAP) from purely sensory portion of the nerve. The sural nerve is purely sensory.

3. Late responses:

       a. F-wave: Motor stimulus travels both ortho- and antidromically. Antidromic stimulus reflected through neuron and back; creates small F-wave seen after first (M) wave. F-wave delayed in proximal neuropathies (e.g., DM, GBS) and also in motor neuron dz and radiculopathy.

       b. H-reflex: CMAP from stimulation of sensory nerve, via monosynaptic reflex arc. Always tested in tibia: dorsal and ventral S1 roots. H-reflex delayed and small if proximal sensory or motor axon damage.

4. Repetitive stimulation: Abnormalities are hallmark of NMJ dz.

       a. Myasthenia: Baseline CMAP normal, but slow repetitive 3-Hz stimulation results in decrement of CMAP if pt. is at rest. With exercise, CMAP can improve for first min, but then worsen in 4-6 min. Abnormal in only half of myasthenics. Single-fiber EMG is more sensitive but less specific.

       b. Lambert-Eaton syndrome: Baseline CMAP small and gets smaller with repetitive 3-Hz stimulation. With exercise, CMAP size greatly increases in a few sec but then worsens in 2-4 min.

       c. Botulism: Baseline CMAP very small; gets smaller with repetitive 3-Hz stimulation; no change with exercise.

C. Electromyography (EMG): AKA single-needle study. Evaluates individual motor units by inserting electrode into muscle.

1. Insertional activity: Brief burst of AP following insertion into resting muscle. Increased in early denervation, some myopathies (especially inflammatory myopathies), myotonia. Decreased in muscle fibrosis, fatty replacement, or periodic paralysis during the paralysis.

2. Spontaneous activity: Normal resting muscle has no spontaneous activity except end-plate noise.

       a. Configuration = duration, amplitude, number of phases

          1) Duration: Long in LMN and neuropathy due to axon sprouting. Short in myopathies and early reinnervation.

          2) Amplitude: High in chronic neurogenic dz.

          3) Polyphasic: Neurogenic and myopathic dz.

       b. Recruitment: Effort recruits additional motor units. Low in LMN or nerve dz. Early recruitment in myopathies. Poor activation has brain cause, e.g., stroke, poor effort.

   c. **Fibrillations:** Spikes, positive sharp waves. Seen 2-3 wk after denervation.
   d. **Fasciculations:** Discharge of an entire MU. Seen in LMN dz.
   e. **Myotonia, myokymia:** Complex repetitive discharges.

ENCEPHALOPATHY, DELIRIUM, AND DEMENTIA

A. **See also:** Metabolic, Toxic, and Deficiency Disorders, p. 69.
B. **Management of agitation:**
   1. **Acute:** See Psychiatric emergencies, p. 97.
   2. **Chronic:** Risperidone (less sedating) or quetiapine (less risk of movement disorder). Although both have black box warnings in the elderly, there are few humane alternatives. Orally disintegrating or depo formulations for pts who cheek pills.
C. **Delirium:** Agitated confusion, usually with the implication of acute metabolic cause. Usually slurred speech, often frank hallucinations, motor signs (tremor, myoclonus, asterixis), rarely seizures.
   1. **DDx:** Hypoxia, hypercapnia, electrolytes, glucose, drug overdose or withdrawal, sepsis, meningitis, encephalitis, high ammonia, uremia, Wernicke's syndrome. Consider also depression, psychosis, thyroid storm, transient global amnesia, nonconvulsive status epilepticus, posterior leukoencephalopathy.
   2. **Tests:** Consider head CT, ABG, EKG, electrolytes, BUN, Cr, Ca, ammonia, toxin screen, CBC, ESR, U/A and other infectious workup, LP, EEG.
D. **Encephalopathy:** Nonspecific term for diffuse brain dysfunction, often from systemic process, that is not a classic dementia.
   1. **Reversible causes of subacute or chronic encephalopathy:**
     a. **The big two:** Addiction (p. 102), pseudodementia of depression/anxiety (p. 104). Ask family members as well as pt. if their mouth says no but their eyes say yes; contact them in private later.
     b. **Others:** Bilateral SDH, NPH, vasculitis, lymphoma, metabolic, tumor (especially falx meningioma), thyroid, B_{12}, thiamine, infection (especially HIV, syphilis, fungal).
   2. **Creutzfeldt-Jakob dz (CJD):** Sporadic, acquired (e.g., bovine spongiform encephalopathy, BSE), or familial buildup of prion protein particles.
     a. **H&P:** Variable combinations of myoclonus, dementia, and ataxia; progresses to death in weeks to 2 yrs. BSE more often begins with psychiatric symptoms.
     b. **Incidence:** Peaks in late 60s for sporadic form, about age 30 for BSE.
     c. **Tests:** Brain biopsy shows spongiform encephalopathy. EEG shows diffuse periodic sharps. MRI shows characteristic DWI changes in the caudate, putamen, and cortical ribbon. CSF has 14-3-3 protein (also high in encephalitis and some gliomas). Brain biopsy shows spongiform encephalopathy.

    d. Precautions: CJD is transmissible only when infected neural tissue contacts an open wound. However, the agent is not inactivated by standard sterilization techniques.

E. Dementia: Chronic selective loss of ≥2 higher cortical functions, especially memory and naming. Pt. may be disoriented acutely at night, but frank hallucinations are rare.

  1. H&P: Education, baseline personality, ADLs, falls, incontinence, drug changes, h/o depression. Check primitive reflexes. See also Mini-Mental Status Exam, p. 98.

  2. Tests: Head CT, CHEM10, CBC, VDRL, ESR, TSH, B$_{12}$. Consider HIV test, LP, EEG, heavy metal screen, brain biopsy.

  3. Potentially reversible causes: See Encephalopathy, above.

  4. Normal pressure hydrocephalus (NPH):

    a. H&P: Frontal gait, incontinence (from abulia or not being able to get to bathroom), dementia (frontal, abulic, vs. Alzheimer's type). No headache or papilledema

    b. Tests: Serial large-volume LPs (not perfectly sensitive, pt can need up to 3 mo of VP shunt before improving). Consider ICP monitor × 48 h to look for plateau waves (V or A). Consider trial of levodopa to rule out Parkinson's dz.

    c. Rx of NPH: Ventriculoperitoneal shunt. Gait apraxia responds best; dementia worst, especially if longstanding. Risk of SDH (vessels already stretched by atrophy).

  5. Irreversible causes:

    a. Alzheimer's dz (AD): Usually with triad of aphasia, apraxia, agnosia.

    b. Lewy body dz: More episodic delirium, psychiatric features (visual hallucinations, depression), and extrapyramidal features than AD. May benefit from low-dose levodopa or a dopamine agonist in combination with an atypical neuroleptic (e.g., quetiapine). Avoid typical neuroleptics.

    c. Frontotemporal dementia (A tauopathy, formerly Pick's disease): More personality change, less aphasia or amnesia than AD.

    d. Cortical vs. subcortical dementia: Latter is more manageable because pt has insight, can use cueing and to-do lists. Often associated with executive dysfunction.

	Subcortical	Cortical
Examples	Basal ganglia dz	Alzheimer's dz
Language	Normal	Impaired
Memory	Bad retrieval	Bad encoding
Memory cues	Cues help	Cues do not help
Processing speed	Slow	Normal
Insight	Normal	Impaired
Basic motor skills	Slow, clumsy	Normal
Ideomotor skills	Normal	Impaired

Table 8. Cortical vs. subcortical dementia.

    e. Mixed: Lewy body disease, Multi-infarct dementia, CJD, MS.
    f. Rx: Social services, treat depression (avoid TCAs), neuroleptics such as haloperidol (see Delirium above re black box warnings), or short-acting benzodiazepines for agitation. Consider donepezil (a cholinergic agonist) or memantine (an NMDA antagonist).

EVOKED POTENTIALS

A. General: AKA evoked responses. They record latency, amplitude, R/L discrepancies from scalp during stimulation of sensory modalities. They can detect clinically silent lesions and give objective proof of sensory deficits, but a positive MRI usually makes EPs unnecessary.

B. Visual evoked potentials (VEP): Stimulate with flashing light or checkerboard pattern. Detects vision when pt. can not communicate; delayed in optic neuritis even after recovery. P100 is prolonged in retinal or optic nerve lesion—need ERGs (electroretinograms) to differentiate between them.

C. Somatosensory evoked potentials (SSEP): Stimulate peripheral nerves (usually median, common peroneal, posterior tibial), record on scalp, sometimes spine. Prolonged if lesion anywhere along nerve, plexus, nerve root, spinal cord, brainstem, thalamus, cortex.

D. Brainstem auditory evoked responses (BAER): Measure function of auditory nerves and brainstem auditory pathways. Peripheral vestibular dz does not affect BAER. There are seven waves, but only I, III, and V are important. I is from CN VIII; III = bilateral superior olive, V = inferior colliculus. IPL = interpeak latency.
    1. All waves absent: Suggests peripheral deafness.
    2. I-III prolonged (or III absent): Suggests pontomedullary junction lesion, e.g., MS, CPA tumor, pontine glioma, brainstem infarct.
    3. III-V prolonged (or V absent): Pons/midbrain lesion, e.g., MS, extrinsic mass compressing brainstem (includes contralateral CPA tumor).
    4. All waves prolonged: Suggests diffuse dz, e.g., MS, big glioma. Not usually metabolic.

EYES AND VISION

A. Vision: <u>Sudden visual loss is an emergency.</u>
    1. H&P: Time course of visual loss, eye pain, headache, fevers, joint pain, DM, check BP, ocular and carotid bruits, fundi (disc pallor, papilledema, retinopathy, arterial occlusion or cholesterol plaque, cherry red spot), red desaturation, pinhole correction, Amsler grid for metamorphopsia, size of blind spot.
        a. Whenever you use dilating drops to examine the fundi, <u>note it clearly in the chart</u> so the next examiner will not think the pt is herniating.
    2. Poor acuity: See eye chart, back endpapers. Suggests eye or optic nerve problem. If acuity corrects to normal with pinhole, the problem is in the media of the eye, not nerve.

3. **Binocular blindness:** Usually from a lesion at the optic chiasm (e.g., pituitary mass) or in both occipital lobes (e.g., bilateral PCA infarcts), or toxic/metabolic/nutritional—unless both eyes have been exposed to the same insult (e.g., shower of emboli).
4. **Monocular blindness:** Transient (TMB) or permanent loss, sudden and nontraumatic.
   a. **Causes:**
      1) **TMB:** Embolus or thrombus, often from carotid lesion. 11% of TMB pts later have stroke, 41% of them within 1 wk. Temporal arteritis or other vasculitis....
      2) **Sudden permanent monocular blindness:** All causes of TMB, plus optic neuritis, intraocular bleed, retinal detachment, acute angle closure glaucoma, infection....
   b. **Types of retinal infarct:**
      1) **Central retinal artery:** Cherry red spot seen in fundus after 6 h.
      2) **Branch retinal artery:** Fundus pallor along that branch.
      3) **Anterior ischemic optic neuropathy:** Often idiopathic; sometimes arteritis.
   c. **Tests:** ESR, CRP, fibrinogen, TEE, temporal artery biopsy (within days of starting steroids). See also Stroke workup, p. 20.
   d. **Rx of TMB:**
      1) **Prednisone:** 60 mg qd until artery biopsy results are back. Vessel inflammation can be patchy, so if clinical suspicion is high, continue prednisone and rebiopsy.
      2) **IV heparin:** See Anticoagulants, p. 160.
      3) **Decrease intraocular pressure** to help move a possible embolus through the eye. Hypercarbia probably does <u>not</u> help.
         a) **Massage eye:** Have pt. press hard × 4 sec; off × 4 sec.
         b) **IV mannitol** 50 g, or IV acetazolamide 400 mg. Watch BP.
         c) **Anterior paracentesis** by ophthalmologist.
   e. **Rx of optic neuritis:** See Demyelinating Disease, p. 33.
5. **Visual field defects:**
   a. **Monocular scotoma:** Prechiasmal lesion, e.g., glaucoma, retinal hemorrhage, optic neuritis, retinal detachment.
   b. **Noncongruent bilateral scotomata:** Chiasm + nerve lesion.
   c. **Bitemporal defect:** Chiasmal lesion, e.g., aneurysm or pituitary mass. Consider glaucoma.
   d. **Homonymous defect** (same side in both eyes): Postchiasmal.
      1) **Sparing macula:** Visual cortex.
      2) **Including macula:** Optic radiations.
      3) **Superior quadrant defect:** Optic radiations in inferior temporal lobe that can be affected by mastoid infection causing cerebritis.
      4) **Inferior quadrant defect:** Optic radiations in parietal lobe.
6. **Higher visual system abnormalities:**
   a. **Anton's syndrome:** Bilateral occipital lesions cause blindness, but pt denies he is blind.
   b. **Bonnet's syndrome:** Visual deprivation hallucinations (formed, stereotyped, no other signs of delirium).
   c. **Motion and visuospatial processing:** Dorsal, occipitoparietal "where" pathway.

      1) **Balint's syndrome:** Visual disorientation (simultanagnosia), optic ataxia (deficit of visual reaching), ocular apraxia (deficit of visual scanning). From bilateral occipitoparietal lesion.

   d. **Object recognition:** Ventral, occipitotemporal "what" pathway lesions cause visual agnosia.

      1) **Prosopagnosia:** Inability to recognize faces; from bilateral inferior visual association cortex lesions.

      2) **Word blindness:** Alexia without agraphia. Seen in left hemisphere lesion near splenium of callosum. Usually with R homonymous hemianopsia and color anomia or achromatopsia.

      3) **Achromatopsia vs. color anomia:** In former, pt. cannot perceive colors; in latter, pt. can perceive them but not name them.

B. Pupils

  1. **Causes of anisocoria:** (unequal pupils)

   a. **Horner's syndrome:** See p. 12.

   b. **Third nerve lesion:**

      1) **H&P:** Unilateral large pupil; also ophthalmoplegia and ptosis. Anisocoria is worse in light (vs. Horner's). Ask about time course, comorbid conditions (e.g., DM).

      2) **DDx:** Aneurysm (especially P-comm) > ischemia (e.g., DM or HTN) > trauma, uncal herniation, tumor, etc. In an alert pt., a fixed dilated pupil is almost never herniation.

         a) **Pupil involvement:** Suggests compression because pupillary parasympathetic fibers are the most superficial.

         b) **Pupil sparing:** Suggests ischemic third nerve. But only consider a lesion pupil sparing if it is otherwise a complete third nerve palsy (ophthalmoplegia and ptosis). Otherwise you may be fooled by an early compressive third.

         c) **R/O P-comm aneurysm:** Immediate CT and LP to r/o bleed, consider angiogram. May not need this if deficit is clearly pupil sparing.

   c. **Drug effects:**

      1) **Dilators** (mydriatics): From sympathetic agonists, e.g., atropine, scopolamine, phenylephrine, tropicamide, albuterol. Test with 1% pilocarpine (a parasympathetic agonist); it will not constrict pupil if the pupil was previously drug dilated, but will in third nerve compression or Adie's syndrome.

      2) **Constrictors:** From parasympathetic agonists, e.g., pilocarpine.

   d. **Acute glaucoma:** Fixed pupil, about 6 mm. Also decreased acuity; red, painful eye; hazy cornea; blurred vision; shallow ant. chamber if side-illuminate with penlight.

      1) **Rx:** <u>Emergent</u> IV acetazolamide or mannitol; topical pilocarpine.

   e. **Adie's (tonic) pupil:** One large pupil, reacts poorly to light, with better constriction to near; then redilates sluggishly. Often sudden, in young woman, with decreased DTRs.

      1) **Test:** Dilute pilocarpine (0.1%) will constrict Adie's pupil but not normal pupil.

    f. Argyll-Robertson: Small, irregular, unequal (sometimes equal) pupils, constrict to near better than light.
      1) DDx: Syphilis, diabetic pseudotabes....
    g. Old ocular surgery or trauma.
    h. Physiologic anisocoria: Should be less than 1 mm difference in both light and dark, briskly reactive.
  2. Causes of bilateral fixed or poorly reactive pupils:
    a. Bilateral large pupils:
      1) Fixed: Death, subtotal medullary lesion, immediately post anoxia or hypothermia, severe hypoglycemia, bilateral or nuclear third palsy, botulism.
      2) Reactive (usually): Anxiety, opiate withdrawal, aerosolized albuterol, overdose of IV dopamine, atropine, aminoglycosides, tetracycline, Mg, amyl nitrite.
    b. Midsized pupils: Dorsal midbrain lesion, e.g., from hydrocephalus. May see sluggish reaction to near, as in Argyll-Robertson pupil.
    c. Pinpoint pupils: Opiates, pontine lesion (usually with skew deviation or ophthalmoplegia), metabolic encephalopathy.
  3. Afferent pupillary defect (APD, Marcus-Gunn pupil): Transient dilation as flashlight moves from good to bad eye. From optic neuritis or retinal lesion.
C. Fundi
  1. Disk edema: Ask about pulsatile tinnitus, gray/blackouts of vision lasting a few seconds, headache, N/V, and diplopia, which are all other signs of increased ICP. Look for venous pulsations, acuity, fields.
    a. Papilledema: Term reserved for disk edema due to high ICP.
    b. Bilateral disk edema: Usually painless. High ICP from intracranial tumors, pseudotumor cerebri, metabolic problems....
    c. Unilateral edema:
      1) Visual loss and pain: Optic neuritis, infection/inflammation, temporal arteritis.
      2) Visual loss, no pain: Ant. ischemic optic neuropathy from temporal arteritis or vascular risk factors.
  2. Optic atrophy: Glaucoma, past neuritis, toxic/metabolic optic neuropathies, chronic papilledema.
D. Eye Movement Abnormalities
  1. See also: Cranial Nerves, p. 32.
  2. Acute extraocular paralysis is an emergency: Consider botulism, myasthenic crisis, P-comm aneurysm, cavernous sinus thrombosis, infection, fistula, variant Guillain-Barré syndrome.
  3. H&P: Direction of greatest deficit, h/o lazy eye, drugs, thyroid dz, pain, alteration with fatigue. Note head tilt (compare with old photo), check Bell's reflex, stereopsis, ocular bruit.
    a. Eye muscles:
    b. Figure shows the main field of action of individual eye muscles. Have pt. track your finger in these directions; also test saccades laterally and vertically.

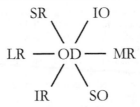

Figure 7. Direction of ocular muscle action, right eye.

   c. **Diplopia without visibly disconjugate gaze:**
     1) **Red glass test:** Convention is to hold it over R eye. Have pt. report relative positions of red and normal images in all directions of gaze. Diplopia is maximal in the field of gaze of the paretic muscle, and the image belonging to the paretic muscle projects peripherally.
     2) **Alternating cover test:** For phoria (latent): shift cover to other eye while fixating. If covered eye moves in, it is exophoria; if out, it is esophoria; if down, it is hyperphoria; if up, it is hypophoria. If eyes are never conjugate (but not paralyzed), it is a tropia, not a phoria.
  4. Causes of eye movement abnormalities: Nerve palsy, brainstem lesion, raised ICP with herniation, strabismus, myasthenia gravis, drugs (especially DPH), multiple sclerosis, Graves' dz, orbital entrapment, trauma, meningitis or other infection, migraine, Wernicke's syndrome, Fisher variant of GBS, mitochondrial dz.
   a. **Causes of painful ophthalmoplegias:** Cavernous sinus tumor, thrombosis, fistula, or dissection; zoster, DM, migraine, infection, Tolosa-Hunt syndrome.
  5. Bilateral conjugate gaze palsies:
   a. **Bilateral fixed eyes:**
     1) **Caloric test:** See p. 222.
     2) **Oculocephalic reflex:** (Doll's eye test is a confusing term.) Do only if C-spine is stable.
   b. **Bilateral upgaze palsy:** The main vertical gaze center is the rostral interstitial nucleus of MLF in dorsal midbrain; there may be another at the cervicomedullary junction.
     1) **Causes:** Can tell supranuclear lesions (e.g., PSP, dorsal midbrain syndrome) from age-related eye muscle weakness by the presence of other deficits and by the following tests:
       a) **Bell's reflex:** Eyes normally roll up when pt tries to close lids against your resistance. This reflex is intact in supranuclear lesions.
       b) **Vertical doll's eyes:** Have pt fix on a target while you move pt.'s head. Intact in supranuclear lesions.
       c) **Light-near dissociation:** Present in pretectal lesions. The pupil constricts better when accommodating near targets than it does to light.
     2) **Dorsal midbrain lesion** (Parinaud's syndrome): Often from basilar stroke or pineal tumor. Upgaze worse than downgaze.

See convergence paresis, retraction nystagmus, and lid retraction ("setting sun eyes") on attempted upgaze. May see skew deviation, light-near dissociation.

c. **Bilateral downgaze palsy:** Early PSP, bilateral ventral midbrain lesions, anoxic coma.

d. **Bilateral lateral deviation:** Contralateral cerebral hemisphere or midbrain lesion; ipsilateral pons lesion.

   1) **Causes:** Lesion of 6th nucleus, pedunculopontine reticular formation (PPRF), parietal neglect, L frontal (in latter two, oculocephalic reflex can overcome gaze paresis).

   2) **Nuclear 6th vs. PPRF lesion:** Although the rostral PPRF is usually affected with the 6th nerve given their close proximity, lesion of the 6th nerve nucleus involves 7th nerve as well (genu of 7th wraps around 6th nucleus), giving an ipsilateral lower motor neuron 7th palsy (forehead spared). A pure PPRF lesion spares 6th nerve function.

e. **Internuclear ophthalmoplegia (INO):**

   1) **H&P:**

     a) **Ipsilateral eye:** Poor adduction to nose.

     b) **Contralateral eye:** Abduction nystagmus (on lateral gaze).

     c) **Convergence paresis:** Except in very caudal lesions.

   2) **Location:** Lesion is on side of the eye with poor adduction, in the MLF, rostral to 6th nerve nucleus (blocks path from 6th to contralateral 3rd), anywhere from pons to midbrain.

   3) **DDx:** The elderly usually have vascular causes; young adults usually MS; children usually pontine glioma. Myasthenia can cause a "pseudo-INO."

f. **One-and-a-half syndrome:** An INO plus horizontal gaze palsy. The ipsilateral eye cannot adduct or abduct. The contralateral eye cannot adduct and has abduction nystagmus. The lesion is lower in the pons than that causing an INO; it is at the level of the 6th nerve nucleus and involves the MLF and PPRF.

g. **Congenital progressive external ophthalmoplegia (CPEO):** See Mitochondrial Disorders, p. 72.

6. **Skew deviation:** A vertical misalignment, seen in posterior fossa and brainstem lesions.

7. **Unilateral ophthalmoparesis:**

a. **Individual muscle palsy:** See Figure 7, p. 48

b. **CN III (oculomotor):** See also Anisocoria (unequal pupils), p. 46.

   1) **H&P:** Fixed and dilated pupil, ptosis, partial ophthalmoparesis. Only lateral gaze is intact, so eye is deviated down and out. Superior trunk controls upgaze and lid; inferior trunk controls downgaze and pupil.

   2) **Causes:** Important to rule out P-comm aneurysm immediately (see p. 47). Midbrain lesion usually has contralateral hemiparesis too. Pupil-sparing palsy (ptosis plus ophthalmoparesis must be present) suggests nerve ischemia usually in setting of diabetes; also temporal arteritis or myasthenia. Often idiopathic.

c. **CN IV (trochlear):**

   1) **H&P:** Diplopia on looking down and in.

2) **Compensatory head tilt:** Away from side of lesion. "<u>GOTS</u> <u>Worse</u>"—<u>G</u>aze <u>O</u>pposite, <u>T</u>ilt <u>S</u>ame makes a 4th palsy <u>Worse</u>.
   a) **Chronic?** Look at driver's license to see if head tilt is old.
3) **Bielshowsky test:** Look for hypertropia and diplopia on straight gaze, R gaze vs. L, and R head tilt vs. L tilt.
4) **Causes:** Closed head trauma > vascular > tumor. Often idiopathic.

d. **CN VI (abducens):**
   1) **H&P:** In a nerve lesion, only the ipsilateral eye cannot look laterally. A nuclear lesion also impairs contralateral eye's ability to look towards the lesioned side.
   2) **Causes:** Tumor (30%) > trauma, ischemic, high ICP, Graves' dz, idiopathic, Wernicke's syndrome....
   3) **Cavernous sinus syndromes:**

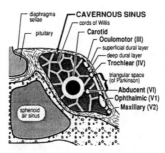

Figure 8. The cavernous sinus. (From Greenberg MS. *Handbook of Neurosurgery.* 3rd ed. Lakeland, FL: Greenberg Graphics; 1994: 103, with permission.)

   a) **H&P:** Variable involvement of CN III, IV, V_{1-2}, VI. An isolated VI palsy with a Horner's syndrome is a giveaway. Often with pain and proptosis.
   b) **DDx:** Carotid artery aneurysm, dissection; venous thrombosis, infection, tumor, Tolosa-Hunt, Wernicke's....
   c) **Tolosa-Hunt syndrome:** Idiopathic granuloma near the superior orbital fissure, causing pain and III, IV, or VI palsies. Responds to steroids but r/o tumors and infection first. Do not confuse Tolosa-Hunt with Ramsay-Hunt syndrome (see p. 93).

8. **Nystagmus:** Although jerk nystagmus is described by the direction of the fast phase, it is always a disorder of slow eye movements.
   a. **H&P:** Note whether nystagmus is present in primary gaze; direction of fast component, whether it extinguishes with fixation. Look for accompanying palatal or facial myoclonus, which suggests denervation of the inf. olive, by damage to the central tegmental tract.
   b. **Causes of nystagmus:** See also Vertigo, p. 127.

1) **Horizontal:**
   a) **Jerk nystagmus:** Saccadic movement in one direction; slow corrective movement in the other. Causes include drugs, cerebellar or brainstem lesion, vestibular dz, congenital syndromes. A few beats of end-gaze nystagmus may be normal.
   b) **Pendular nystagmus:** Slow movements in both directions. Drugs and vestibular causes are uncommon (unlike jerk nystagmus). Seen in congenital blindness.
2) **Downbeat:** Often craniocervical junction problem causing ant. cerebellar vermis lesion, e.g., with Chiari malformation. Also MS, drugs, Wernicke's syndrome....
3) **Upbeat:** Often medullary lesion; also MS, drugs, Wernicke's....
4) **Rotatory:** If in combination with horizontal nystagmus and vertigo, usually a peripheral, vestibular lesion. If pure rotatory, usually medullary or diencephalic.

9. **Other ocular oscillations:**
   a. **Square wave jerks:** Small-amplitude macrosaccades on attempted fixation. Causes: Often cerebellar or demyelinating dz.
   b. **Ocular bobbing:** Constant, conjugate down and up oscillations—fast down, then slow drift back to midposition 2-12 $\times$/min, with horizontal gaze paralysis. Should distinguish it from vertical nystagmus. Causes: Often pontine lesion; sometimes metabolic or from hydrocephalus. Consider also vertical nystagmus.
   c. **Ocular dysmetria:** Eye over- or undershoots target, then makes refixation saccades. Causes: Often cerebellar dz. Distinguish from hypometric saccades, in which eye always undershoots; a sign of extrapyramidal bradykinesia.
   d. **Ocular flutter:** Rapid bursts of horizontal oscillations in primary gaze. Similar causes to opsoclonus.
   e. **Opsoclonus:** Continuous, conjugate, multidirectional saccades. Often from paraneoplastic syndrome; MS, postviral opsoclonus-myoclonus; encephalitis, drugs, tumors.

E. **Lids**
   1. **Ptosis:** (lid droop)
      a. **Unilateral ptosis:** Horner's, third nerve palsy, myasthenia (varies with fatigue), trauma. Sag from 7th nerve palsy can mask ptosis. 7th nerve palsy can imitate a contralateral ptosis because it widens the ipsilateral palpebral fissure.
      b. **Bilateral ptosis:** Nuclear third lesion, myasthenia, progressive external ophthalmoplegia, age-related periorbital atrophy, redundant lid tissue, oculopharyngeal dystrophy, bilateral third palsy.
   2. **Blink rate:** Decreased in extrapyramidal bradykinetic syndromes. These pts often cannot suppress blinks to repeated forehead tap (Myerson's sign) and may have blepharoclonus (lid fluttering) with eyes closed.
   3. **Lid retraction:** Consider dorsal midbrain syndrome; hyperthyroidism (often with lid lag as pt looks down), chronic steroids.

F. **Exophthalmos:** (AKA proptosis)
   1. **DDx:** Carotid cavernous fistula (usually pulsatile), tumor, hyperthyroidism, infection, inflammation, hemorrhage, 3rd nerve palsy (via rectus relaxation), carotid sinus occlusion.

G. Horner's syndrome:

1. **H&P:**
   a. **Ptosis:** An ID photo can show if it is old.
   b. **Miosis** (small pupil): Worse in dark because the abnormal pupil fails to dilate (vs. 3rd nerve lesion, which is worse in light). There should be a dilation lag when lights are turned off.
   c. **Anhidrosis:** Seen if lesion is in nerve before the sweat afferents leave with ext. carotid artery. Wipe on iodine bilaterally and let it dry; then put starch from a glove on top. Sweat will turn it purple.

2. **Tests for localization:**
   a. **Cocaine test** confirms Horner's: dilates normal pupil only. Blocks reuptake, so no effect unless norepinephrine being released at pupil.
   b. **Apraclonidine** is a readily available alternative to cocaine. It dilates Horner's pupil only. It is a weak α_1-agonist.
   c. **Hydroxyamphetamine test** dilates Horner's pupils only if 3rd-order neurons are intact because it is an indirect agonist that releases norepinephrine from the intact terminal.

3. **Causes of isolated Horner's syndrome:**
   a. **3rd-order lesion:** Usually idiopathic (if congenital, iris is often heterochromic) but r/o carotid dissection (no anhidrosis if internal carotid).
   b. **1st- and 2nd-order:** Tumor (including Pancoast) > cluster HA > vascular (dissection, cavernous thrombosis, ischemia) > cervical disk > trauma (including thoracic surgery) > meningitis > PTX > intrinsic brainstem lesion (usually with other findings).

HEADACHE

A. H&P: Similarity to previous HAs, onset and time course, N/V, photophobia, neck pain, trauma, fever, neurological aura, change in sx with position, h/o cancer, family history of aneurysms or migraine, what drugs work for pain. Cranial or sinus tenderness, eye changes, focal neurological signs.

B. Causes:
1. **Sudden paroxysmal headache (HA):** Intracranial hemorrhage (especially subarachnoid), arterial dissection, benign orgasmic HA, thunderclap migraine, hypertensive crisis....
2. **Subacute progressive HA:** Posterior fossa stroke, cerebral vein thrombosis, temporal arteritis, tumor, obstructive hydrocephalus, CSF leak (e.g., post LP), meningitis, sinusitis, or other infection, vascular malformations, glaucoma....
3. **Recurrent or chronic HA:** Migraine, neck arthritis, postconcussive syndrome, pseudotumor cerebri, neuralgia, temporal arteritis, temporomandibular syndrome, drugs (stimulants, solvents, alcohol withdrawal)....

C. Tests:
1. **Sudden or subacute headache (HA):** CT without contrast to r/o bleed, or with contrast to r/o tumor.
   a. **Consider also:** MRA to r/o vascular malformations, dissections, aneurysm. LP to r/o SAH, meningitis, or leptomeningeal carcinomatosis.

    2. Recurrent or chronic HA: Can usually be diagnosed without tests. Consider ESR.
D. Cluster HA:
    1. H&P: Occur at the same time each day, nonthrobbing, uniorbital, ipsilateral running nose, red eye, red cheek, tender temporal artery, lasts 10 min to 2 h, up to 8 times a day, sometimes with Horner's. Alcohol can trigger. Unlike migraneurs, cluster headache sufferers do not lie still, but may walk restlessly. Youngish men.
    2. DDx: Migraine, trigeminal neuralgia, sinus tumor, Tolosa-Hunt....
    3. Rx: Ergot, 100% O_2, methysergide, prednisone taper (can cause rebound). Prophylaxis is more effective than treating acute attack; try calcium channel blocker or lithium.
E. Postconcussive HA: See Concussion, p. 119.
F. LP HA: From continued CSF leak. Worse when standing.
    1. Rx: Lie flat × 24 h; aggressive fluids (especially carbonated, caffeinated drinks), pain drugs. Consider blood patch, IM steroids, abdominal binder.
G. HIV HA: See p. 55.
H. Occipital neuralgia: Pain in occiput, usually with trigger point along superior nuchal line. Injection of local anesthetic and steroids may help.
I. Migraine:
    1. H&P: Unilateral (but not <u>always</u> same side), throbbing, N/V, photophobia, phonophobia, often preceded by visual or other neurologic change.
    2. Rx of acute migraine:
        a. Treat nausea: E.g., with phenothiazine like metoclopramide 10 mg PO/IM/IV.
        b. Triptans: $5-HT_1$ serotonin receptor agonists. E.g., sumatriptan (Imitrex). SC: 6 mg. PO: 25 mg test; if partial relief in 2 h, try up to 100 mg PO; no more than 300 mg qd. Nasal spray 5-20 mg into one nostril, q2h if needed; no more than 40 qd.
            1) Contraindications: Ergots within 24 h, possible CAD.
        c. NSAID: E.g., naproxen 500 mg PO. Beware of short-acting NSAIDS or quick tapers because of rebound HA.
        d. Ergots:
            1) Contraindications: CAD, HTN, hemiplegic or aphasic migraine (ergots are vasoconstrictors).
            2) Dihydroergotamine (DHE): Put pt on a cardiac monitor for first DHE dose. Give metoclopramide 10 mg IV 10 min beforehand, then 1 mg DHE; repeat in 1 h prn; then q6h prn. If it works, try DHE nasal spray, or Cafergot PO.
            3) Cafergot: Ergotamine and caffeine. Give 2 tabs, then 1 q30min, max 6 in 24 h.
        e. Midrin: A sympathomimetic amine with a sedative. Give 2 tabs, then 1qh to relief; max 5 in 12 h.
            1) Contraindications: HTN, glaucoma, renal failure, MAOIs.
        f. Fioricet: 1-2 tabs q4h, for attacks fewer than 3 ×/month. Beware rebound HA.
        g. Opiates: Danger of rebound HA and addiction.
        h. Steroids: For status migrainosus.

3. **Prophylaxis of migraine** (if having migraines more than 3 ×/month):
   a. **TCAs:** Amitriptyline is the only one with proven efficacy, although nortriptyline is probably also effective and better tolerated.
   b. **Propranolol:** Start 10-20 bid. Avoid in asthma, CHF.
   c. **5-HT antagonists:** E.g., methysergide. Need test dose. Danger of retroperitoneal fibrosis.
   d. **Calcium blockers:** E.g., verapamil.
   e. **ACDs:** E.g., valproate 250-500 mg tid.
J. **Rebound HAs:** Common after stopping opiates, Fioricet, NSAIDs. Can cause vicious cycle of analgesic use.

HEARING

A. **Weber's test:** Tuning fork on vertex.
   1. **Conductive (middle ear) deafness:** Fork is louder in affected ear.
   2. **Perceptive (inner ear) deafness:** Fork is louder in good ear.
B. **Rinne's test:** Tuning fork on mastoid first; when no longer heard, hold it in air by ear.
   1. **Normal:** Air conduction heard twice as long as bone conduction.
   2. **Conductive deafness:** Air conduction briefer than bone conduction.
   3. **Perceptive deafness:** Test is normal (air conduction heard longer).
C. **Causes of deafness:**
   1. **Middle ear:** Wax, foreign body, trauma, infection, otosclerosis.
   2. **Cochlea:** Ménière's dz, inflammation, trauma, tumor, toxin (aminoglycoside, cisplatin), vasculitis, internal auditory artery occlusion.
   3. **Retrocochlear:** Cerebellopontine angle mass (acoustic Schwannoma, meningioma, aneurysm, dermoid, epidermoid), multiple sclerosis, brainstem glioma, syringobulbia, inflammation (zoster), brainstem infarct (especially AICA).

INFECTIONS, CNS

A. **Abscess and focal cerebritis:**
   1. **H&P:** Headache, focal deficits, altered mental status. Seizures occur in 40%. Fever, neck stiffness, vomiting, and papilledema are uncommon. Look for other infections, especially ear, nose, mouth, lung, and heart. Ask about HIV risk factors.
   2. **DDx:** Tumor, granuloma.
   3. **Causes:** Anaerobic streptococci are most common. Posttraumatic or surgical cases are more likely to be *Staphylococcus* or Enterobacteriaceae. Many abscesses are polymicrobial.
   4. **Tests:** CT or MRI with contrast should show ring-enhancing cavity, edema, mass effect. Blood cultures, CXR, consider echocardiogram. LP is contraindicated.
   5. **Rx:**
      a. **Surgery:** Needle aspiration or excision of abscess, ideally before Abx initiated.

    b. Abx: Treat for ≥ 6 wks. Adjust Abx on basis of abscess cultures.

        1) Ear or unknown source: Ceftriaxone 2 g IV q12h (or cefo-taxime 2 g IV q4-6h) + metronidazole 500 mg IV q6h. Some also use penicillin 4-5 MU IV q4-6h.

        2) HIV-positive: Add coverage for toxoplasmosis; see below.

        3) Post head trauma or surgery: Vancomycin 1 g IV q12h + ceftazidime 2 g IV q8h or cefepime 2 g IV q12h.

    c. Steroids: Only if severely high ICP because steroids may decrease antibiotic penetration.

B. Cryptococcosis: A fungus, *Cryptococcus neoformans*, the most common cause of fungal meningitis. Cryptococcal meningitis <u>may be an emergency</u> because pts can die suddenly from high ICP.

    1. H&P: HIV, immunosuppression, pigeon exposure. Headache, fever, meningeal signs, confusion, signs of high ICP. Seizures uncommon.

    2. DDx: Other meningitides.

    3. Tests: CSF (see p. 19). CSF India ink stain is positive in 75%. Serum and CSF cryptococcal Ag. CT/MRI usually normal.

    4. Rx: Regimens vary; consider amphotericin B and flucytosine, then fluconazole. Consider serial LPs for high ICP.

C. Cysticercosis: A helminth, the pig tapeworm *Taenia solium*.

    1. H&P: Country of origin, seizures, headache, signs of raised ICP.

    2. DDx: Other parasitic dz.

    3. Tests: Stool ova and parasites. Blood serology better than CSF, but slow. Consider long-bone x-ray series to look for calcified muscle cysts. CT/MRI appearance depends on stage. Chronic, inactive lesions are calcified, nonenhancing, usually at gray-white junction. Active, degenerating cysts enhance and have edema.

    4. Rx: Albendazole 15 mg/kg qd for 8 d. Regimens vary; praziquantel 50 mg/kg divided tid for 12-14 d is an alternative. Consider steroids because dying cysts cause inflammation. Surgery for cyst removal or shunting is often necessary for posterior fossa or intraventricular cysts. If cysts are inactive, rx may not help. Treat seizures.

        a. Macular cysts: Rule them out <u>before</u> albendazole (check acuity and fundi).

        b. Ventricular cysts: Consider surgery.

        c. ID consult is often helpful.

D. Empyema, CNS: An <u>IMMEDIATE SURGICAL EMERGENCY</u>. Usually see HA out of proportion to neurological deficit.

    1. Brain subdural empyemas: Frequently from sinusitis or trauma. Unlike subdural blood, they are better seen on MRI than CT (restricted diffusion). Consult ENT preoperatively for sinus drainage during the same procedure. Watch for sinus thrombosis.

    2. Spinal cord empyemas: Never do an LP in a pt. with fever and back pain until you have ruled out empyema with MRI.

E. Human immunodeficiency virus (HIV): See also Infection, p. 219.

    1. Incidence: 50% of HIV pts. have a CNS or PNS problem; this can be the presenting complaint.

    2. Headache: Have a very low threshold for MRI + gadolinium and LP. All pts. with HA and fever should get both.

3. **Focal brain sx:** Consider toxoplasmosis, lymphoma, progressive multifocal leukoencephalopathy (PML), *Cryptococcus*, VZV encephalitis, tuberculoma, neurosyphilis, clot, bleed, bacterial abscess.
4. **Nonfocal/encephalitic sx:**
   a. **HIV dementia complex:** Subcortical dementia with psychomotor slowing; often psychosis, frontal, corticospinal, or basal ganglia signs.
   b. **Encephalitis:** CMV, HSV, HIV.
   c. **Metabolic encephalopathies.**
5. **Meningeal sx:** Meningitis from HIV (primary infection), *Cryptococcus*, TB, syphilis, bacterial, lymphomatous.
6. **Cranial neuropathy:** CNS lesion, meningitis, peripheral neuropathy.
7. **Spinal cord sx:** B_{12} deficiency, HTLV-1, HSV or VZV myelitis; vacuolar myelopathy.
8. **Peripheral nerve sx:** Can be immune mediated, drug induced, or infectious (e.g., CMV or VZV radiculopathy).
   a. **Lumbosacral polyradiculopathy** (cauda equina syndrome): Subacute leg weakness with inability to walk ± back pain, early bowel and bladder problems.
      1) **DDx:** Usually CMV. Consider also lymphomatous meningitis, neurosyphilis, spinal cord mass.
      2) **Tests:** LP shows >100 WBCs/μL (often with high PMNs), high protein, normal or low glucose. EMG shows axonal and demyelinating lesion.
      3) **Rx:** Ganciclovir or foscarnet.
   b. **Distal symmetric peripheral neuropathy (DSPN):** From nucleoside reverse transcriptase inhibitors (NRTIs), e.g., didanosine (ddI) or zalcitabine (ddC), or from Kaposi's chemotherapy (vincristine, cisplatin).
9. **Myopathy:** From zidovudine (AZT).

F. **Lyme dz:**
1. **H&P:**
   a. **Early** (3 d-1 mo): Erythema migrans in ~70%.
   b. **Middle** (up to 9 mo): Heart block ± myocarditis, recurrent arthritis, recurrent meningitis, radiculoneuritis and cranial neuritis (especially peripheral 7th-nerve lesion).
   c. **Late:** Fatigue, mild encephalopathy, MS-like lesions on MRI, neuropathy, seizures.
2. **Tests:** CSF Lyme Ab titer (only test CSF if seropositive).
3. **Rx:**
   a. **Isolated 7th palsy or mild neuropathy:** Doxycycline 100 mg bid × 21-28 d or amoxicillin 500 mg tid × 21-28 d.
   b. **More serious neurological sx:** Ceftriaxone 2 g IV q12h × 2-6 wk.

G. **Meningitis:**
1. **Bacterial meningitis is an emergency:** It may be necessary to give IV Abx empirically before the LP. LP can be done up to 2 h after first dose without destroying culture results.
2. **H&P:** Prior focal signs, earache, cough, gastroenteritis, immunosuppression, trauma. HA, fever, stiff neck, rash, photophobia, fundi, stiff neck, runny ear or nose.

    a. Brudzinski's sign: Bending chin to chest → hips and knees flex.

    b. Kernig's sign: Pain on straight leg raise. Could also be nerve compression.

3. **Tests:** CT (consider contrast), LP (technique, p. 224; CSF findings, p. 19), blood cultures, CBC, HIV test, CXR. Consider testing nasal discharge for glucose, chloride to r/o CSF leak.

4. **DDx of meningitis:** Tumor + fever, abscess, toxic exposure.

5. **Bacterial meningitis:**

    a. Respiratory precautions if you suspect *N. meningitidis.*

    b. Dexamethasone 20 min before, or at least with, the first Abx dose, at 0.15 mg/kg every 6 h for 2-4 d, or until pathogen determined. Helps *H. influenzae* primarily. No point in starting it after the first dose of Abx.

    c. Empiric Abx: These suggestions do not apply outside the US and are heavily influenced by vaccine use. Adjust on basis of culture and sensitivities.

Patient	Likely Pathogens	Antibiotics
18-50 yr	Pneumococcus, meningococcus	Vancomycin 0.5 g IV q6h + ceftriaxone 2 g IV q12h
>50 yr	Pneumococ., meningococ, gram-neg bacilli, *Listeria*	Vancomycin 1 g IV q6h + ceftriaxone 2 g IV q12h + ampicillin 2 g IV q4h
Immunocompromised	*Listeria*, pneumococ., *H. influenzae*	Vancomycin 1 g IV q 6h + ceftriaxone 2 g IV q12h + ampicillin 2 g IV q4h
Head trauma, surgery, shunt	*Staphylococcus*, gram-neg. bacilli, pneumococ.	Ampicillin 2 g IV q4h + vancomycin 1 g IV q12h + cefepime 2 g IV q12h

Table 9. Empiric antibiotics for bacterial meningitis. (Adapted from Tunkel AR, et al. *Clin Infect Dis.* 2004;39:1267-1284.)

6. **Viral meningoencephalitis:**

    a. Herpes simplex encephalitis:

        1) HSV encephalitis is an emergency: Acyclovir should be started empirically before HSV PCR is back.

        2) H&P: Viral prodrome; then rapid progression of floridly abnormal behavior, amnesia, seizures, hemiplegia, coma.

        3) Tests: HSV PCR in CSF; high CSF RBCs, monocytes, and protein. MRI may show ant. temporal lobe edema, uncal herniation. EEG often shows periodic lateralized epileptiform discharges.

        4) Rx: Acyclovir 10 mg/kg IV q8h for 7-10 d. Watch closely for signs of uncal transtentorial herniation.

b. **Others:** Varicella, enterovirus, mumps, arboviruses (e.g., eastern equine encephalitis, St. Louis encephalitis), rabies.

7. **Tuberculous meningitis and tuberculomas:**
   a. **H&P:** Recent TB exposure. HIV risk factors. Slow onset of headache, low-grade fever, then meningismus and focal neurological signs. In young pts. but not in secondary reactivation, it is usually associated with disseminated dz.
   b. **Tests:** CSF shows lymphocytosis, low glucose, high protein, and positive AFB cultures (after 4-6 wk). AFB stain is frequently negative. PPD is negative in 1/3 of pts.; CXR shows pulmonary TB in about 75%. Molecular tests are controversial.
   c. **Rx:** If suspicious, must start rx before CSF cultures come back. Check with an ID specialist for current recommendations, but typical practice starts with isoniazid, rifampin, pyrazinamide, and ethambutol. Give pyridoxine supplements; watch for hypersensitivity, liver dysfunction, and neuropathy. Steroids are sometimes used if there is high ICP, encephalopathy, or evidence of vasculitis.

8. **Chronic or recurrent meningitis:**
   a. **DDx of chronic meningitis:**
      1) **Noninfectious:** Neoplasm, sarcoid, vasculitis, lupus, Vogt-Koyanagi-Harada syndrome, Behçet's dz, chronic benign lymphocytic meningitis, Mollaret's meningitis, chemical meningitis, post-SAH . . . .
      2) **Infectious:** TB, fungal, cysticercosis, HACEK organisms, Lyme, brucellosis, syphilis.
   b. **Tests:**
      1) **Blood:**
         a) **General:** Electrolytes, LFTs, CBC, ESR, ANA, RF, ACE, SIEP, VDRL.
         b) **Antibodies** to *Brucella*, toxoplasmosis, *Cryptococcus*, Lyme, histoplasmosis, coccidiomycosis.
         c) **Antigen:** *Cryptococcus*.
      2) **CSF:**
         a) **Cultures:** Bacterial, mycobacterial, fungal cultures. Consider volume, >10 cc; prolonged (HACEK organisms), CO_2 (*Brucella*), or anaerobic (*Actinomyces*) incubations.
         b) **Assays:** Cryptococcal Ag and Ab, India ink prep for fungi, AFB, VDRL, HSV PCR.
         c) **Cytology:** Mollaret's cells, flow cytometry.
      3) **Imaging:** MRI for parameningeal abscess; consider CXR, spine, skull films.
      4) **Other:** PPD, sputum AFB, stool fungi, meningeal biopsy.

H. **Progressive multifocal leukoencephalopathy (PML):** Hemiparesis, visual field cut, ataxia, cognitive changes over days to weeks. From JC virus infection; usually with HIV. Usually no mass effect or enhancement, unlike lymphoma, toxo). No specific rx; HIV rx helps some.

I. **Syphilis:** A spirochete, *Treponema pallidum*.
   1. **H&P:** Other sexually transmitted dz, genital lesions, HIV.

      a. Early meningitis: 6-12 mo after primary infection.
      b. Meningovascular: Cranial neuropathies, especially 7th and 8th, arteritis, stroke.
      c. Tabes dorsalis: Sharp leg pains, Argyll-Robertson pupils, proprioceptive ataxia, overflow incontinence, dropped reflexes.
      d. General paresis of the insane: May present with any psychiatric sx. Tabes and meningovascular syphilis are uncommon. Often see brisk DTRs, expressionless face, dysmetria.
  2. DDx: Cryptococcal, TB, or carcinomatous meningitis, CNS sarcoid, Lyme, vasculitis.
  3. Tests: Serum fluorescent treponemal absorption test positive in 90%. RPR and serum VDRL may be negative. CSF VDRL nearly always positive, with high protein and lymphocytes. HIV test.
  4. Rx: 24 MU penicillin G IV, 3-4 MU × 10-14 d.
J. Toxoplasmosis: An intracellular protozoan, *Toxoplasma gondii*.
  1. H&P: Immunosuppression, focal deficits, HA, confusion, fever, seizures.
  2. DDx: Lymphoma, bacterial abscess, viral or fungal encephalitis, PML.
  3. Tests: CT/MRI—enhancing, usually ring enhancement, with edema. LP (see p. 19). Toxoplasmosis titer (Ab not usually useful). HIV test, CD4 count.
  4. Rx (often empiric for 2 weeks before brain bx): Acutely, pyrimethamine 200 mg PO × 1; then pyrimethamine 50-75 mg PO qd + leucovorin 10-20 mg PO qd + sulfadiazine 1-1.5 g PO q6h × >6 wk, then half-dose pyrimethamine + sulfa indefinitely.

INFLAMMATORY DISORDERS

A. See also: Demyelinating Disease (p. 33), myositis (p. 83).
B. Vasculitis: Angiitis and vasculitis are synonyms. Arteritis is vasculitis restricted to arteries.
  1. Angiitis, primary CNS: Small-medium arteries.
      a. CNS sx: HA, encephalopathy, stroke/bleed.
      b. PNS sx: None.
      c. Systemic sx: None.
      d. Tests: Angiogram, MRI, bx (leptomeninges and cortex).
      e. Rx: High-dose steroids ± cyclophosphamide.
  2. Angiitis, hypersensitivity: Small vessels.
      a. CNS sx: Variable.
      b. PNS sx: Asymmetrical, painful distal sensorimotor neuropathy, mononeuritis multiplex.
      c. Systemic sx: Purpura.
      d. Tests: Evaluate potential causes (drugs, infections, cancer, connective tissue dz, cryoprotein).
      e. Rx: Treat cause.
  3. Arteritis, giant cell (temporal arteritis): Extracranial branches of the aorta.
      a. CNS sx: HA (esp. unilateral temporal), ischemic optic neuropathy, transient monocular blindness, TIA/stroke.
      b. PNS sx: None.

   c. **Systemic sx:** Jaw claudication.
   d. **Tests:** ESR (often >100 mm/h), D-dimer, fibrinogen, CBC (anemia common), temporal artery bx.
   e. **Rx:** Prednisone 60 mg/d. Start at clinical suspicion—short-term use will not affect bx results.
4. **Arteritis, Takayasu's:** Extracranial branches of the aorta.
   a. **CNS sx:** TIA/stroke (due to large-vessel stenosis).
   b. **PNS sx:** None.
   c. **Systemic sx:** None.
   d. **Tests:** Aortic angiography.
   e. **Rx:** Steroids.
5. **Polyarteritis nodosa:** Small-medium arteries.
   a. **CNS sx:** Cranial neuropathies, stroke/hemorrhage, encephalopathy, seizures.
   b. **PNS sx:** Mononeuritis multiplex, polyneuropathy.
   c. **Systemic sx:** Any organ, esp. kidney.
   d. **Tests:** p-ANCA, MRI, visceral angiogram, EMG, nerve/muscle bx.
   e. **Rx:** Cyclophosphamide.
C. **Connective tissue dz:**
1. **Behçet's syndrome:** Small vessels. Higher prevalence along old silk route in Near East.
   a. **CNS sx:** Subacute brainstem dysfunction (cranial nerve palsies, cerebellar dysfunction, long-tract signs), HA, MS-like sx.
   b. **PNS sx:** None.
   c. **Systemic sx:** Uveitis, erythema nodosum, skin lesions, oral/genital ulcers.
   d. **Tests:** MRI often shows brainstem and subcortical nuclei lesions.
2. **Rheumatoid arthritis:**
   a. **CNS sx:** Atlantoaxial subluxation with cord compression, vasculitis (rare).
   b. **PNS sx:** Compression neuropathies.
   c. **Systemic sx:** Arthritis, cardiac complications.
   d. **Tests:** Rheumatoid factor, MRI.
   e. **Rx:** NSAIDS, TNF-α inhibitors, steroids, methotrexate.
3. **Systemic lupus erythematosus:**
   a. **CNS sx:** Psychiatric sx, cognitive deficits, seizures, cranial nerve palsies, HA, myelitis, stroke/bleed, MS-like sx, vasculitis.
   b. **PNS sx:** Polyneuropathy.
   c. **Systemic sx:** Inflammation of joint, skin, heart, lungs, kidney.
   d. **Tests:** ANA (high sensitivity, low specificity), anti-dsDNA (low sens, high spec), antiphospholipid antibodies, MRI.
   e. **Rx:** Steroids, cyclophosphamide; warfarin or aspirin for thrombotic events due to antiphospholipid syndrome (q.v. p. 192).
4. **Sjogren's syndrome:**
   a. **CNS sx:** MS-like disease, vasculitis (rare).
   b. **PNS sx:** Dorsal root ganglionopathy (may lead to sensory ataxia), polyneuropathy.
   c. **Systemic sx:** Dry eyes, dry mouth.

        d. Tests: ANA, anti-Ro, anti-La (not sensitive or specific); antiphospholipid antibodies, Schirmer's lacrimal flow test, salivary gland bx.

        e. Rx: High-dose steroids ± cyclophosphamide.

    5. Wegener's granulomatosis: Small-medium arteries.

        a. CNS sx: Cranial neuropathies, basilar meningitis, optic nerve sx, pituitary sx, stroke/bleed, seizures.

        b. PNS sx: Polyneuropathy.

        c. Systemic sx: Lung and kidney.

        d. Tests: MRI, c-ANCA, bx.

        e. Rx: Cyclophosphamide.

        f. Rx: High-dose steroids ± cyclophosphamide ± other immunosuppressants.

INSTANT NEUROLOGICAL DIAGNOSIS

Onset	Focal	Diffuse
Acute	Vascular	Toxic/metabolic
Subacute	Inflammatory	Inflammatory
Chronic	Tumor	Degenerative

Table 10. Instant neurological diagnosis. Courtesy of James Albers, MD, and Roger Albin, MD.

INTRACRANIAL HEMORRHAGE

A. See also: CT signs of intracranial hemorrhage, p. 180; arterial diagrams in Cerebrovascular Ischemia, p. 20.

B. Epidural hematoma:

    1. H&P: Typically, head trauma with brief LOC; then lucid interval, then obtundation, contralateral hemiparesis, and ipsilateral pupil dilatation.

    2. Cause: Injury to the meningeal artery or its branches.

    3. Rx: <u>Epidural hematomas should go to the OR immediately.</u>

C. Subdural hematoma (SDH):

    1. DDx: Epidural hematoma, subdural empyema, cerebral atrophy.

    2. Causes:

        a. Acute SDH: Usually follows trauma (injury to the bridging veins).

        b. Chronic spontaneous SDH: In the elderly, especially with cerebral atrophy, alcoholism; or poor hemostasis.

    3. Rx of SDH:

        a. Symptomatic SDH should be surgically drained.

        b. Asymptomatic SDH may be watched.

        c. Seizure prophylaxis: If acute, s/p seizure, or s/p surgical intervention. Often started on AED for ~3 wk, then d/c if no seizures.

D. Subarachnoid hemorrhage (SAH):

    1. Traumatic vs. spontaneous SAH: <u>Nontraumatic SAH is an emergency;</u> needs immediate angiogram to r/o aneurysm. Traumatic SAH can usually be watched. Make sure the head trauma preceded LOC, not vice versa.

2. **H&P in spontaneous SAH:** Sudden, severe HA—"worst HA in my life." N/V, LOC, stiff neck, cranial nerve deficits (especially third nerve), obtundation, ocular hemorrhage.

3. **Causes of SAH:**
   a. **Trauma:** Most SAH are traumatic.
   b. **Aneurysms:** 75% of spontaneous SAH are ruptured aneurysms.
      1) **Location:** 75% anterior circulation; 25% posterior. 25% have multiple aneurysms.
      2) **Associations with aneurysms:** Polycystic kidney dz, fibro-muscular dysplasia, AVMs, Ehlers-Danlos syndrome type IV, Marfan's, aortic coarctation, Osler-Weber-Rendu syndrome.
   c. **Idiopathic:** 15% of all spontaneous SAH. Associated with cigarettes, oral contraceptives, HTN, alcohol.
   d. **Other:** AVMs, vasculitis, carotid/vertebral artery dissection.

4. **Tests in spontaneous SAH:**
   a. **Blood:** CBC, PT, PTT, blood bank sample with 6 units held for OR, DPH level if pt has received it.
   b. **EKG:** For arrhythmia, MI, cerebral Ts, long QT, U waves.
   c. **Head CT:** See p. 180 for CT appearance.
   d. **LP if CT negative:** See CSF table (Table 3, p. 19). SAH has high opening pressure, blood that does not clear in successive tubes, xanthochromia if bleed >6 h. WBC may be secondarily high.
   e. **Emergent angiogram:** For spontaneous SAH, to r/o correctable aneurysm. Consider calling angiographers to prepare them when you first know of pt. Angiogram and early intervention are especially indicated in pts with Hunt-Hess (H-H) grade 1-3 because of good prognosis. For H-H 4-5, prognosis is poor; thus, reassess frequently and consider treatment if pt improves after ventriculostomy.
      1) **Angiogram-negative spontaneous SAH:** Repeat angio in 2 wk.

5. **Prognosis in SAH:**
   a. **Mortality:** 30% die before reaching hospital; 10% more in first few days. 50% total in first month.

H-H Grade	SAH Symptoms	Tests and Prognosis
0	Unruptured aneurysm (incidental finding)	F/u MRIs, ~1% a yr rupture
1	Mild HA, stiff neck	Emergent angiogram, good prognosis with intervention
2	Severe HA/stiff neck ± cranial nerve sx	
3	Drowsy/confused ± mild focal deficit	
4	Stupor, hemiparesis, ± mild decerebration	Angio only if pt better after EVD
5	Deep coma, decerebrate posturing	Poor; usually palliative care

Table 11. Hunt-Hess clinical grading scale, diagnostic testing, and prognosis for subarachnoid hemorrhage.

   b. Morbidity: 50%-60% have serious deficit even with successful clipping.

   c. Rebleeding risk: With unclipped aneurysm, 15% rebleed in 14 d, 50% in 6 mo, then 3%/yr. Hypertension greatly increases rebleed risk.

   d. Hunt-Hess (H-H) grading in SAH: Guides prognosis and rx.

6. Rx of spontaneous SAH:

   a. Immediate SBP control:

      1) Place arterial line in the ER: SBP goal <140, MAP 70-100.

      2) Nimodipine: 30 mg q2h to a total dose of 180 mg/d, as tolerated. Can use nicardipine drip for better control.

      3) Other BP agents: Labetalol, nicardipine, or nipride. If pt. is also having an MI, consider nitroglycerine $\pm$ labetalol.

   b. Oxygenation: If needed for airway protection, intubate pt after baseline exam. All other pts should get supplementary oxygen.

   c. Monitoring: Cardiac monitor, arterial and central line, NG tube if altered consciousness. Neuro checks q1h. ABG, coags, glucose, electrolytes, and CBC qd. Euvolemia. (strict I&Os). Daily CXR: until stable to r/o neurogenic pulmonary edema.

   d. Avoid all anticoagulants: Consider DVT prophylaxis after SAH stabilized/source treated (o/w, TEDs/P-Boots).

   e. Vasospasm prophylaxis: Nimodipine 60 mg q4h PO (from 30 mg q2h, see above) $\times$ 21 d, gentle volume expansion (e.g., D5NS + 20 KCl at 100 cc/h), but not at expense of keeping SBP low.

   f. Seizure prophylaxis: DPH load 1 g, then 100 mg tid. If patient never had a seizure and has good mental status exam and aneurysm is secured, may d/c ACD.

   g. ICU orders: Bedrest with HOB >30 degrees, pain drugs, normothermia, TEDs and airboots, stool softener. Minimize stimulation. Keep Na >135, Mg >2.0, glucose <120 (with IV insulin if necessary). Gastric prophylaxis. Ondansetron for N/V. No free water.

7. Complications of SAH:

   a. Vasospasm:

      1) Signs of vasospasm: Delayed neurological deficit, ~day 6-10; often abulia, poor attention, LE $>$ UE weakness.

      2) Tests: ABG to r/o hypoxia, electrolytes to r/o low Na, stat head CT, bedside transcranial ultrasound (TCD).

         a) Consider repeat angiogram: ~day 6-7 in all pts. whose exam has worsened. Based on its results, consider hypertensive or endovascular treatment with nicardipine or milrinone, or angioplasty.

      3) Triple-H therapy of vasospasm: Hypertension, hypervolemia, and hemodilution. Arterial line, MAP goal 70-120 (SBP 160-200). D/c antihypertensives, give blood (keep Hct <40%), albumin (q6h for CVP <8), then phenylephrine (neosynephrine), then fludrocortisone 0.2 mg bid.

        a) **Contraindications:** Unclipped aneurysm, severe brain edema or infarct, cardiac instability.

        b) **If poor exam** (Fisher grade 2 or 3): Get angiogram on day 6 or 7. Based on the results, consider albumin (1 bottle q6h for CVP <8), HT treatment, angioplasty, or endovascular treatment with nicardipine or milrinone.

        c) **Other:** Oxygen, consider ICP monitor, bid serum and urine electrolytes.

    b. **Hydrocephalus:** EVD (q.v., p. 86) in the EW for all pts with H-H > grade 3. Others receive it as sx and scan warrant. See Rx of ICP, p. 68. Beware of lowering ICP quickly; it can cause rebleeding. Keep EVD at 18 cm above EAM (20 cm while aneurysm not secured), then can lower for ICP issues.

    c. **For focal signs of elevated ICP:** Mannitol 1 g/kg (usually, 50-100 g) IV bolus, then 25 mg q6h for osms <310/serum Na <160, osmolal gap <10 (gap between serum osmolality and calculated serum osmolarity). Consider hypertonic NaCl (3% infusion or 23% bolus prn). Beware of lowering intracranial pressure quickly; it can cause rebleeding.

    d. **Hyponatremia:**

        1) **Cause:** Usually cerebral salt wasting (see p. 197), not SIADH.

        2) **Rx:** For Na goal >140, hydration with NS → salt tablets (up to 2 g tid) → 3% NaCl → 23% NaCl, as necessary. Florinef will help to retain Na and expand intravascular volume.

    e. **Ocular hemorrhage:** Consult ophthalmology to follow intraocular pressures.

E. **Parenchymal hemorrhage:** AKA intracerebral (vs. intracranial) hemorrhage.

    1. **H&P:** <u>An acute parenchymal bleed is an emergency.</u> Most significantly expand within 1st 1-3 h after onset (38% of hematomas expand; of those, 26% within 1 h vs. 12% within 1-24 h).

    2. **Tests:** Stat noncontrast head CT, PT, PTT, INR, platelets, D-dimer, fibrinogen, electrolytes, BUN/Cr, glucose, LFTs, blood bank sample.

        a. **If alternative etiology** is suspected (i.e., atypical for HTN ICH), consider further imaging when pt is stable [CTV/MRV to rule out venous sinus thrombosis; MRI w/susceptibilities to evaluate for CAA; with gadolinium to evaluate for tumor (but may need to delay up to 3 months)].

    3. **Causes:** Location is guide to cause; see Ct signs of intracranial hemorrhage, p. 180.

        a. **Most common:** Trauma, hypertensive bleed, amyloid angiopathy.

        b. **Hemorrhagic metastasis:** Melanoma, renal clear cell CA, thyroid, choriocarcinoma....

        c. **Hemorrhagic transformation of infarct:**

        d. **Other:** Aneurysm, AVM, cavernous malformation, coagulopathy, cocaine, infection, vasculitis, vasculopathy (e.g., moya-moya), venous thrombosis.

    4. **Prognosis:** Outcome depends on age, Glasgow Coma Scale (GCS) at presentation, and hematoma volume.

	Parenchymal Bleed	Hemorrhagic Infarct
Symptoms	Progressive	Max. at onset
CT appearance	Dense, homogeneous	Mottled, "petechial"
Onset of blood	At time of first deficit	Often days to weeks after
Ventricular blood	Common	Rare
Mass effect	Usually milder	Prominent

Table 12. Distinguishing a primary parenchymal bleed from a hemorrhagic infarct.

1) **ABC/2 estimate of bleed volume:** On head CT, let A = largest diameter of hematoma in cm, B = diameter perpendicular to A, C = 1/2 of the # of CT scan slabs with blood in them (each CT slab is ~0.5 cm). An ellipsoid approximation gives bleed volume $\approx$ ABC/2.

GCS	ICH Vol (cc)	30-Day Mortality (%)
	<30	19
≥8	30-60	46
	>60	75
	<30	44
<8	30-60	74
	>60	91

Table 13. ICH volume predicts mortality. (Adapted from Broderick J, et al. *Stroke.* 1993;24:987-993.)

2) **Bleed volume is best mortality predictor:**
3) **Modifiers:** Intraventricular bleed or hydrocephalus makes prognosis worse.
4) **In anticoagulated pts,** ABC/2 tends to overestimate bleed size; best to use ABC/3.
5. **If risk of vascular anomaly:** (Pt young, without traditional risk factors, bleed is near Sylvian fissure, has SAH component, has heterogeneous appearance, etc.) Get stat CTA of head and neck and neurosurgery consultation.
6. **Rx of parenchymal bleed:**
   a. **SBP control:** Usual SBP goal ~140-160; however, official guidelines recommend MAP <130, SBP <180 (more liberal to prevent drop in CBF and further ischemia). Treat hypotension aggressively with fluids or vasopressors (if SBP <90 or CPP <60).
   b. **Correct coagulopathy:** Stat reversal of anticoagulation with FFP (2-4 U) and IV vit K (10 mg × 1) for goal INR <1.3. If pt is on warfarin and ASA, give 6 U of platelets. Check coags q4h for 24 h, and repeat FFP/vit K as needed. For other coagulopathies, use institutional protocols, i.e., consult hematology/transfusion

medicine services for help (e.g., heparin/LMWH – protamine; direct thrombin inhibitors – ε-aminocaproic acid; etc.). For platelet disorders, transfuse as needed.

c. **Consider early hemostatic Rx:** Recombinant activated factor VII (rFVIIa) is currently available, although expensive. Consider thrombotic risk.

d. **Rx of mass effect:** If evidence of secondary hydrocephalus, midline shift, poor neuro exam, acute deterioration, significant IVH, pt will require stat:
   1) **EVD placement** by neurosurgery: Goal CPP >70, ICP <20 (adjust EVD settings accordingly). Prophylactic antibiotics while EVD is in place (cefazolin or vancomycin).
   2) **If mass effect progresses after EVD:** Hypertonic agents (mannitol, 3% and 23% NaCl), hyperventilation, or even hemicraniectomy with clot removal (especially if R-sided). But no data that hemicraniectomy helps anyone but young pts with superficial clots, especially if cerebellar bleeds >3 cm.
   3) **Monitoring:** If neuro exam unrevealing, follow with serial head CTs.

e. **Normoglycemia**, **normothermia**, **euvolemia:** May need insulin drip, acetaminophen, cooling blanket, NS, strict I&Os.

f. **DVT prophylaxis:** Pneumo-boots (after leg ultrasounds if in hospital >24 h); can use SQ heparin in ~48 h.

g. **Seizure prophylaxis:** Controversial; not necessary for small, deep bleeds without subarachnoid component.

h. **Steroids:** Useless in management of swelling from hemorrhage.

i. **Disposition and outcomes:** Neuro-ICU with frequent neuro checks, close EVD management. Discuss prognosis with family depending on exam, bleed volume, clinical course (secondary events).

F. Vascular malformations:
   1. **Arteriovenous malformations (AVM):** Congenital direct connection between arteries and veins. CNS sites: intraparenchymal > subarachnoid (~5% of all SAH) > intraventricular > subdural.
      a. **H&P:** Hemorrhage (~4%/yr; rarely associated with early rebleeding or vasospasm), seizures, headache, focal deficits, cranial bruits.
      b. **Tests:** May be seen on MRI (susceptibilities/gradient echo series) or MRA, but arteriogram is needed to characterize an AVM's blood supply.
      c. **Rx:** Endovascular embolization, XRT, or surgery.
   2. **Venous angiomas:** No arterial inputs. Lower bleed risk than with AVMs. Usually seen on MRI.
   3. **Cavernous malformations:** Sinusoidal vessels without intervening neural tissue. Present with seizures, focal neurological deficit, HA. Often <u>not</u> seen on angiogram because of low flow and presence of thrombosis.
   4. **Dural-based AV fistulae:** Vascular malformations in one of the major venous sinuses. Typically acquired due to change in cerebrovascular hemodynamics or intracranial pressure changes. Sx depend on lesion site (papilledema with superior sagittal sinus involvement; pulsatile tinnitus in transverse/sigmoid sinus; seizures in cortical lesions). Angiogram w/external carotid artery injection is diagnostic.

G. Intraventricular hemorrhage: Usually hypertensive, possible other small-vessel arteriopathy (CAA, AVM) or aneurysm. Prognosis is worse due to risk of hydrocephalus; pt will usually need an EVD.

INTRACRANIAL PRESSURE

A. See also: CT appearance of herniation, p. 180.
B. Sx and progression of herniation:
  1. Central supratentorial herniation: Usually subacute, from tumor. Diencephalon is forced down through tentorium.
     a. Diencephalic stage (reversible): Small pupils with light-near dissociation, roving eyes with decreased upgaze, obtundation, yawning. Progresses to Cheyne-Stokes breathing and decorticate posture.
     b. Pontine stage (not reversible): Midsized fixed pupils (even though pontine lesions cause pinpoint nonreactive pupils). Cheyne-Stokes progresses to tachypnea. Decreased doll's eyes and calorics. Disconjugate gaze ± intranuclear ophthalmoplegia. Decorticate posture becomes decerebrate, then flaccid.
     c. Medullary stage: Dilated pupils. Slow, irregular respirations.
  2. Uncal supratentorial herniation: Usually rapid, often from hematoma of temporal lobe, malignant cerebral edema following an acute ischemic stroke, encephalitis (e.g., HSV).
     a. First stage: Unilateral pupil dilation often before mental status change. Uncal herniation can pinch off PCAs.
     b. Second stage: Ophthalmoplegia and hyperventilation. May see Kernohan's false localizing sign: ipsilateral hemiplegia as contralateral peduncle is compressed.
     c. Third stage: Midposition pupils and decerebrate posture.
     d. Fourth stage: Sx of central herniation (see *above).
  3. Cingulate herniation (subfalcine): Often seen in malignant cerebral edema of ischemic stroke, ICH, GBM. Can pinch off ACA and present with abulia, poor concentration, LE weakness.
  4. Subtentorial herniation: Often presents with respiratory arrest, so prophylaxis is more useful than monitoring. Rapid and devastating; often requires emergent neurosurgical intervention (suboccipital decompression).
     a. Upward cerebellar herniation: May see dorsal midbrain syndrome.
     b. Tonsillar herniation: Compresses medulla.
C. Causes of high ICP: Mechanism determines rx.
  1. Mass lesion: E.g., blood, tumor, trauma. Use osmolar agent, mass resection, EVD, VP shunt.
  2. Poor CSF resorption: E.g., pseudotumor cerebri (see p. 69). Rx with acetazolamide (decreases CSF production), osmolar agent, shunt.
  3. Cerebral edema:
     a. Vasogenic: From tumor, abscess. Use steroids, osmolar agent, resection, shunt.
     b. Ischemic (cytotoxic): From stroke, trauma (diffuse axonal injury). No role for steroids. Use osmolar agent, shunt, resection.
     c. Granulocytic: From infection.
     d. Interstitial: From obstructive hydrocephalus.

D. Tests to assess ICP:
  1. **CT:** See p. 180 for CT appearance of high ICP.
  2. **CSF pressure:**
     a. **Methods:** See neurosurgical decompression techniques, p. 85.
        1) **LP is often <u>contraindicated</u>** if you suspect high ICP from mass lesion, posterior fossa process, or obstructive lesion in spinal canal. Okay to assess pseudotumor.
        2) **External ventricular drain (EVD):** Allows pressure measurements as well as CSF drainage.
        3) **ICP monitor:** (AKA bolt, subarachnoid screw) Allows only pressure measurements and short-lived measurement capacity (~5 d).
     b. **Values:** Normal <7 mm Hg (100 mm water). Needs rx if >18 mm Hg (200 mm water). Life threatening if >25 mm Hg (350 mm water) and mean arterial pressure <85.
     c. **Conversions:** 1 mm water = 0.07 mm Hg.
     d. **Cerebral perfusion pressure (CPP)** = MAP (mean arterial pressure) − ICP (intracranial pressure).
E. Rx of acute ICP:
  1. **Guidelines for hyperosmolar therapy:** Monitor the following features:
     a. **Exam:** Tie therapy to clear change in exam, e.g., dilated pupil or decreased consciousness.
     b. **ICP:** Keep ICP <18-20 mm Hg, CPP >70 mm Hg.
     c. **Blood:** Check electrolytes and serum osmolality q6h while on an agent. Hold the next dose for Na >160, serum osm >310, or osmolal gap (measured minus calculated serum osmolality) >10.
  2. **Miscellaneous:** HOB up 30 degrees, airboots or SQ heparin.
  3. **Mannitol:** Tolerance may develop to mannitol after ~48 h of use; thus, some advocate delay in use.
     a. **Dose:** 25-100 **g** (not mg) IV bolus for average-sized person, or 0.25-1 g/kg. Then 25-50 g q4h.
     b. **Contraindications:** Low BP, severe hyponatremia (will initially lower Na, then increase it), serum osm >310. If there is a large volume of damaged blood-brain barrier, there is little effect from mannitol. Rebound is rare; never use rebound as a reason not to give mannitol.
     c. **To discontinue mannitol:** Typical taper is 25 g q6h × 1 d, 25 q8h × 1 d, 25 q12h × 1 d, 25 q24h × 1 d, then stop.
  4. **Hypertonic saline:** Well tolerated; does not cause initial hyponatremia.
     a. **Contraindications:** Na >160.
     b. **Infusion:** 3% NaCl, ~40-50 cc/h; can go through peripheral IV for up to 12 h, then needs central line.
     c. **Bolus:** 23% NaCl, 15-30 cc q6h via central line.
     d. **D/c:** Requires taper to prevent rebound.
  5. **Dexamethasone:** Helps if high ICP is from tumor or some infections, not stroke or head trauma. 10 mg IV, then 4 mg q6h.
  6. **Hyperventilation:** Last-ditch, temporary effect. Keep pCO_2 ~30.
     a. **Danger of ischemia:** pH >7.5 transiently decreases cerebral blood flow through vasoconstriction.
     b. **Danger of rebound:** Can occur when you raise pCO_2 after pH has compensated, so wean slowly (increase pCO_2 range by 5 U q8h).
  7. **Barbiturates:** Raise brain perfusion by lowering ICP more than BP. Often require IV pressors. They also lower brain metabolism.

8. **Surgery:** E.g., EVD, VP shunt, hemicraniectomy. See neurosurgical decompression techniques, p. 85.
9. **Choice of antihypertensives when ICP is high:**
   a. **Avoid:** Nitroprusside, nitroglycerine, hydralazine, and Ca channel blockers, which raise ICP via vasodilation and, therefore, decrease cerebral perfusion.
   b. **Use:** β-blockers or ACE-I for BP control. Nicardipine is one Ca channel blocker that is well tolerated and effective.

F. **Pseudotumor cerebri** (benign intracranial hypertension):
   1. **H&P:** Headache, papilledema, constricted visual fields. More common in obese young women or pts with rapid weight gain.
   2. **Tests:** LP shows high opening pressures, symptom relief after large-volume tap. Pt should have periodic visual field checks.
   3. **Causes:** Obesity, steroid use, hyper-/hypovitaminosis A, drugs [tetracycline, nitrofurantoin, isotretinoin (Accutane)], anemia.
   4. **DDx:** Dural sinus thrombosis, mass lesion, meningitis, inflammation (SLE, sarcoid, Behçet's dz).
   5. **Rx:** Primary goal is preventing visual loss. Acetazolamide 250-1000 mg PO qd-tid (check electrolytes); repeated LPs, weight loss. Consider VP shunt or optic nerve fenestration. The latter protects against visual loss better but is less effective at controlling CSF pressure and HA.

METABOLIC, TOXIC, AND DEFICIENCY DISORDERS

A. **Metabolic disorders:** E.g., electrolyte disorders (see p. 195), glucose disorders (see p. 199), hepatic encephalopathy (see p. 202), thyroid dz (see p. 200), uremic encephalopathy (see p. 214).
B. **Drugs:**
   1. **Alcohol:**
      a. **Dependence:** Consider it especially in pts with depression, unexplained neuropathy, frequent falls, liver abnormalities. Talk to pt and family members separately; assess impact on job, etc.
      b. **Withdrawal:**

Do you ever think about **C**utting down on your drinking?
    Do you ever feel **A**ngry when people ask about it?
Does it make you feel **G**uilty?
    Do you ever have an **E**ye-opener?

Table 14. The CAGE screening questions for alcoholism.

1) **Hx:** Ask time of last drink, h/o withdrawal and nonwithdrawal seizures, detox programs. Focal seizures are rarely alcoholic; does pt have a h/o head injuries?
2) **PE:** Stage withdrawal severity by tremor, anxiety, level of confusion, pulse, N/V, sweatiness.
3) **Tests:** Chem 20, CBC, PT, PTT, ammonia, B_{12}.
4) **All potentially withdrawing pts should get:**

a) **Vitamins:** Thiamine 100 mg IM/IV qd, folate, MVI.
b) **IV fluids:** No glucose until thiamine given. D5 1/2 NS + KCl at 150 cc/h.
c) **Replete electrolytes:** KCl, Ca/Mg/Phos.
d) **GI prophylaxis:** Ranitidine or sucralfate. Guaiac stools.

5) **Rx of withdrawal seizures:**
   a) **Acute:** Diazepam 5-10 mg IV, or lorazepam 1-2 mg if pt. has liver dz or if drug must be given IM.
   b) **Chronic:** ACD prophylaxis does not help unless pt also has seizures from TBI, etc.

6) **Rx of acute withdrawal:** Sx include ANS instability. Doses based on VS, agitation, sweating, tremor, seizures.
   a) **Benzo:** Diazepam 15 mg q4h–20 mg q15min, OR lorazepam 3 mg q4h–4 mg q15min. Hold for somnolence, RR <12, SBP <100.
   b) **β-blocker** or clonidine for altered VS.
   c) **Consider haloperidol IV/PO:** Check EKG for QTc.
   d) **Taper:** When VS and sx are stable for 24 h, then taper over 4-7 d.

7) **Withdrawal prophylaxis:** For pts with behavioral sx but stable VS. Treat like acute withdrawal but with shorter taper and lower doses. Treat pts with more RFs (e.g., previous DTs, szs, >65 yr) more aggressively.

c. **Delirium tremens:** Severe withdrawal. 5%-10% mortality. Autonomic instability (tachycardia, HTN, sweating, fever); hallucinations, seizures, tremor.

d. **Wernicke's syndrome:** See p. 72.

e. **Hepatic encephalopathy:** See p. 202.

f. **Alcoholic cerebellar degeneration:** Truncal ataxia evolves over weeks or months. Nystagmus and limb ataxia are rarer. Sagittal CT shows vermis atrophy.

g. **Alcoholic neuropathy:** Sensory > motor neuropathy, often painful. Vibration sense is lost first.

h. **Marchiafava-Bignami dz:** Corpus callosum degeneration, associated with red wine consumption. Presents as a frontal lobe dementia.

i. **Tobacco-alcohol amblyopia:** Bilateral optic neuropathy, may progress to blindness over a few weeks. Treat with B vitamins.

2. **Intravenous drugs:** Neurological complications of IV use include:
   a. **Cerebral complications of endocarditis:** Abscess, mycotic aneurysm, bacterial meningitis.
   b. **Neuropathies:** Mononeuropathy 2-3 h after injection, various polyneuropathies and Guillain-Barré syndrome.
   c. **Transverse myelitis:** Often with reuse after 1- to 6-mo abstinence; mechanism unclear.
   d. **Toxic amblyopia:** Probably from quinine contamination.

3. **Opiates:** See p. 156.

4. **Stimulants:** E.g., cocaine, amphetamines.
   a. **Direct effects:** Agitation, progressing to motor stereotypy, psychosis, seizures, coma, malignant hyperthermia, death.
   b. **Vascular effects:** Cerebral bleeds. Occasionally ischemic stroke in intranasal but not IV users. Small-vessel cerebral vasculitis

from cocaine; multiorgan necrotizing vasculitis (like polyarteritis nodosa) from amphetamines.

c. Exogenous toxins:

1. **Carbon monoxide:**
   a. **H&P:** Exposure; HA, N/V, confusion—cherry red lips, cyanosis, and retinal hemorrhages are rare. Globus pallidus necrosis when severe. Delayed neuropsychiatric sx in 10%-30% that resolve after a year in 50%-75%.
   b. **Rx:** 100% O_2. In coma, persistent sx, or pregnancy, consider hyperbaric O_2.

2. **Heavy metals:** Arsenic, lead, mercury, and thallium poisoning produce encephalopathy, neuropathy. Large doses of other metals can cause neuropathy, but usually systemic signs predominate.
   a. **Tests:** 24-h urine analysis; blood lead levels.
   b. **Rx:** For arsenic, lead, or mercury, use penicillamine 250 mg PO qid; for thallium, use diphenylthiocarbazone or sodium dicarbamate.

3. **Organophosphates:** In pesticides, flame retardants. Inhibit acetylcholinesterase. Depressed levels of RBC indicate recent exposure.
   a. **Acute effects:** Respiratory and neck weakness, up to 2 wk.
   b. **Delayed effects:** May see central-peripheral axonopathy 1-3 wk after exposure, with paresthesias, distal to proximal weakness.

	Exposure	Symptoms
Arsenic	Insecticide, Paris green	Sensory > motor neuropathy, red hands, burning feet, hyperhidrosis
Lead	Paint, gas, batteries	Adults: neuropathy, painful joints; children: cerebral edema, encephalopathy, low IQ
Mercury	Industrial, polluted fish	Severe arm and leg pain, dementia with primarily motor neuropathy
Thallium	Insecticide, rat poison	Stocking-glove sensorimotor neuropathy, with alopecia

Table 15. Heavy metal toxicity.

D. Vitamin deficiencies:

Sign	Deficiency
Encephalopathy	B_{12}, folate, nicotinic acid, thiamine
Seizures	Pyridoxine
Myelopathy	B_{12}, folate, vitamin E
Myopathy	Vitamin D, E
Neuropathy	Thiamine, B_{12}, folate, pyridoxine, vitamin E
Optic neuropathy	B_{12}, folate, thiamine, other B vitamins

Table 16. Neurological signs of vitamin deficiency.

1. **Vitamin A:** Deficiency causes night blindness and optic atrophy. Excess >50,000 IU qd causes pseudotumor cerebri.
2. **Thiamine (B_1) deficiency:**
   a. **Wernicke's syndrome:**
      1) **H&P:** Most common in alcoholics, poor nutrition, hyperemesis. Onset may be subacute or acute. See ophthalmoplegia (often bilateral 6th palsy, nystagmus), confusion, truncal ataxia, sometimes signs of alcohol withdrawal.
      2) **Rx:** Thiamine 100 mg IM/IV × 5 d, then PO. Avoid glucose until the first dose of thiamine is given.
      3) **Prognosis:** Death, if untreated. With rx, ocular abnormalities resolve within hours to days; confusion within days to weeks; ataxia within months. Korsakoff's syndrome: anterograde and retrograde amnesia with prominent confabulation, retained attention and social behavior.
   b. **Beriberi:** Rare in developed countries. See sensorimotor polyneuropathy and cardiomyopathy.
3. **Pyridoxine (B_6):** In adults, both excess (>500 mg qd for several wks) and deficiency cause peripheral neuropathy. Excess causes dorsal root ganglionopathy. Deficiency is usually from isoniazid, hydralazine, or penicillamine. Some infants are genetically pyridoxine dependent and require high doses to prevent seizures.
4. **Vitamin B_{12} deficiency:**
   a. **H&P:** Usual presentation is distal paresthesias, then weak, unsteady gait. Sometimes confusion, psychiatric sx, or poor vision is first. Exam shows polyneuropathy, myelopathy, or both. There may be central scotomata, brainstem, or cerebellar signs. H/o GI malabsorption, anemia.
   b. **Tests:** Macrocytic anemia is not always present. B_{12} levels are usually low, but elevation of metabolites methylmalonic acid and homocysteine are more sensitive. Perform a Schilling test for pernicious anemia if suspicion is high, even if B_{12} levels are normal.
   c. **Rx:** Oral B_{12} is as well absorbed as IM, even in pernicious anemia. Oral: 2000 μg qd for 1-2 wk, then 1000 μg qd for life. IM: 100-1000 μg IM qd × 2 wk, then 1000 μg IM q mo. Do not give folate until B_{12} has been repleted for 1-2 wk.
5. **Vitamin E deficiency:** Often from fat malabsorption. See spinocerebellar degeneration, often with peripheral neuropathy, sometimes pigmentary retinopathy, nystagmus, ophthalmoplegia, and proximal weakness.
6. **Folate deficiency:** In alcoholism, pregnancy, DPH use. Can cause B_{12}-like syndrome but not dementia. In first trimester of pregnancy, causes spina bifida.

MITOCHONDRIAL DISORDERS

A. **H&P:** Stroke-like episodes, migraines, developmental delay, encephalopathy, failure to thrive, hypotonia, ataxia, weakness, exercise intolerance, lethargy, muscle cramps, hearing loss, blindness, glucose intolerance, seizures, constipation, GERD. Family history.

B. Tests:
  1. **For crisis:** Infectious workup, brain MRI/MR spectroscopy, EEG, serum lactate, pyruvate, lytes, LFTs, NH_3, ABG (pH), U/A. CSF lactate, pyruvate, EKG.
  2. **Diagnostic workup:** Above plus serum ketones, lactate and pyruvate (more sensitive after a crisis), quantitative amino acids, 3-methylglucaconic acid, carnitine, urine organic acids, very long–chain fatty acids, WBC lysosomal enzymes. EMG, EKG, echocardiogram. Muscle biopsy (try weakest muscle), mitchondrial DNA analysis. CSF alanine, glycine.
C. Cause: Inherited or spontaneous mutations in mtDNA or nuclear DNA. Genocopies (extreme clinical heterogeneity with identical mutations) and phenocopies (different mutations with same disease) are the rule. MtDNA varies within cells and between cells (heteroplasmy).

	CPEO	MERRF	MELAS
Weakness	±	+	+
Ragged red fibers	+	+	+
Short stature	+	+	+
Deafness	+	+	+
Dementia	+	+	+
Spongy brain degen.	+	+	+
Ophthalmoplegia	+		
Retinal degeneration	+		
Heart block	+		
CSF protein >100 mg/dL	+		
Myoclonus			
Ataxia	±	+	
Seizures		+	+
Vomiting			+
Cortical blindness			+
Hemiparesis			+

Table 17. Symptoms of mitochondrial disorders. See text for abbreviations.

D. Congenital progressive external ophthalmoplegia (CPEO): AKA Kearns-Sayre syndrome. See Table 17; also see bilateral ptosis, mild proximal myopathy.
E. Leber's hereditary optic neuropathy: Progressive blindness from optic atrophy.
F. Leigh's dz (Subacute necrotizing encephalomyelopathy): Usually pediatric, with hypotonia, developmental delay, apneic episodes; sometimes seizures, ataxia, neuropathy, ophthalmoplegia.
G. MERRF (myoclonic epilepsy with ragged red fibers): See Table 17.
H. MELAS (mitochondrial encephalopathy with lactic acidosis and stroke-like episodes): See Table 17.

I. **Neuropathy, ataxia, and retinitis pigmentosa:** Also see growth retardation, dementia.
J. **Treatment:**
   1. **General:** Avoid extreme temps, toxins (ETOH, cigarettes, ASA), meds that compromise mitochondria (DPH, phenobarbital, valproate, tetracycline). Coenzyme Q_{10} 4 mg/kg/d, "B50" complex (B_1, B_2, etc.), vitamin E 100–400 IU/d, L-carnitine 100 mg/kg/d.
   2. **Crisis:** Hydrate, treat infection and seizures. Add vitamin C 1,000 mg/d, zinc 30 mg/d, biotin 10 mg/d, α-lipoic acid 10 mg/kg/d.

MOVEMENT DISORDERS AND ATAXIA

A. **See also:** Pediatric movement disorders, p. 145.
B. **Terminology:** "Movement disorders" tends to include only problems with a presumed basal ganglia cause. "Extrapyramidal" is a term used mostly by psychiatrists to distinguish from pyramidal, corticospinal sx.
C. **Movement disorder consult service jingle:** "Jerky or stiff?/We're there in a jiff./Trouble with tone?/Call us on the phone."
D. **H&P:** What tasks are difficult? Nature and frequency of falls. Associated depression, dementia, incontinence. Alcohol, benzodiazepine, or neuroleptic use. Assess facial expression, saccades, voice, handwriting, involuntary movements, speed, amplitude, tone, ability to rise from a chair, posture, postural reflexes, gait base, arm swing, festination, freezing, turning Romberg sign, weakness, ataxia.
E. **Gait disorders:**

	Description	Typical Cause
Akinetic	Stoops, shuffles, many falls	PD syndromes, meds, NPH
Choreic	Postures, writhes, few falls	DA meds, TD, HD
Ataxic	Wide-based, lurches, few falls	Alcoholism, Cb CVA, mass
Spastic	Leg stiff, circumducts	CST CVA, mass; CP
Neuropathic	Steps high, foot slaps	DM, alcohol, PNS lesion
Myopathic	Waddling, lordotic	Myositis, steroids, alcohol
Antalgic	Limps, winces, groans	Arthritis, trauma
Orthostatic	Sways when stands/turns	Meds, ANS failure, dehydr.
Psychogenic	Wild movements but few falls	Somatoform disorder

Table 18. Common gait disorders.

F. **Ataxia and dysmetria:** Ataxia, dysmetria; inaccurate movement targeting and coordination, from cerebellar or brainstem disorder. Dysmetria (AKA intention tremor) is an oscillation that worsens as the limb approaches the target. In postural muscles, it is called ataxia; in eye movements, nystagmus.
   1. **Acute:** Often with vertigo, nystagmus, N/V. From drugs, post fossa bleed/stroke. Secondary edema may need rapid decompression.
   2. **Subacute:** From drugs, tumor, postinfectious cerebellitis, vasculitis.

3. **Chronic progressive:** Alcoholism, Wilson's dz, drugs, toxins, CJD, hereditary, hereditary metabolic dz, paraneoplastic syndromes.
4. **DDx:** Action tremor; other gait disorders (see above).

G. **Hereditary ataxias and movement disorders:** leaves out most recessive dzs, genes for dzs that are usually sporadic (e.g., PD), and very, very rare dzs (all are rare).

1. **Trinucleotide repeat diseases:** Typically adult onset. Dzs caused by CAG repeats sometimes show anticipation; in successive generations, repeat length is longer, age of onset is younger, and severity is greater.
2. **Genetic testing:** Pts often request testing of at-risk relatives. Especially in dzs where preventive rx is not available, strongly urge, even insist, that they see a professional genetic counselor first to discuss emotional and economic risks (e.g., that a positive test may affect health insurance access).

Disease[1]	Sx[2]	Triplet?	Transmitted[3]	Comments
Friedreich's	A	+	AR	Heart, DM
Huntington's	M,P	+	AD	First[1] sx may be psych.
SCA1	A,W,N,P	+	AD	Usually pure ataxia
SCA2	N,P	+	AD	Slow saccades
SCA3 (MJD)	A,N	+	AD	Dystonia, spasticity
SCA6 (SBMA)	A	+	AD	Usually pure ataxia
SCA7 (OPCA)	A,N	+	AD	Retinal degeneration
DRPLA	A,M,P	+	AD	Pedi myoclonic epilepsy
Myotonic dyst.	W,P	+	AD	Heart, DM
Fragile X	P	+	XL	Long face, big testes
Wilson's	A,M,P	–	AR	Liver dz
DRD	M	–	ADi	Sx best in AM
DYT-1	M	–	ADi	Pure dystonia

[1]SCA = spinocerebellar ataxia; MJD = Machado-Joseph's disease; SBMA = spinobulbar muscular atrophy (Kennedy's syndrome); OPCA = olivopontocerebellar atrophy; DRPLA = dentatorubral - pallidoluysian atrophy; DRD = dopa - responsive dystonia; DYT - 1 = primary dystonia.

[2] A = ataxia; M = Mvt disorder; W = weak; P = psychological/cognitive.

[3]AD = autosomal dominant; ADi = with incomplete penetrance; AR = autosomal recessive; XL = X - linked

Table 19. Hereditary disorders causing ataxia, chorea, or weakness.

H. **Basal ganglia movement disorders:** Impair starting, stopping, sequencing.

1. **Hypokinetic disorders:** Slow movements; subcortical cognitive problems (q.v. Table 8, p. 43), poor motivation, depression.
   a. **Causes:** Decreased dopamine or lesion of the direct pathway (excitatory) through the internal pallidum.

    b. Sx: Rigidity, bradykinesia, rest tremor.

    c. Rx: Dopaminergics, anticholinergics

  2. Hyperkinetic disorders: Excessive, rapid movements; also delusions, agitation, impulsivity.

    a. Causes: Lesions that raise dopamine or that affect the indirect (inhibitory) pathway through the external pallidum.

    b. Sx: Chorea, dyskinesia, tics, athetosis, akathisia.

    c. Rx: Typical neuroleptics (D2-blockers).

  3. Mixed disorders: Dystonia

I. Akathisia: Motor restlessness. May be excruciating. Often a transient neuroleptic SE or after neuroleptic d/c. Try benztropine 0.5-1 mg bid, propranolol 10-20 mg tid, clonidine 0.1 mg bid, or clonazepam 0.5-1.0 mg bid.

J. Asterixis: Irregular, slow, tremor-like flapping of hands, trunk, from temporary lapses of tone. Treat underlying cause—usually metabolic, e.g., liver failure.

K. Choreoathetosis: Chorea is involuntary, rapid movements, often incorporated into voluntary movements. Athetosis is slower, more writhing.

  1. Causes of choreoathetosis:

    a. Chemicals: Especially neuroleptics.

    b. Immune-mediated: Sydenham's, SLE, chorea gravidarum....

    c. Hereditary disorders:

      1) Huntington's dz: Autosomal dominant CAG sequence repeat, genetic test available. Presents usually in adulthood with chorea or psychiatric sx.

    d. Other: Huntington's, Wilson's, Hallervorden-Spatz dz, idiopathic torsion dystonia....

  2. Rx of choreoathetosis: Typical neuroleptics (via D2 receptor antagonism), e.g., haloperidol: start 0.5 mg bid, up to 8 mg bid. Atypical neuroleptics work only to the extent of their D2 antagonism, so you usually need higher dose.

L. Dyskinesia: Reserved for chorea caused by dopamine receptor hypersensitivity. See Parkinsonian dyskinesias (p. 77); Tardive dyskinesia (p. 171).

M. Dystonia: Involuntary maintenance of abnormal posture, expression, or limb position. Often task dependent and relieved by sensory tricks (*gestes antagonists*).

  1. DDx: Spasticity, musculoskeletal lesion....

  2. Acute dystonia: Reaction to antiemetic or neuroleptic, carbon monoxide, stroke, etc. Rx: diphenhydramine 50 mg IV/IM.

  3. Chronic dystonia:

    a. Focal: Torticollis, blepharospasm, writer's cramp, spasmodic dysphonia (q.v.), Meige's syndrome (lip smacking and blepharospasm)....

      1) Rx: Botulinum toxin injections q 3-4 mo; perhaps clonazepam or anticholinergic.

    b. Generalized: See Causes of choreoathetosis, above; pediatric dystonia, p. 146. Genetic tests available. Rx:

      1) Always try levodopa/carbidopa to r/o dopa-responsive dystonia.

      2) Anticholinergics: E.g., trihexyphenidyl. Start 0.5 mg qhs, may need 20-50 mg tid.

      3) Other: Baclofen, clonazepam, pallidal deep brain stimulator.

N. Myoclonus: Brief, monophasic, irregular jerks in different body parts. Often triggered by sensory stimuli.

   1. DDx: Tics, myoclonic epilepsy, periodic limb movements of sleep, tremor, chorea.

   2. Causes: Metabolic or hypoxic encephalopathy, seizure, benign essential myoclonus, physiological myoclonus (sleep jerks), drugs (e.g., opiates)....

   3. Rx: Clonazepam: start 0.5 mg tid, to 2 mg tid. Valproate ER: start 250 mg qhs, to 500-1,000 mg bid.

O. Neuroleptic-induced movement disorders: See p. 170.

P. Serotonin-induced movement disorders: See p. 164.

Q. Idiopathic Parkinson's dz (IPD): Must distinguish IPD from atypical parkinsonism, below.

   1. H&P: Bradykinesia, rigidity, tremor are cardinal. Falls, stooping, festination, response to carbidopa/levodopa, depression, cognitive changes, hallucinations, orthostasis, autonomic dysfunction.

   2. Tests: Levodopa/carbidopa challenge is nearly diagnostic for IPD. MRI only rules out rare causes. Fluorodopa PET is rarely done.

   3. Cause: Dopamine idiopathic Parkinson's dz (IPD). Must distinguish IPD from atypical parkinsonism, below.

   4. Rx of early/moderate dz: Start all meds slowly, with meals, to avoid N/V. See also Dopaminergic Drugs, p. 169.

     a. Medication-induced nausea: Take meds with meals. Extra carbidopa 25 mg, or ondansetron 1 mg, before dose. AVOID metoclopramide, prochlorperazine, etc. Med nausea passes in months.

     b. Precursor: Levodopa/carbidopa 25/100 mg tid, or much higher.

       1) Levodopa does not worsen dz progression but is commonly perceived to.

       2) Minimize dose fluctuations to decrease receptor hypersensitization and dyskinesias.

     c. COMT inhibitors: E.g., entacapone; prolong DA half-life.

     d. Dopamine agonists: E.g., pramipexole. More sedation and hallucinations but longer half-life and less link to dyskinesias than levodopa.

     e. MAO-B inhibitors: E.g., selegiline, rasagiline. Safer than the MAO-A inhibitors used as antidepressants.

     f. Antioxidants: Initial studies show sx slowed by coenzyme Q_{10} at doses >1,200 mg divided daily. No evidence for vitamin E.

   5. Rx of complications:

     a. Constipation: Bowel stimulant, e.g., senna, milk of magnesia.

     b. On-off dose fluctuations: Use smaller, more frequent levodopa doses, partial replacement with an inhibitor or agonist.

     c. Meal-related changes: Take levodopa on an empty stomach, and avoiding its CR form, to enhance absorption.

     d. Dyskinesias: Amantadine 100 mg tid, or clozapine.

     e. Off-phase dystonia: Artane 2 mg tid.

     f. Hallucinations or nightmares: Quetiapine 25 mg qhs, but it may worsen severe rigidity. Clozapine 12.5-25 mg qhs is safe and underused.

   g. Orthostatic BP: Consider high-salt diet, head of bed up 10 degrees (place bricks under bed), fludrocortisone 0.1 mg qd, or midodrine 10 mg tid.

   h. Subthalamic nucleus deep brain stimulator (DBS): Actually, the current DBS inhibits or jams STN function to decrease PD sx. Pts can turn on/off and sometimes adjust the current DBS. For questions, call 1-800-328-0810.

      1) Indication: Medical rx failed. Strong levodopa effect is best prognostic sign—DBS does not help PD-plus. Alzheimer's type cortical dementia is a contraindication, but PD-related executive dysfunction (see p. 150) is not.

      2) If pt is too rigid: Have them check if DBS is on; increase voltage using their access device, increase PD meds.

      3) If pt is dyskinetic/dystonic: Decrease or turn off DBS; decrease PD meds.

      4) MRIs with DBS: Voltage must be turned to zero by a trained provider—not just turned off by the pt. Can only do head scans on some scanner brands and can never do body scans.

      5) EKGs with DBS: If there is interference, have pt shut off DBS with their access device.

      6) Surgery with DBS: Usually safe, use bipolar cautery with pad far from head.

6. DDx:

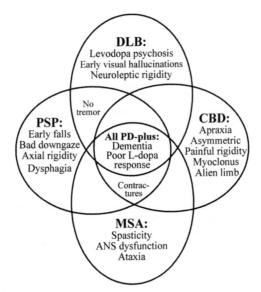

Figure 9. Symptom overlap in syndromes of atypical parkinsonism. Abbreviations are defined in the following text.

    a. Atypical parkinsonism, AKA "Parkinson's plus syndromes": All share poor levodopa response, early dementia.
        1) Major subtypes: In clinical practice, the symptom complexes overlap. See Figure 9. Progressive supranuclear palsy (PSP), diffuse Lewy body dz (DLB), corticobasoganglionic degeneration (CBD), and multiple systems atrophy (MSA).
        2) MSA subtypes: MSA itself includes Shy-Drager syndrome (more ANS dysfunction), striatonigral degeneration (more spasticity), and olivopontocerebellar atrophy (more ataxia).
        3) Rx: Symptomatic. High-dose levodopa may help for awhile.
    b. Drug-induced parkinsonism: All neuroleptics except clozapine—and this includes most antiemetics except ondansetron—cause reversible parkinsonism and may unmask latent true IPD.
    c. Chemicals: Rotenone, manganese, carbon monoxide, and others can cause irreversible parkinsonism.
    d. Other: NPH, essential tremor, depression, arthritis, focal basal ganglia lesions, spasticity, postencephalitic, CJD. . . .

R. Tone:
    1. Rigidity: "Lead-pipe" resistance to passive movement, from basal ganglia lesion. Rigid pts are strong, if given enough time to reach full power.
    2. Spasticity: "Clasp-knife" stiffness, weakness, and spasms. From corticospinal tract lesions.

S. Tics: Quick, repetitive, coordinated movements or vocalizations, driven by urge, partly repressible.
    1. DDx: Tourette's syndrome, Sydenham's chorea, Wilson's dz, Lesch-Nyhan's syndrome, myoclonus. . . .
    2. Rx: (generally not well tolerated)
        a. Clonidine (central α-agonist): Start 0.05 mg qd, to 2 mg bid.
        b. Pimozide (or other D2-blocker): Start 0.5 mg qhs, to 8-16 mg qd.

T. Tremor: Oscillation from alternating contraction of antagonist muscles.
    1. Tests: TSH; consider copper studies.
    2. DDx: Focal seizure, segmental myoclonus, chorea.
    3. Rest (parkinsonian) tremor: 3-5 Hz, decreases during movement, often asymmetric, "pill-rolling."
    4. Action tremors: Worse with movement.
        a. Physiologic tremor: 8-13 Hz, low amplitude. Normal. Worse with adrenergic stimulation (anxiety, caffeine, hyperthyroidism, sedative withdrawal, etc.).
        b. Essential (benign) tremor: 4-8 Hz. Genetic. Rx includes:
            1) Propranolol: Start 10-20 mg tid, to 60-200 mg qd.
            2) Primidone: Start 50 mg qd, to 125 tid.
            3) Surgery: Thalamic deep brain stimulator.
        c. Cerebellar tremor: Strictly, dysmetria. Oscillations worsen as limb approaches target.
        d. Rubral tremor: Midbrain tremor would be a better term. Violent beating or flapping.
        e. Hemiballism from a subthalamic nucleus lesion. Looks rubral. Often from small stroke.

    f. **Anxiety/depression and tremor:** Mirtazapine (Remeron) is one of the few antidepressants that does not worsen tremor.

    g. **Bipolar or mood lability:** Change lithium, valproate, or lamotrigine to carbamazepine, gabapentin, or Topamax or, in severe cases, clozapine (can suppress tremor and raise mood).

    h. **Epilepsy and tremor:** Valproate, carbamazepine, gabapentin.

NEUROMUSCULAR DISORDERS

A. See also: Neuromuscular Disorders; Weakness, p. 129.

B. Presenting clinical features:

	Ant. Horn Cell	Neuropathy	NMJ dz	Myopathy
Weakness	Asymmetric	Symmetric, distal	Eyes, face, proximal	Symmetrical, limb > face
Atrophy	Marked, early	Moderate	None	Slight early, marked late
Sensory loss	None	Yes	None	None
Classic features	Fasciculations, cramps, tremor	Sensory and motor	Diurnal fluctuation	Weakness, sometimes pain
Reflexes	Increased or decreased	Lost early	Normal	Decreased if severe weakness

Table 20. Presenting features of neuromuscular diseases.

C. Abnormal muscle activity:

    1. **Clonus:** Repetitive unidirectional contraction of a muscle group.

    2. **Fasciculations:** Random twitching of a muscle fiber group.

    3. **Fibrillations:** Random single-fiber twitching.

    4. **Myotonia:** Delayed muscle relaxation, often triggered by percussion. Worse in cold, improves with exercise.

    5. **Myokymia:** Repetitive, undulating fasciculations.

D. Pulmonary function in neuromuscular dz: Characterized by decreased vital capacity (VC), hypercarbia. A bedside test of VC is to have the pt count aloud while maximally exhaling: normal >40. Consider intubating if <20, or for VC <18 mg/kg. Oxygen saturation monitors are not adequate tests, as desaturation may only occur late. For Pulmonary function test findings, see p. 219.

E. Amyotrophic lateral sclerosis (ALS):

    1. **H&P:** Weakness without cognitive, sensory, or ANS dysfunction. Combination of upper and lower motor neuron signs. Often asymmetric onset, hand atrophy, foot drop, leg spasticity, bulbar sx, fasciculations, cramps. Ask about family history.

2. **DDx:** CIDP, other motor system atrophies (dystrophies, spinal muscular atrophy), cervical spinal cord injury, syringomyelia, MS, myasthenia, paraneoplastic syndrome, multifocal motor neuropathy with conduction block, heavy metal poisoning, HIV, HTLV, Lyme, diabetic amyotrophy, postpolio syndrome....

3. **Tests:**
   a. **Consider peripheral neuropathy workup:** See p. 93.
   b. **EMG:** Much denervation and reinnervation (fasciculations, fibrillations, polyphasic increase in amplitude of motor units, normal conduction speed).
   c. **Biopsy:** Usually not indicated. Shows neurogenic atrophy.

4. **Rx:**
   a. **Riluzole** (Rilutek): 50 mg PO bid. Slightly slows progression.
   b. **Supportive:** E.g., splints, G-tube, ventilator, antispasmodics, control saliva....

F. **Botulism:** Preformed toxin blocks acetylcholine (ACh) release from NMJ. Infantile form from infection (honey).
   1. **H&P:** Bradycardia, ocular, bulbar, respiratory, and somatic paralysis with intact thought and sensation. For EMG findings, see p. 41.
   2. **Treatment:** Supportive, antitoxin. Slowly improves over weeks.

G. **Lambert-Eaton myasthenic syndrome:** Blockage of presynaptic ACh release by antibodies to a voltage-gated calcium channel. 90% of pts. have detectable Ab, 50% have an underlying cancer (small-cell lung, transitional cell).
   1. **H&P:** Unlike myasthenia, often begins with proximal limb rather than cranial nerve weakness, and may transiently improve rather than worsen weakness. Respiratory muscles not usually affected. Significant ANS sx.
   2. **Tests:** Similar to myasthenia, *below, plus workup for occult cancer.
   3. **Rx:** Treat underlying cancer. 3,4-Diaminopyridine (DAP) 5-25 mg bid or qid, steroids, azathioprine. PEx or IVIg for intractable dz. Pyridostigmine is not as effective as it is in myasthenia. Avoid drugs that affect the neuromuscular junction (see p. 82).

H. **Myasthenia gravis:** Most caused by antibodies to the acetylcholine receptor (measurable in 85% of pts.). Half of "seronegative" cases have muscle-specific kinase (MuSK) Ab. 10% of pts have a thymoma. Rarely congenital.
   1. **H&P:** Ask if sx worse at end of day or after repeated use, diplopia, dyspnea, recent infection, or med change. Check vital capacity (see Pulmonary function in neuromuscular dz, p. 80), sustained eye elevation, neck strength, repeated standing. Ice pack on eyelid may improve myasthenic ptosis. Pt. should have normal pupils, sensory, and reflex exam (but reflexes may be depressed if limbs are very weak).
   2. **DDx:** Guillain-Barré syndrome, CIDP, botulism, motor neuron dz, organophosphate poisoning, myopathy, muscular dystrophy, thyroid dz.
   3. **Tests:** Edrophonium test (if pt currently symptomatic), ACh receptor Ab, MuSK Ab, EMG with 3-Hz repetitive stimulation and single-fiber studies (see p. 41), chest CT for thymoma, electrolytes, Ca/Phos/Mg, CPK, ANA, RF, TSH, antithyroid Ab.

    a. Edrophonium test (Tensilon test): A short-acting cholinesterase inhibitor. 1-2 mg IV. If no change, give additional 8 mg (i.e., total 10 mg). Need double-blind, placebo control. Do not perform if pupils miotic (suggests cholinergic crisis). Perform with a cardiac monitor if the pt is elderly. Have atropine ready for bradycardia.

4. Myasthenic crisis and cholinergic crisis: Both present with weakness. <u>Both are emergencies</u> because of the danger of respiratory collapse. May have both at once.

	Myasthenic Crisis	Cholinergic Crisis
Heart rate	Tachycardic	Bradycardic
Muscles	Flaccid	Flaccid, + fasciculations
Pupil	Normal or large	Small
Skin	Pale, sometimes cool	Red, warm
Secretions	No change	Increased
Edrophonium test	Improves strength	Increases weakness

Table 21. Distinguishing myasthenic and cholinergic crises.

    a. Tests: Bedside vital capacity, cardiac monitor.
    b. Rx of myasthenic crisis:
       1) Cholinergics: Prostigmine 0.5 mg IV push, then pyridostigmine 24 mg in 500 mL D5 1/2 NS.
       2) Respiratory support: Admit to ICU, monitor vital capacity, intubate if it is <15-18 mL/kg or if aspiration risk. Remember that O_2 saturation is not sensitive; pt will become hypercarbic before becoming hypoxic.
       3) Remove precipitants: Drugs, infection, heat.
       4) Plasmapheresis: ~6× in 2 wk.
       5) Steroids: Consider methylprednisolone 60 mg IV qd. Steroids may acutely worsen weakness; monitor closely.
    c. Rx of cholinergic crisis: Similar to myasthenic crisis since pyridostigmine overdose is usually a response to worsening myasthenia.
       1) Atropine: 2 mg IV for nonmuscle effects.
       2) Ipratropium inhaler: For bronchospasm.
5. Outpatient rx of myasthenia:
    a. Pyridostigmine (Mestinon): Start 30-60 mg q4-6h. SEs: diarrhea, urinary frequency, bradycardia, cholinergic crisis.
    b. Prednisone: Pt may worsen for first few weeks. Start 10 mg qd as outpt, or admit for more aggressive load. Increase slowly.
    c. Azathioprine: Start 50 mg q AM; increase to 150 mg q AM over 3 wk. Takes months to affect symptoms. Monitor LFTs/CBC weekly × 2 months, then monthly.
    d. Thymectomy: In young pts, or if thymoma. Works better if done early.
    e. Other: Cyclophosphamide, cyclosporine, tacrolimus, mycophenolate.

6. **Drugs to avoid in myasthenia and Eaton-Lambert syndrome:**
   a. **Anticholinergics.**
   b. **Cardiovascular:** Beta-blockers, antiarrhythmics (these can sometimes cause transient drug-induced myasthenia).
   c. **Antibiotic:** Gentamicin, tetracycline, clindamycin (penicillin and erythromycin are better).
   d. **Neurological:** DPH, lithium, neuroleptics, muscle relaxants....
   e. **Antimalarial:** Chloroquine.

I. Myopathy:
1. **H&P:** Swallowing, diplopia, symmetry of weakness, proximal vs. distal, difficulty with stairs or reaching overhead, tripping, myalgia, myotonia (cannot release grip), Gower's maneuver, rash (violet lids, subungual telangiectasias), edema. Bowel, bladder should be normal.
2. **DDx:** Muscular dystrophy, myasthenia, MS, metabolic, infection (HIV, syphilis, TB, parasites), drugs (steroids, HAART), lupus, sarcoid, amyloidosis, cord lesion, ischemia, polymyalgia rheumatica, diabetic amyotrophy, Behçet's, rhabdomyolysis, glycogen storage dz....
3. **Tests:** CPK, EMG, ESR, ANA, TSH, MCV, muscle biopsy.
4. **Types:**
   a. **Inflammatory (myositis):** Myalgias, CPK moderately high.
      1) **Dermatomyositis:** Associated with carcinoma in 20%, butterfly rash, Jo-1 Ab. Rx:
         a) **Steroids:** Prednisone 60-100 mg qd until improvement, then 40 qd × several months. If pt is already on steroids, try tapering them because it may be steroid myopathy.
         b) **Immunosuppression:** Follow WBC, LFTs q week, then q month.
         c) **Azathioprine:** Effects take months. Start 50 qd × 1 wk, then 100 qd × 1 wk, then 150 qd.
         d) **Methotrexate:** 0.4 mg/kg/treatment IV at first treatment, increasing to 0.8 mg/kg in 3 weeks. Dose weekly at first, then every 2-3 wk.
      2) **Inclusion body myositis:** Most common myopathy in age >50. Quads and deep flexors affected early. No response to rx.
      3) **Overlap syndromes:** With collagen vascular diseases (e.g., MCTD, SLE).
   b. **Polymyositis:** Less common, less pain.
   c. **Dystrophies:** Hereditary disturbance of structural protein, extremely high CK. Dystrophin deficiency (Duchenne's, Becker's), limb-girdle muscular dystrophies (LGMD), congenital dystrophies....
   d. **Myotonic dystrophies:** Classic dive-bomber EMG, multisystem abnormalities. Most common dystrophy in adults, three types, all AD inheritance, triplet repeat expansion.
   e. **Channelopathies:** Range from myotonia to periodic paralyses. Na, Cl, Ca, and K channel abnormalities. Hyper-and hypokalemic periodic paralysis, paramyotonia congenital....
   f. **Metabolic:** Thyroid, carbohydrate, and lipid metabolism deficiencies....

NEUROSURGICAL PROCEDURES

A. See also: Trauma, p. 119; Intracranial Hemorrhage, p. 61; Intracranial Pressure, p. 67; Spinal Cord, p. 113; Tumors of Brain, p. 120; PEDIATRIC Tumors, p. 151; PEDIATRIC Head Circumference, p. 137.

B. Neurosurgery pre-op orders:
1. **NPO except meds after midnight:** IV fluids (D5NS); NGT to suction if urgent case.
2. **Compression boots on call to OR.**
3. **Void on call to OR.**
4. **Pre-op meds:** Consider:
    a. **Steroids:** E.g., dexamethasone 10 mg PO qhs, 10 mg IV on call. For pts on chronic steroids, give stress-dose steroids (see p. 173).
    b. **Prophylactic Abx:** E.g., 1 g cefazolin or vancomycin on call.
    c. **GI prophylaxis:** E.g., ranitidine 150 mg PO qhs, 50 mg IV on call to OR.
    d. **Seizure prophylaxis:** Phenytoin 100 mg tid for craniotomy/hemicraniectomy, large/superficial ICH/tumor resection, seizure on presentation, etc.
    e. **Sleeping pill:** Beware of benzodiazepines in pts who are elderly or encephalopathic. Consider quetiapine.

C. Pre-op check: The pre-op note should document:
1. **Vital signs and neuro exam.**
2. **Tests:** Chem 10, CBC, platelets, PT, PTT, ACD levels, UA, EKG, CXR.
3. **Blood:** Type and hold 2 units (4 for vascular cases).
4. **Pt consent.**
5. **Plan.**

D. Post-op orders:
1. **Admit:** To postanesthesia care unit, transfer to ICU when stable.
2. **Vital signs:** Every 15 min × 4 h, then q1h; temperature q4h × 3 d, then q8h; craniotomy checks.
3. **Activity:** Bedrest, HOB elevated 20-30 degrees for craniotomies. Compression boots or TED hose. Incentive spirometry q2h while awake (<u>except</u> if posttranssphenoidal).
4. **Diet:** NPO except meds.
5. **I/Os:** Hourly. If no bladder catheter, straight catheter q6h prn.
6. **IV fluids:** E.g., NS + 20 mEq KCl/L at 75 cc/h.
7. **O_2:** E.g., 2 L per nasal cannula.
8. **Meds:** Consider same options as pre-op; also BP meds, analgesic, and fever prophylaxis.
9. **Postanesthesia rigors:** Too soon for post-op infection. Meperidine or buspirone can help.

E. Post-op check: Document events, VS, I/Os, exam, wound check, labs, plan.

F. Post-op deterioration:
1. **Emergent CT for all altered mental status.**
2. **DDx:** Hemorrhage, infarction, seizure, tension pneumocephalus, infection, cardiac or pulmonary event, persistent anesthetic effect (unlikely in a pt who was initially doing well post-op).
3. **Seizures:** Intubate pts who have labored breathing or do not quickly regain consciousness. Draw ACD levels and then bolus with additional ACDs; do not wait for levels.

G. Craniotomy:

1. **Frontal, temporal, parietal, and occipital craniotomies:** For access to cortical and subcortical lesions; also for access to the ventricles. Transcallosal approaches have increased risk of venous infarction; usually require pre-operative angiogram.

2. **Posterior fossa (suboccipital) craniotomy:** Used to reach the cerebellopontine angle, one vertebral artery, or as an extreme lateral approach to the anterolateral brainstem. In addition to the routine post-op issues described above.

   a. **Closely monitor respirations:** Pts may benefit from 24-48 h post-op intubation since posterior fossa complications often have respiratory arrest as the presenting sign.

   b. **Keep SBP <160:** With nicardipine, labetalol, or nitroprusside if necessary. Sudden BP change suggests hematoma or edema.

   c. **Posterior fossa hematoma or edema:** Presents with sudden changes in breathing or BP; pupils, consciousness, and ICP are not affected until late. Rx is rapid intubation, ventricular drainage (through prophylactically placed burr hole, if possible), and immediate reoperation. An emergent CT scan may be informative but may dangerously delay treatment.

   d. **Watch for CSF leak through wound or nose:** See p. 20.

   e. **If corneal reflex is poor** due to 5th or 7th nerve injury, protect eye with drops, ointment, or patch.

3. **Pterional craniotomy:** To reach anterior circulation and basilar tip aneurysms, cavernous sinus, and suprasellar tumors. The craniotomy is centered over the depression of the sphenoid ridge. When the sella is accessed, consider post-op complications of transsphenoidal surgery, below.

H. Transsphenoidal surgery: Used for sellar tumors without significant suprasellar extension.

1. **Post-op complications:** DM (see p. 199), adrenal insufficiency, hypothyroidism, hypogonadism, secondary empty sella syndrome (visual loss from chiasm retracting into sella), infection, CSF leak (p. 20), carotid artery rupture, nasal septal perforation.

2. **Post-op orders:**

   a. **I/Os q1h,** with urine specific gravity q4h and electrolytes with osmolarity q6h.

   b. **IV fluids:** D5 1/2 NS + 20 mEq KCl/L at 75-100 mL/h, plus replace urine output mL for mL.

   c. **Abx:** Continue pre-op regimen until nasal packs removed.

   d. **Steroid taper:** E.g., hydrocortisone 50 mg IM/IV/PO bid, taper 10 mg/dose/d. Test AM cortisol 24 h after stopping steroids.

   e. **Activity:** No incentive spirometry or drinking through a straw, to avoid aspirating the sinus fat graft.

I. CSF access and decompression techniques: All increase risk of CNS infection.

1. **External ventricular drain:** AKA intraventricular catheter or ventriculostomy. For temporary ICP monitoring and CSF drainage. May be inserted at the bedside, if anterior approach. Usually done in non-dominant hemisphere.

    a. Orders: Hang bag 15 cm above ear (EAM − external auditory meatus); drain for pressure >15 cm ("EVD @ 15 and open"). If need to withdraw more fluid, first lower the bag (e.g., to 10 cm). Empiric nafcillin 2 g IV q4h, cefazolin, or vancomycin.

    b. Weaning: Can sometimes wean even if output is high (~150 cc qd). Clamp; open if pressure >20; then leave open until it decreases to 15. Pts. who do not tolerate clamping may need a shunt.

2. Ventricular shunts: Usually ventriculoperitoneal; occasionally ventriculoatrial, ventriculopleural, or lumboperitoneal. For permanent CSF drainage. Inserted in OR.

    a. Hardware: May contain valves to prevent overshunting, reservoirs to allow CSF taps, or tumor filters to prevent seeding.

    b. Complications: Infection, undershunting or occlusion, overshunting (can cause headache or SDH).

3. Shunt or reservoir tap: To access the reservoir, shave scalp, iodine prep for 5 min, and insert a 25-gauge butterfly needle at an oblique angle.

4. Ommaya reservoir: An indwelling reservoir attached to a ventricular catheter. It allows intrathecal chemotherapy or Abx, or recurrent CSF aspiration.

5. Lumbar drain: Temporary catheter placed to lower CSF pressure, usually to treat postoperative CSF leak or before VP shunt for presumed NPH. Pt should be on Abx while drain is in place.

PAIN

A. H&P: Location, quality, duration, intensity, aggravating and relieving factors, h/o trauma, disability, litigation, drugs tried, other treatments, imaging work, psychiatric history, strength, range of motion, straight leg raise, pin prick and light touch sensation, skin color and temperature, dystrophic skin changes.

B. Common MD false beliefs about pain:

1. Masking: Pain meds dangerously mask important sx?
No—you can continue the workup with pt comfortable.

2. Physical signs: Pain correlates with VS, ability to sleep?
No—ANS activation varies widely.

3. Addiction: Addicts overreport pain because they are addicted?
No—opiate receptor downregulation physiologically worsens pain.

4. Dosing: In treating addicts, keep med doses as low as possible?
No—they have opiate tolerance, so need more.

5. Emotion: Pain only appears to worsen with stress?
No—it actually worsens it through physiological mechanisms.

6. Chief complaint-ism: Treat the true CC, whether pain or emotion?
No—treat both. Treat anxiety even when it is secondary. Conversely, pts. who irrationally fear a brain tumor may not let go of that until you treat their HA.

C. Common pt pain myths: Address these directly and sympathetically.

1. Masking: Pain meds dangerously mask my important sx. *See above.*

2. Fear of med dependence: Needing a med ≡ physical tolerance ≡ addiction. *Explain the difference and that <1% of pts. who take meds for pain abuse them. But also ask if relatives have addictions.*

3. Ignoring mood: Pain is the main cause of my suffering. *Describing the physiological effects of stress may help pts. take mood seriously.*

4. **Stoicism:** Pain complaints are for the weak. ("That which does not kill me makes me strong"—Nietzsche.) *Point out that pain saps strength whether you complain or not.*

D. Pain rx by comorbidity:
1. **Acute physical injury or surgery:** NSAIDS or opiates.
2. **Depression:** Duloxetine; TCAs (beware of TCA SEs).
3. **Depression and somatization:** Duloxetine.
4. **Epilepsy:** Valproate, carbamazepine.
5. **Mood lability:** Valproate, carbamazepine.
6. **Substance abuse:**
   a. **Acute pain:** Use opiates as needed, but <u>higher</u> dose (see above).
   b. **Chronic pain:** Avoid opiates. If you must, use fentanyl patch (hard to abuse) or <u>methadone</u>—much cheaper, easier to titrate.

E. Pain rx in substance abusers:
1. **Sx of prescription substance abuse:** Pt requests early refills, gets them from other MDs, relatives (talk to them alone!) report confusion.

F. Pain rx by cause:
1. **Bone pain:** NSAIDS (especially aspirin) + acetaminophen are selectively good for bone pain; also steroids, opiates. XRT or strontium-90 for metastases. A corset may help compression fractures.
2. **Complex regional pain syndrome** (includes sympathetically mediated pain or reflex sympathetic dystrophy): Look for altered color or temperature of skin, burning pain, skin hypersensitivity to light touch, trophic changes, stiff joints.
   a. **Lidocaine patch or ointment:** May help skin hypersensitivity.
   b. **IV phentolamine test:** Can help predict the effect of sympathetic nerve block. Check EKG first.
3. **Sympathetic nerve block:** May help if signs of sympathetically mediated pain (e.g., skin cold, damp).
4. **Gout:** NSAIDS or colchicine; allopurinol (not in acute flare), keep pt hydrated; avoid loop diuretics.
5. **Organ metastases:** Steroids.
6. **Mouth pain from ulceration:** 1:1:1 ratio of diphenhydramine, Xylocaine, and Kaopectate liquids, give 15 cc q3h prn.
7. **Needles, splinters, etc.:** In pain-sensitive children and opiate addicts, lidocaine ointment 30 min before the needle.
8. **Neuropathic pain:**
   a. **Drugs:** Duloxetine, nortriptyline, or ACDs.
   b. **Treat accompanying depression:** See Table 25, p. 100.
   c. **Surgery:** Nerve decompression may help if movement worsens paresthesias.
9. **Thalamic pain syndrome** (Déjèrine-Roussy syndrome): Hypersensitivity after thalamic stroke. Rx rarely successful.
10. **Trigeminal neuralgia:** Lancinating, often with trigger points. Often associated with MS. Rarely from dental dz or brain tumor. Try carbamazepine 100-400 tid, gabapentin, pregabalin, baclofen, or lamotrigine. Consider surgery or radiofrequency ablation.
11. **Zoster (shingles):**
    a. **Acute:** If pt. over 50 or lesions last >72 h, give antiherpetic (e.g., famciclovir). Try lidocaine cream.

    b. Postherpetic pain:
       1) Early nerve blocks.
       2) Constant pain: Try a TCA.
       3) Lancinating: Try gabapentin or other ACD.

PARANEOPLASTIC SYNDROMES

A. Incidence: Although rare (1% of cancer pts.), paraneoplastic syndromes precede the diagnosis of cancer in about 60% of cases.

Syndrome	Clinical Features	Antibody	Typical Cancer
Brain Sx			
Brainstem encephalitis	Ataxia, cranial n. or motor dysfunction, abnl CSF	Ma1, Ma2	Small-cell lung cancer (SCLC), testicular
Limbic encephalitis	Depression, confusion, abnl CSF	Hu, others	SCLC
Subacute cerebellar degen.	Ataxia, dysarthria, nystagmus, nl CSF	Yo (AKA Purkinje cell)	Breast, ovary; SCLC
Opsoclonus, myoclonus	Jerky eye and limb movement	Ri	Lung, breast
Isolated CNS angiitis			Hodgkin's
Retinal degeneration	Loss of vision	Retinal	SCLC, melanoma
Spinal Cord Sx			
Necrotizing myelopathy	Weakness, sensory loss	?	SCLC
Motor neuron disease	Weakness, fasciculations	?	Various lymphomas and carcinomas
Stiff person syndrome	Painful spasms	Amphiphysin, GAD	Lung, lymphoma, breast, thymoma
Peripheral Nerve Sx			
Subacute sensory neurop.	Sensory ataxia, gait instability, dysesthesias	Hu, others	SCLC, plasma cell dyscrasias
Gammopathy-assoc. neurop.	Sensory loss, weakness, areflexia	Monoclonal Ig	Myeloma, Waldenstrom's, lymphoma
Guillain-Barré (AIDP)	Rapid weakness, areflexia	?	Lymphoma
Neuromuscular Junction Sx			
Lambert-Eaton	Proximal weakness, areflexia, eyes spared	Calcium channel	SCLC (1%-3% of pts.)
Myasthenia gravis	Weakness, areflexia, eyes often involved	ACh receptor	Thymoma (15% of pts.)
Muscle Sx			
Dermato- or polymyositis	Weakness, high CPK	Muscle	Breast, lung, GI, uterine, ovarian, Hodgkin's

Table 22. Paraneoplastic syndromes.

PERIPHERAL NERVE ANATOMY

A. See also: Peripheral Neuropathy p. 93.
B. Spinal level by disc:

Disc	Root	Motor	Sensory	Reflex
C5-6	C6	Biceps, wrist ext.	Med. arm and hand	Biceps
C6-7*	C7	Triceps, wrist flex.	Middle finger	Triceps
C7-T1	C8	Finger flex.	Lat. hand	Finger
L3-4	L4	Quadriceps	Med. calf	Knee
L4-5*	L5	Dorsiflexors	Med. foot	
L5-S1	S1	Plantar flexors	Lat. foot	Ankle

Table 23. Symptoms of disc herniation. *Most common syndromes.

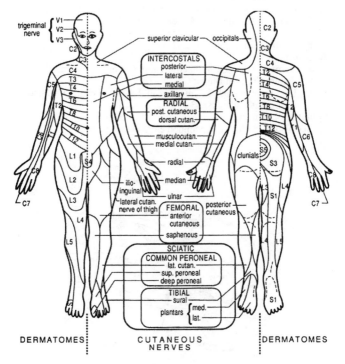

Figure 10. Dermatomes and peripheral nerve territories. (From Patton HD, et al. *Introduction to Basic Neurology*. Philadelphia: Saunders; 1976, with permission.)

C. Spinal level by function:
   1. Movement:
      a. Neck: C1-4.
      b. Diaphragm: C3-5.
      c. Shoulder: Abduction and lateral rotation are C5. Adduction and medial rotation are C6-8.
      d. Elbow: Flexion is C5-6. Extension is C6-8.
      e. Wrist: C6-8. Extension = radial n. Flexion = median + ulnar n.
      f. Hand: Finger abduction and adduction are ulnar nerve (C8-T1). Grip is median nerve. Finger extension is radial nerve.
      g. Thumb test: Can tell radial, median, and ulnar nerve lesions by thumb movements. Mnemonic is <u>RUM</u>: <u>R</u>adial extends, <u>U</u>lnar adducts, and <u>M</u>edian abducts. Flexion + extension = in plane of the palm; abduction + adduction = at right angles to the palm.
      h. Intercostals: T2-9.
      i. Abdominals: Upper is T9-10. Lower is T11-12.
      j. Hip: Flexion is L2-4, adduction is L3-4, abduction is L5-S1.
      k. Knee: Extension is L2-4; flexion is L4-S1.
      l. Foot: Dorsiflexion is L4-S1; plantar flexion is S1-2.
      m. Bladder, anal sphincter: S2-4.
   2. Sensation:
      a. Arm: Shoulders: C4; inner forearm: C6; outer forearm: T1; thumb: C6; fifth finger: C8.
      b. Leg: Front of thigh: L2; medial calf: L4; lateral calf: L5; fifth toe: S1; midline buttocks: S3.
D. Spinal level by nerve:
   1. See also: p. 95 for sx of common entrapment syndromes.

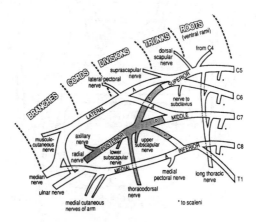

Figure 11. The brachial plexus. (From Warwick R, Williams P. *Gray's Anatomy*. 35th ed. London: Churchill Livingstone; 1973, with permission.)

2. **Brachial plexus:** C5-T1.
   a. **Plexi:**
      1) **Upper plexus:** C5-6. Deltoids, biceps, supra- + infraspinatus.
      2) **Middle plexus:** C7.
      3) **Lower plexus:** C8-T1.
   b. **Cords:** Upper-mid-lower plexi recombine to form three cords; lateral and medial cord then recombine to form median nerve.
      1) **Lateral cord** (from upper + middle plexus) forms musculocutaneous nerve, lateral anterior thoracic nerve, median nerve.
      2) **Posterior cord** (from upper, middle, and lower plexus) forms radial nerve, axillary nerve, and subscapular nerve.
      3) **Medial cord** (from lower plexus) forms ulnar nerve, medial cutaneous nerve, median nerve.
3. **Nerves of arm:** Note that any weakness of both flexors and extensors or of all intrinsic hand muscles implies that the lesion cannot be a mononeuropathy.
   a. **Long thoracic nerve:** C5-7. Serratus anterior. Test: scapula wings when pt presses arm forward against a wall.
   b. **Axillary nerve:** <u>C5</u>-6. Deltoid, etc. Test: abduct arm >90 degrees.
   c. **Musculocutaneous nerve:** <u>C5</u>-6. Biceps.
   d. **Radial nerve:** C5-8, esp. <u>C7</u>. Extensors (triceps, wrist, and finger), supinator, brachioradialis.
   e. **Median nerve:** C6-T1. Flexors except ulnar: most forearm flexors, flex. dig. superior; all pronators. Hand: LOAF muscles (<u>L</u>umbricals 1 and 2, <u>O</u>pp. pollicis, <u>A</u>bd. poll. brev., <u>F</u>lex. poll. brev.).
   f. **Ulnar nerve:** C8-T1. Flexor digitorum profundus 3 and 4, flexor carpi ulnaris. Most of intrinsic hand (except LOAF muscles above): thumb adductors and flexors, interossei, lumbricals 3 and 4, hypothenar muscles.
4. **Leg:**
   a. **Femoral nerve:** L2-4.
      1) **Function:** Extend knee.
      2) **Muscles:** Iliopsoas, quadriceps, sartorius, rectus femoris.
   b. **Obturator nerve:** L2-4.
      1) **Function:** Adduct leg.
      2) **Muscles:** Adductor longus, brevis, and magnus; gracilis, pectineus....
   c. **Sciatic nerve** (tibial and peroneal nerve): L4-S2.
      1) **Function:** Extend and abduct hip, flex knee, all foot mvts.
         a) **Deep peroneal nerve:** Extends toes and ankle.
         b) **Superficial peroneal nerve:** Everts foot.
         c) **Tibial nerve:** Superficial tibial flexes foot; deep tibial flexes toes.
      2) **Muscles:** Semitendinosus and semimembranosus, biceps femoris, gastrocnemius, soleus, foot muscles....
E. **Spinal level by reflex:**
   1. **Cervical:** Biceps is C5-6. Supinator is C5-6. Triceps is C6-8.
   2. **Thoracic:** Scratch towards navel. Contraction with scratching above navel is T8-10; below navel is T10-12.
   3. **Lumbar:** Knee is L2-4. Ankle is S1-2. Babinski is L4-S2.

PERIPHERAL NEUROPATHY

A. See also: Periperhal Nerve Anatomy, p. 89; Weakness, p. 129.

B. H&P: Ask about weakness, paresthesias, numbness, distal vs. proximal, symmetric vs. focal, ANS sx, limb injuries, alcoholism, DM, medications, HIV status, hepatitis, FH, reflexes.

C. DDx: CNS lesion; myopathy, NMJ dz, metabolic (e.g., paresthesias from alkalosis)....

D. Tests: EMG/NCS, KCl/Ca/Mg/Phos, CPK, B_{12}, MCV, ESR, TSH, hemoglobin A1c, Lyme titer, syphilis, SPEP/UPEP, LFTs, HIV, ANA. Consider ANCA, ALA, ACE level/chest film, heavy metals, fat pad biopsy for amyloid, HCV, HBV, cryoglobulins.

E. Types of neuropathy: Polyneuropathy (usually axonal degeneration or demyelination); mononeuropathy or mononeuropathy multiplex (usually entrapment, trauma); sensorimotor; motor; sensory.

F. Causes of neuropathy:
   1. **A mnemonic:** DANG THERAPIST: DM, Alcohol, Nutritional, GBS, Trauma, Hereditary, Endocrine/Entrapment, Renal/Radiation, AIDS/Amyloid, Paraprotein/Porphyria, Infectious (e.g., leprosy), Systemic/Sarcoid, Toxins.
   2. **Causes categorized:** By acuity, distribution, and EMG finding:
      a. **Acute, generalized:**
         1) **Axonal degeneration:**
            a) **Infections:** Lyme, HIV, EBV, hepatitis, CMV.
            b) **ICU neuropathy:** Proximal, sensorimotor, in setting of SIRS, multiorgan failure.
            c) **Misc:** Porphyria, "axonal Guillain-Barré syndrome."
         2) **Demyelination:** Guillain-Barré syndrome, arsenic, infections, e.g., HIV and diphtheria.
      b. **Chronic, generalized:**
         1) **Axonal degeneration:** Dying back, stocking-glove pattern.
            a) **Nutritional:** Alcohol, folate, vitamin B_{12} or E deficiency, B_6 toxicity.
            b) **Toxic:** DPH, vincristine, heavy metals (thallium, mercury, lead, arsenic), antiretrovirals, acrylamide, etc.
            c) **Endocrine:** DM, hypothyroidism.
            d) **Infectious:** HIV, Lyme.
            e) **Genetic:** Charcot-Marie-Tooth (CMT) type II, familial amyloidosis, Friedreich's ataxia, etc.
            f) **Lipid problems:** Fabry's dz, Tangier dz, Bassen-Kornzweig dz.
            g) **Other:** Uremia, liver disease, vasculitis, sensory neuropathy (anti-Hu paraneoplastic, Sjögren's), lipid dzs (Fabry's, Tangier, Bassen-Kornzweig).
         2) **Demyelination:**
            a) **Uniform slowing on EMG:** CMT types 1A, 1B, and X; myelin dysmetabolism, e.g., metachromatic leukodystrophy, Refsum dz, Krabbe dz.
            b) **Nonuniform slowing:**
               i. **Infectious or inflammatory:** HIV, CIDP, multifocal neuropathy with conduction block.

   ii. **Paraprotein:** Lymphoma, myeloma, Waldenstrom's, cryoglobulinemia, POEMS syndrome (Polyneuropathy with Organomegaly, Endocrinopathy, M-protein, and Skin changes), MGUS (Monoclonal Gammopathy of Uncertain Significance).

 c. **Mononeuropathy multiplex** (multifocal or asymmetric):
  1) **Axonal:**
   a) **Vascular:** DM, vasculitis, connective tissue dz, subacute bacterial endocarditis.
   b) **Infectious or inflammatory:** HIV, Lyme, leprosy, VZV, hepatitis A, sarcoid.
   c) **Neoplastic:** Neurofibromatosis, lymphoma, leukemia, direct local invasion.
   d) **Miscellaneous:** Genetic, e.g., inherited brachial plexus neuropathy; traumatic, e.g., multiple compressions.
  2) **Demyelinating:**
   a) **Inflammatory:** Guillain-Barré; multifocal motor neuropathy with conduction block.
   b) **Genetic:** HNPP: hereditary neuropathy with liability to pressure palsies.
   c) **Multiple compressions.**

G. Specific neuropathies:

 1. **Inflammatory demyelinating polyneuropathies:** E.g., Guillain-Barré syndrome, CIDP. See p. 36.
 2. **Charcot-Marie-Tooth dz:** The most common hereditary neuropathies. CMT-1 is demyelinating, CMT-2 is axonal. Both start in the feet, usually before age 20, with weakness, numbness, pes cavus.
 3. **Cranial neuropathies:** Important to distinguish central from peripheral neuropathies. See also individual nerves or sx.
  a. **Cranial polyneuropathy syndromes:**
   1) **Cavernous sinus syndromes:** See p. 50.
   2) **Basilar meningitis.**
   3) **Jugular foramen syndromes:** Variable compression of the lower four cranial nerves. Look for corticospinal signs or Horner's syndrome as evidence for brainstem compression.
   4) **Polyneuritis cranialis:** A variant of Guillain-Barré syndrome; see p. 37.
   5) **Myasthenia gravis:** See p. 81.
   6) **Botulism.**
  b. **Bell's palsy:** Idiopathic CN VII palsy. R/o secondary palsies.
   1) **H&P:** Pressure/pain behind ear, hyperacusis, decreased taste, subjective but not objective numbness. Unilateral face weakness including brow, eye closure (can see eye roll up, Bell's phenomenon). Examine eardrum to rule out Ramsay-Hunt syndrome (geniculate VZV reactivation affecting CN VII and VIII)—unrelated to the Ramsay-Hunt syndrome of myoclonus and spinocerebellar atrophy (see Eponym rant, p. 28).
   2) **Rx:** Eye protection (drops during day, ointment and patch at night). Consider PO prednisone and valacyclovir/acyclovir if within 1 wk of symptom onset.

     3) **Tests:** Consider Lyme Ab, CBC, ESR, ANA, ANCA, chest film (to r/o TB, sarcoid, adenopathy), ACE, HIV, UBJ/SPEP if elderly, MRI, CSF if suspect carcinomatous meningitis.

4. **Diabetic neuropathy:** By far the most common cause of neuropathy. Can affect any nerve.
   a. **Polyneuropathy:** Distal, sensory > motor, axonal degeneration on EMG. R/o tarsal tunnel syndrome.
   b. **Autonomic neuropathy:** Gastroparesis, orthostasis, burning pain, erectile dysfunction, sphincter involvement.
   c. **Diabetic amyotrophy:** Asymmetric painful lumbosacral plexopathy. Recovers spontaneously.
   d. **Mononeuropathy:** E.g., pupil-sparing third nerve palsy (see p. 46). Also CN IV, VI, VII. Usually recovers. DDx: Entrapment neuropathies.
   e. **Rx:** See Neuropathic pain, p. 87, and Diabete mellitus, p. 199.
5. **Neuropathy in kidney failure:** Uremia causes a dying-back neuropathy and increases risk of compression neuropathies.
6. **Plexopathies:**
   a. **Brachial plexopathy:** See Figure 11, p. 90.
      1) **H&P:** Sudden, severe shoulder pain, worse with arm movement, then weakness of shoulder, arm, hand. Often with numbness on upper arm. Ask about previous viral syndrome; smoking history. Look for Horner's syndrome.
      2) **DDx of brachial plexopathy:** Pancoast tumor, post radiation therapy, DM, Lyme, vasculitis, trauma (p. 94), idiopathic brachial neuritis (Parsonage Turner syndrome)....
      3) **Tests:** CXR, glucose, ANA, ESR; EMG (not positive <3 wk after sx start), MRI with contrast of shoulder. CSF nl.
      4) **Rx:** Steroids do not help idiopathic cases.
      5) **Prognosis:** Idiopathic cases usually start to recover in 4 wk; upper plexus may fully recover by 1 yr; lower plexus may take 2-3 yr.
   b. **Lumbosacral plexitis:** Rarely idiopathic.
      1) **H&P:** Sudden leg pain, then weakness, paresthesias but little objective sensory loss. Straight leg raise may be positive, but there should be no back pain or exacerbation of pain by Valsalva maneuver. Pt. needs pelvic and rectal exams.
      2) **DDx:** Pelvic mass, DM, Lyme, vasculitis, femoral neuropathy, radiculopathy, cauda equina syndrome, post-XRT....
      3) **Tests:** Consider CEA, PSA, glucose, ANA, ESR, pelvic CT. EMG not positive <3 wk after sx start but is crucial for dx: should see at least two spinal levels involved, with sparing of the paraspinal muscles. MRI with contrast of pelvis.
      4) **Rx:** Steroids do not help.
      5) **Prognosis:** Pain gets better before strength; only slow, incomplete recovery.
7. **Entrapment neuropathies and traumatic nerve injuries:**
   a. **H&P:** Ask about worsening at night; repetitive stresses, e.g., typing; comorbid dz, e.g., alcoholism, DM, hypothyroidism, acromegaly, arthritis, cancer; previous entrapments (consider hereditary neuropathy with pressure palsies). Light touch is often

lost before pin prick (opposite to spinal cord injuries). Pain may be referred; e.g., pain above wrist from carpal tunnel syndrome.

b. Tests for compression: See syndromes below. Consider EMG if surgery is an option. EMG may be normal for the first 2-4 wk after onset of sx.

c. Rx of entrapment: Splint, NSAIDS, gabapentin, duloxetine; consider surgery if weak.

d. Brachial plexus trauma: See Figure 11.

  1) Upper plexus lesion: Erb-Duchenne palsy. Often from trauma pulling head away from shoulder.

   a) Motor: Bellhop's tip position: internal rotation at shoulder, with elbow extension. Weak shoulder abduction and extension, weak biceps and triceps.

   b) Sensory: Numb over deltoid, radial forearm.

  2) Lower plexus lesion: Déjèrine-Klumpke palsy. Often from forced arm abduction or lung apex tumor (pancoast tumor; often with Horner's syndrome). See claw deformity similar to ulnar neuropathy, below.

e. Common entrapment syndromes: (See also Spinal level by nerve, p. 90.)

  1) Median nerve entrapment:

   a) Anterior interosseous nerve syndrome: Branches just distal to elbow. Decreased flexion of D1-2 causes weak pinch. No sensory loss.

   b) Carpal tunnel syndrome (CTS):

    i. H&P: Tingling or numbness in D1-4 (through medial but not lateral ring finger). Pain may radiate above wrist, but not to neck. Pain awakens pt from sleep. Exam is not that sensitive. May see weak grip, thenar atrophy.

    ii. Phalen's sign: 60 sec of wrist flexion → paresthesias.

    iii. Tinel's sign: Tapping on wrist causes paresthesias.

    iv. DDx: Cervical radiculopathy, thoracic outlet syndrome, pronator teres syndrome, de Quervain's dz....

  2) Radial nerve entrapment:

   a) Mid-upper arm compression (Saturday night or honeymoon palsy): See wrist and finger drop; no triceps weakness.

   b) Forearm compression: Finger drop without wrist drop. Consider surgery for entrapment.

  3) Ulnar nerve entrapment: Ulnar claw deformity: fingers 4 and 5 have metacarpal hyperextension with finger flexion.

   a) Wrist (Guyon's canal) vs. elbow compression: Make a fist; if poor flexion of 4 and 5, then lesion is above wrist.

   b) Elbow compression: Cubital tunnel syndrome (under arcuate ligament) vs. ulnar groove.

  4) Thoracic outlet syndrome:

   a) Compression of the brachial plexus by a cervical rib or elongated transverse process of C7. However, cervical ribs are common in normal persons. Maneuvers to look for obliteration of radial pulse have very low specificity.

b) **Droopy shoulder syndrome:** Usually young women. Pulling down on arm worsens sx.

5) **Peroneal nerve palsy:** From calf compression or long bed rest. See foot drop, steppage gait. Numb lateral calf and foot dorsum. Weak foot inversion suggests L5 root lesion. In trauma, anterior compartment syndrome, which requires <u>immediate</u> fasciotomy, can cause peroneal palsy.

6) **Meralgia paresthetica:** Lateral femoral cutaneous nerve compression, often from weight change, causes thigh tingling.

7) **Tarsal tunnel syndrome:** "CTS of the foot." Posterior tibial nerve compression causes sole paresthesias.

PREGNANCY AND CHILDBIRTH

A. Neurological complications of pregnancy:

1. **Cerebral hemorrhage:** The risk increases with each trimester.
   a. **Causes:** AVMs and aneurysms are most common; also DIC, anticoagulants, placental abruption, mycotic aneurysm, metastatic choriocarcinoma, and eclampsia.
   b. **Rx:** Hyperventilation, hypothermia, and steroids are safe; try to avoid mannitol. Surgery is based on same criteria as nonpregnant pts.

2. **Cerebral infarction:** About 1 in 3,000 pregnancies. 70% are arterial occlusion, 30% secondary to cerebral venous thrombosis.

3. **Cerebral venous thrombosis.**

4. **Chorea gravidarum:** Rare. Usually starts after first trimester, remits after delivery. See Choreoathetosis, p. 76, for DDx. Haloperidol is a relatively safe rx.

5. **Eclamptic encephalopathy:** Associated with hypertension, proteinuria, edema, oliguria, hyperreflexia, and seizures. Usually young primigravidas, >20 wk gestation. Give magnesium 4 g IV over 15 min, then 1-2 g/h, along with Ringer's lactate. Seizures may also be treated with diazepam or DPH.

6. **Neuropathies of pregnancy:** Bell's palsy, carpal tunnel syndrome, and meralgia paresthetica are most common.

7. **Obstetrical palsies:** From fetal head, forceps, or leg holders. Most common is L4-5 palsy, compressed by fetal brow as it crosses the pelvic rim.

8. **Pseudotumor cerebri:** Usually presents around week 14 and spontaneously resolves in 1-3 mo.

B. Effects of pregnancy on neurological conditions:

1. **Migraine:** Most migraineurs improve during pregnancy, but migraines may also begin during pregnancy, especially in the first trimester. Acetaminophen, barbiturates, and low-dose opiates are the safest analgesics. Avoid serotonin agonists, ergots, and propranolol. Amitriptyline may be acceptable but should be stopped 2 wk before delivery.

2. **Multiple sclerosis:** Flares are less likely during pregnancy but more likely postpartum. Epidural anesthesia is okay in MS.

3. **Myasthenia:** Avoid magnesium sulfate, scopolamine, large amounts of procaine. Watch for neonatal myasthenia for 72 h. Myasthenia often flares postpartum.

4. **Neuropathy:** CIDP and Charcot-Marie-Tooth dz may worsen.
5. **Tumors:** Most enlarge during pregnancy and shrink a little afterwards. Increased ICP may be an indication for termination of the pregnancy. ICP generally does not increase during labor, however.
6. **Seizures:** ACDs may harm the fetus, although so may seizures. Birth defect rate is as high as 10%.
    a. **Before pregnancy:** Give <u>all</u> young women folate 1 mg qd. Carbamazepine decreases oral contraceptive levels.
    b. **During pregnancy:** Keep ACD doses as low as possible. Monitor free levels since plasma proteins change in pregnancy.
    c. **Postpartum:** Seizure incidence increases 10-fold during the first 24 h after delivery. If doses are increased in pregnancy, return them to initial postpartum levels to avoid toxicity.

PSYCHIATRIC DISORDERS

A. **Psych-neuro overlap:** You can rarely treat one without treating—or causing—the other.
B. **Psychiatric emergencies:** Pts. who are suicidal, violent, or who attempt to leave the hospital without the capacity to make decisions may need restraint. However, restraints are terrifying, humiliating, and will permanently hurt the pt's likelihood of seeking medical care. Be aware of regulations governing use of restraints.
    1. **Calm pt down verbally:** Soothing tones can backfire. Instead, mirror pts.' arousal to nonverbally show you are not ignoring them. Do not yell back, of course; yell *with* them, e.g., "How upsetting!" Once they sense you are resonating with them, it is easier to redirect them. It can help to say their behavior frightens you and the staff—they may calm down, having achieved their goal.
    2. **Chemical restraint:** Pt more often accepts oral meds if you offer a "choice" between oral and IM.
        a. **Oral:** Olanzapine 5-10 mg (wafer) or haloperidol or benzo.
        b. **IM:** Haloperidol 5 mg, lorazepam 2 mg, Benadryl 50 mg.
        c. **IV:** Fewer extrapyramidal sx from IV haloperidol than IM. 2.5 mg (mild agitation) to 10 mg (extreme); 1-2 mg lorazepam.
    3. **Physical restraint:** Usually 4-point (all limbs). Consider 5-point (strap across chest) for big young pts. Although soft restraints may be enough for frail demented pts, they usually have hidden reserves of strength and ingenuity. No one should be in physical restraints for more than a short time without sedation. Consider requesting sitters.
C. **Psychiatric mental status exam:**
    1. **Activation/energy:** Excited, placid, sleepy....
    2. **Appearance:** Disheveled, bizarre clothing choice....
    3. **Behavior:** Cooperativity, restlessness....
    4. **Speech:** Volume, rate, latency, prosody, vocabulary and education.....
    5. **Affect:** Restricted, labile, irritable, sad....
    6. **Mood:** Many pts deny their depression but respond to questions such as: Is the stress of your illness a burden? How are your spirits? Can you still feel pleasure when something good happens?

Depression Criteria: SIGECAPS	Mania Criteria: DIGFAST
Low mood <u>or</u> anhedonia, + 4 of 8 sx:	Irritability + 4 sx, <u>or</u> euphoria + 3 sx:
Sleep change	**D**istractibility
Interest lower (anhedonia)	**I**njudicious behavior
Guilt feelings excessive	**G**randiosity
Energy lower	**F**light of ideas
Concentration lower	**A**ctivity increased
Appetite change	**S**leep need decreased
Psychomotor slowing/agitation	**T**alkativeness
Suicidal thoughts	

Table 24. Criteria for depression and mania.

7. **Perception:** Hallucinations. Auditory ones suggest schizophrenia or bipolar depression. Visual ones suggest delirium. Taste, smell, or touch suggests temporal lobe epilepsy.
8. **Cognition:**
   a. **Thought content:** Suicidal or homicidal thoughts, delusions. Delusions of guilt or somatic problem (e.g., body is rotting) suggest depression. Paranoia is more often bipolar or schizophrenic.
   b. **Thought process:** Ruminative, slow, tangential.
   c. **Mini-Mental State Exam:** Formerly reproduced widely as a rough estimate of cognitive impairment. Now, its copyright is controlled by a company called Psychological Assessment Resources (PAR), Inc. which, for $58, will sell you a pad of 50 one-use-only test sheets.
   d. **Quick Confusion Scale.** A free alternative replacement for the Mini-Mental. Takes about 2.5 min vs. about 10 min for the MMSE, so you'll have time to add a clock draw, object naming, making change, listing f-words, reading/writing.

Item	Scoring		Max Score
A. What year is it now?	2 if correct, 0 if wrong	=	2
B. What month is it?	2 if correct, 0 if wrong	=	2
C. Say to pt.: "Repeat this phrase after me and remember it:			
'<u>John</u> <u>Brown</u>, <u>42</u> <u>Market Street</u>, <u>New York</u>.'"			-
D. About what time is it?	1 if correct within an hr	=	1
E. Count backwards 20→1	2 if no errors, 1 if 1, 0 if ≥2	=	2
F. Say the months in reverse	2 if no errors, 1 if 1, 0 if ≥2	=	2
G. Repeat memory phrase	1 for each underlined phrase	=	5

Table 25. The Quick Confusion Scale. Max score = 14. Score <11 = likely cognitive impairment; score <7 = substantial impairment. (From Irons MJ, *et al.,* *Acad Emerg Med,* 2002;9:989–994.

D. Anxiety disorder and panic attacks:
  1. **DDx:** Heart or lung event, drugs (e.g., steroids, marijuana, cocaine), hyperthyroidism, labyrinthitis, temporal lobe epilepsy, mania.
  2. **Tests:** TSH, consider EKG or ABG during an attack.
  3. **Acute rx:** Lorazepam 0.5-1 mg, repeat after 30 min, or clonazepam. Not good maintenance therapy—need an antidepressant.
  4. **Chronic rx:** Antidepressant (SNRIs are slightly better than SSRIs); cognitive-behavioral therapy.
E. Attention-deficit/hyperactivity disorders:
  1. **Sx:** Significant impairment from inattention, impulsivity, excessive motor activity. Adults are less often hyperactive. Impairment is largely relative to demands of environment—that's why so many of your busy colleagues say they have it.
  2. **Onset:** In childhood. Acute onset suggests mania, delirium, etc.
  3. **Rx:** DA and NE reuptake blockers—Dexedrine, Ritalin, Strattera.
F. Capacity determination: (Competence is a legal decision.) Although psych consults help in assessing capacity, you can do it too.
  1. **Capacity** = The ability to convey a consistent choice; understand its nature and consequences, its relevance to self, and rationally manipulate evidence.
  2. **"Sliding scale":** When health stakes are high, pts. should be held to a higher standard of response.
  3. **Documentation:** "Based on my evaluation of this pt, he/she does/does not have a factual understanding of the current situation [give example], can/cannot rationally manipulate information to make a decision [give example] and does/does not express a choice. Therefore, this pt has/lacks the capacity to make this medical decision."
      a. **If capacity is present, note:** "We should respect the patient's right to make this decision."
      b. **If lacking:** Defer medical decisions to the health care proxy. If none exists, the family or state should pursue guardianship.
G. Depression: Pts. who smile or laugh can still be depressed. Screen <u>all</u> your pts., including stoic or high-functioning ones.
  1. **H&P:**
      a. **SIGECAPS criteria:** See, p. 98.
      b. **Somatic signs of mood disorder:** See "Psychosomatic Neurology", p. 102.
      c. **History:** Stressful events, family hx, previous antidepressant response, careful screen for previous manic sx.
      d. **Suicidality:** Ask whether life feels worth living before moving to more direct questions. Has pt imagined a concrete plan? Previous attempts? Is pt. impulsive? Urging an ER visit may reassure pts. of your concern, and their response will help you assess their level of distress. Remember, a pt.'s "contract for safety" is worth the paper it is written on.
      e. **Psychotic depression:** Suggests bipolar > unipolar depression.
  2. **Neurological DDx/comorbidity:** Up to 50% incidence in stroke, Alzheimer's, Parkinson's. Consider hypothyroidism, low testosterone, menopause.
      a. **"I'm depressed because I'm sick!":** Tell pts. that reactive, "rational" depression is still depression and that its treatment will help them fight their primary illness.

3. **DDx of depression:** Apathy/abulia, fatigue, anxiety, dysthymia (chronically depressed mood with only two SIGECAPS criteria), grief, dysphoric mania. A h/o lability or agitation, especially while on antidepressants, suggests bipolar disorder.
4. **Rx of depression:**
   a. **Compliance:** See p. 105. Depressed pts. may forgo rx because they lack hope they will work or because they lack the energy to fill prescriptions.
   b. **Drugs:** See also Antidepressants, p. 164.

Comorbidity	First Choice	Relatively Bad Choice
No comorbidity		
None	Bupropion, SSRIs	TCAs
Psychiatric		
Anxiety	Duloxetine, venlafaxine	TCAs
Low motivation	Bupropion	SSRI
Mania, impulsivity	Mood stabilizer	Antidepressant alone
OCD tendencies	High-dose fluoxetine	TCAs, bupropion
Psychosis	SSRI + antipsychotic	TCAs, bupropion
Somatization	Duloxetine	TCAs
Neurological		
Abulia (frontal)	Bupropion, dexedrine	TCAs, paroxetine
Delirium, dementia	Citalopram, trazodone	TCAs, bupropion
Fatigue	Bupropion, fluoxetine	TCAs, paroxetine
Insomnia	Trazodone, mirtazapine	TCAs, fluoxetine
Pain	Duloxetine, nortriptyline	SSRIs
Parkinsonism	Bupropion, mirtazapine	Sertraline, TCAs
Seizures	SSRIs, lamotrigine	Bupropion
Tremor	Mirtazapine	SSRIs
Stroke	Citalopram	TCAs
Vertigo	Fluoxetine	TCAs
Medical		
Advanced age	Citalopram, bupropion,	TCAs
Constipation	Bupropion, SSRIs	TCAs
Diarrhea	Mirtazapine, TCAs	SSRIs, bupropion
Diabetes (DMII)	Bupropion, SSRIs	TCAs, paroxetine
Glaucoma (narrow)	Bupropion, SSRIs	TCAs
Heart disease	SSRIs	TCAs, mirtazapine
Hypertension	Mirtazapine	Bupropion, SNRIs
Hypotension	Bupropion, SNRIs	TCAs
Kidney failure	Bupropion	Fluoxetine
Liver failure	Bupropion, citalopram	Duloxetine
Nausea, GERD	Selegiline patch	Paroxetine, venlafaxine
Overweight	Bupropion	TCAs
Pregnancy	SSRIs	TCAs
Sexual dysfunction	Bupropion	Paroxetine, other SSRIs
Smoker	Bupropion	TCAs
Urine retention	Bupropion, SSRIs	TCAs

Table 26. Choice of antidepressant by comorbid condition.

      1) **Who should prescribe?** Many pts. who resist antidepressants will accept them if the neurologist presents them as treatment for a comorbid problem, e.g., duloxetine for pain. Thus, it is sometimes better to curbside a psychiatrist than refer to one. Potentially bipolar pts are the chief exception.

      2) **Choice:** Neurologists often underprescribe bupropion and overprescribe TCAs. Table 25 follows current practice but is not entirely evidence based.

  c. **Psychotherapy:** Cognitive-behavioral psychotherapy has a synergistic effect with meds and also boosts compliance.

  d. **Electroconvulsive therapy:** In the elderly, often safer than meds. Good for catatonic depression; may help parkinsonism. Brain tumor or high ICP is a contraindication. Note: epilepsy and h/o stroke are <u>not</u> contraindications. Stop ACDs the day before.

H. Catatonia: Sustained postures with mutism, waxy flexibility, often echo phenomena and automatic obedience. Can shift between stupor and agitation. More common in bipolar depression than in schizophrenia. Treat with lorazepam, other benzodiazepines, ECT.

I. Mania and bipolar disorder: Many manic pts. appear agitated, not happy. More than 2 wk of irritability + 4 of the DIGFAST criteria (see Table 23), or euphoria + 3 of the DIGFAST criteria.

  1. **Bipolar I vs. II:** While the former pts have had at least one manic episode, the latter have had only hypomanic (i.e., mild) episodes. However, most episodes are depressed in both disorders.

  2. **Secondary mania ("organic"):** Usually R temporal or frontal lesion, or drug.

  3. **Acute rx:** Neuroleptics, e.g., olanzapine, or clonazepam.

  4. **Chronic rx:** Valproate, lithium, neuroleptics.

J. Obsessive-compulsive disorder: An anxiety disorder. Pts. with contamination fears may have great trouble taking pills.

  1. **H&P:** Ask about ritual touching, counting, checking, hand washing; hours per day spent on rituals. Distinguish between obsessions (thoughts) and compulsions (behavior).

  2. **DDx:** Also seen in degenerative dz, grief, Tourette's syndrome, anoxic encephalopathy, magnesium and carbon monoxide poisoning, Sydenham's chorea.

  3. **Rx:** High-dose Prozac, exposure and response prevention therapy, neuroleptics.

K. Personality disorders and rx compliance: These traits have implications for MD–pt relations in the general population.

  1. **See also:** Compliance, p. 105.

  2. **AKA axis II disorders** vs. axis I major mental illnesses: While character disorders are often called "nonbiological," they are on a spectrum with axis I disorders. The chief difference is that people with axis II disorders think their behavior is adaptive, and it responds poorly to rx.

  3. **Cluster A, odd or eccentric:** Shares traits with schizophrenia.

    a. **Paranoid:** Suspicious, poor trust. Litigious.

    b. **Schizoid:** Reclusive, detached. Poor medical f/u.

    c. **Schizotypal:** Bizarre, magical thought. May self-treat in odd ways.

    4. Cluster B, dramatic or emotional: Shares traits with axis II bipolar, but the latter's personality issues resolve between mood episodes.

       a. Antisocial: Ruthless. Be careful with these.

       b. Borderline: Unstable relationships. Set clear MD–pt boundaries. Associated with somatization.

       c. Histrionic: Dramatic. Easy to overtreat their sx. Associated with somatization.

       d. Narcissistic: Big frail ego. If you puncture it, they may end rx.

    5. Cluster C, anxious or fearful: Shares traits with axis II depression and anxiety syndromes.

       a. Avoidant: Shy, oversensitive. Be reassuring but not intrusive.

       b. Dependent: Passive, suggestible. Do not overlook pt.'s real needs.

       c. Obsessive-compulsive: Perfectionist, rigid. Wants rigid guidelines. Fear of contamination, taking pills.

       d. Not otherwise specified: Includes passive-aggressive, masochistic. PD-NOS label is used too broadly for pts. who annoy the MD.

    6. Secondary personality change ("organic"): Causes include focal lesions (trauma, strokes, tumors, epilepsy), degenerative dzs, drugs and toxins, infections (HIV, syphilis)....

       a. Frontal lobe damage:

         1) Orbitofrontal: Disinhibition (unlike mania, not very goal directed).

         2) Dorsolateral prefrontal: Executive dysfunction—poor sequencing, perseveration, trouble multitasking.

         3) Medial frontal: Apathetic, akinetic, incontinent, weak leg.

       b. Temporal lobe damage: Problems with memory, labile moods, pressured speech or expressive aphasia, hypergraphia, philosophical or religious preoccupations, new artistic interests, paranoia, altered sexuality.

L. Psychosis: Hallucinations and delusions.

    1. Causes: Type helps diagnosis.

       a. Visual: Drugs; temporal lobe lesions; degenerative dz, e.g., Alzheimer's; sensory deprivation, e.g., blindness.

       b. Auditory: Schizophrenia, bipolar depression.

       c. Somatic delusions: E.g., of body rotting. Psychotic depression.

       d. Olfactory, gustatory, or tactile: Temporal lobe epilepsy.

    2. DDx: Fluent aphasia, delirium tremens, SLE, Huntington's, Wernicke-Korsakoff's syndrome, endocrine dysfunction.

    3. Rx: Neuroleptics, esp. atypical.

    4. Schizophrenia: Neuroleptics help hallucinations and delusions more than the apathy and cognitive deterioration.

    5. Schizoaffective disorder: Psychosis persists between mood episodes. Do not confuse with schizoid or schizotypal personality disorder (see above).

M. Substance abuse: For pain control in, see p. 87.

"PSYCHOSOMATIC NEUROLOGY"

A. Definition of psychosomatic: Here used broadly to include:

    1. Somatic manifestations of mood disorders.

    2. Somatoform disorders: Somatization, conversion dis., chronic pain dis., hypochondriasis, body dysmorphic dis., factitious dis.

    3. Compliance problems that cause or perpetuate physical sx.

B. Psychosomatic sx are real: We just understand their physiology less. E.g., fMRI shows R parietal activation, opposite of neglect syndromes. Bereavement activates brain regions that regulate physical pain. Stress causes itching in part because endorphins are as pruritic as morphine.

C. Psychosomatic sx are treatable: E.g., conversion paralysis on average causes more disability than an "organic" one but has a better prognosis.

D. H&P: Ask tactfully about recent or childhood severe illness or trauma; stress, litigation. While female sex is a risk factor, somatization is greatly underdiagnosed in men.

    1. MADISON scale for emotional overlay. (There is often an "organic" underlay.)

        M = **M**ultiple unrelated sx

        A = **A**uthenticity of sx emphasized

        D = **D**enial of any association with stress

        I = **I**nterpersonal interactions visibly worsen symptoms

        S = **S**ingularity—sx are 'worst imaginable'

        O = **'O**nly you'—doctor as savior

        N = **'N**othing makes it better,' yet things make it worse

    2. Maybe it's you: An MD's breezy or dismissive reassurance may make a pt. exaggerate real sx in order to be heard, making the MD more dismissive.

Your Perception of Patient	Alternate Possibility
Too many complaints	Pt. is very ill
Reads too much med lit	Pt. reads more than you
Personality disorder	You don't like them
Nonanatomic deficit	Results confuse you
Noncompliant	Treatment is worse than the dz

Table 27. MD characteristics influence who gets called psychosomatic.

    3. Physical signs of conversion disorder: In general, conversion sx are more common on the nondominant side. Some pts may overgeneralize or misreport a complicated real deficit, e.g., a crossed face and body numbness, as in brainstem syndromes or MS. None of the following tests are perfectly sensitive or specific.

        a. Psychosomatic paralysis:

            1) "Give-way" weakness: May see jerky relaxation in weak limb when test both limbs together. But this is also seen with poor proprioception, e.g., MS.

            2) Hoover's sign: Have pt lie down; hold your hand under the good heel while pt. raises the weak leg against resistance. In psychosomatic weakness, pts. do not push down into your hand with the good leg. In somatic weakness, they do.

b. **Psychosomatic numbness:** Numbness may stop at hairline. Pt. may feel vibration more strongly on one side of forehead than the other, or have normal manipulation in numb hand.
c. **Psychosomatic blindness:** Pt. may blink to threat or have normal nystagmus to a moving optokinetic strip (successive black and white squares).
d. **Psychosomatic vertigo:** Very often a med SE, or panic disorder. Ask about palpitations, paresthesias; see if you can reproduce the sensation with hyperventilation or treat it with rebreathing.
e. **Psychosomatic gait** (AKA astasia-abasia): See Table 17.
f. **Nonepileptic spells:** No abnormal EEG during the spell. 30%-50% of pts. with pseudoseizures also have real seizures.

	Epileptic Seizure	Nonepileptic Spell
Clonic limb mvt.	In phase bilaterally	Out of phase
Vocalization type	"Epileptic cry"	Moans, screams
Vocalization timing	Mid-seizure	Start of seizure
Head turning	Unilateral	Violent side-to-side
Eyes	Open	Closed
Postictal	Disoriented, HA	Weeping, anxious
EEG *during* spell	Epileptiform EEG	Muscle artifact only

Table 28. Differentiating epileptic and pseudoseizures.

4. **Somatic signs of mood disorder:**
   a. **Not strictly somatoform:** These resolve when the mood sx do. But in some pts. (e.g., Parkinson's and the elderly) and cultures, depression more often presents with somatic sx than mood sx.
   b. **Common organs:** Heart, gut, and skin are the organs most directly influenced by limbic tone.
   c. **Thorough ROS is crucial:** The more positives, the firmer the dx. Ask about dizziness; blurry or spots in vision; memory loss; fatigue; change in sleep, weight, bowel; N/V; belly pain; migraines; back pain; palpitations; dyspnea; tremor; weakness; numbness (especially bilateral lips and hands).
   d. **Pseudodementia of depression/anxiety:** Typically, pts are disturbed by their cognitive sx much more than family/coworkers. Attention is the primary impairment. Recall cues help (vs. Alzheimer's); naming is intact. Pseudodementia in the elderly is a risk factor for true dementia, but best not to emphasize that fact to depressed pts.
   e. **R/o bipolar II:** Pts. with bipolar depression are more likely than unipolar depressives to have migraine, back pain, and other somatic sx. Probe for hypomanic episodes ("Was there ever a time when, despite your health, you managed to start many new projects or go without sleep?"). Consult a psychiatrist; avoid SSRIs; favor mood-stabilizing pain meds, e.g., gabapentin, lamotrigine.

E. Dx:

1. **DDx:** SLE, MS, dystonia, and thyroid dz often cause sx that appear "nonneurological." Rarer examples include porphyria, carcinoid.
2. **Avoid dismissive reassurance:** Rather than telling the pt., "It's just anxiety," consider how severe that anxiety must be to cause such sx.
3. **Explain psych sx medically:** E.g., "You have excess adrenaline release that causes your palpitations and lightheadedness. Clonazepam can decrease this."

F. Rx:

1. **Treat potential psych issues early:** Addressing them while medical workup continues feels less dismissive to patients.
2. **Do not turf:** Many pts. who will not see a psychiatrist will accept an antidepressant if it is also prescribed for a neurological indication.
3. **Use medications with dual indications:** Pts resist psych meds less when they also have somatic indications. See also Table 25, which lists choice of antidepressants by comorbid condition (p. 100). The belief that we should treat only conditions with known etiology contributes to the relatively low success rate of neurological rx compared with other specialties ("Diagnose, adios").

Comorbid Conditions		Treatment Suggestions
Pain	Depression	Cymbalta, perhaps TCA
	Somatization	Cymbalta
	Mood lability, mania	ACDs, e.g., Depakote
Fatigue	Medication SEs	Provigil
	Anxiety	SNRIs (Effexor, Cymbalta)
	Apathy	Dexedrine, Wellbutrin
	Depression + sleepiness	Wellbutrin, Effexor
	Depression + insomnia	Remeron, Paxil
Tremor	Mood disorder	See p. 79

Table 29. Treating comorbid psychiatric and somatic sx. See also Table 26.

4. **Referral to psychotherapy:** Present this as a way to help the pt manage the stress of their illness, not as treatment for their psychosomatic sx.
5. **Compliance:** Selecting the right rx is only 1/3 of the battle; the other 2/3 is helping the pt to adhere to it.
   a. **Time course noncompliance:** Can be a clue to its cause. Often these are mixed, however.
      1) **Rx stopped within days for a soft SE:** If cause is a soft SE (dizzy, "felt like a zombie," etc.), pt. may be anxious and hypervigilant.
      2) **Rx stopped within weeks to months for no benefit:** Suggests nocebo effect.
      3) **Rx taken erratically:** Attentional/cognitive problems, or barely tolerable SEs.

    b. DDx of noncompliance:
      1) Poor access to medications.
      2) Confusion: Dementia, delirium, or poor understanding of rx.
      3) Self-medication of psychiatric and other problems.
        a) Depression/anxiety/stress → attempt at chemical coping.
        b) Personality disorder → impulsive, emotionally driven drug taking. See p. 101.
      4) Pseudo-addiction: I.e., inadequate symptom relief.
      5) Addiction.
      6) Criminal intent: Not common.
    c. Rx of compliance problems:
      1) Treat the true chief complaint.
      2) Fight nocebo effect: Previous med failures make pt. expectations negative, blocking even powerful drug effects.
        a) Use distinctly new Rx modality, e.g., a transdermal rather than oral analgesic; may block nocebo effect.
        b) Nocebo wears off just as placebo does, so urge pt. to continue.
      3) Warn pt of discontinuation syndromes: Pts. who stop meds suddenly are at risk for rebound sx, esp. from ACDs, SSRIs, SNRIs, benzodiazepines.
      4) Encourage pt's sense of control: Do not fight pts. who self-experiment; rather, guide them to help you fine tune their regimen. However, self-experimentation and prns work poorly for demented and psychotic pts.

RADIATION THERAPY

A. Gray = 100 rads (1 centigray = 1 rad)
B. Indications: Tumor; sometimes inoperable AVMs.
C. Doses: Risk of radiation necrosis varies with total dose.
    1. Primary tumors: 60 Gy to "involved field" over 6-8 wk (5×/wk).
    2. Metastases: 30 Gy to whole brain over 2 wk.
D. SEs:
    1. Acute: N/V, worsened deficits. Seizures rare; usually from edema. Increase steroids.
    2. Subacute (weeks to months): Lethargy from brain XRT, Lhermitte's sign from spine radiation therapy.
    3. Late (months to years):
      a. Sx: Dementia, focal deficits, endocrine changes.
      b. Causes: Radiation necrosis, leukoencephalopathy, pituitary insufficiency, new tumors (gliomas, GBM, meningiomas, nerve sheath tumors), radiation myelopathy (usually from cervical > thoracic radiation therapy).
      c. Tests: PET, SPECT, or MRS to tell recurrent tumor from radiation necrosis. May need biopsy.
      d. Rx: Both recurrence and necrosis respond to surgery; only recurrence responds to more XRT and chemotherapy.
E. Stereotactic radiosurgery: Uses convergent beams to deliver a high radiation dose to a small volume, sparing surrounding brain.

	Compliance Problem	Treatment Strategies
Pt.'s relation to sx	**Poor reporters of symptoms**	
	Stoics	Present illness as a challenge, not a weakness
	Dementia, psychosis, apathetic depression	Ask caretaker; follow PE/labs
	Language barrier (*all* pts have this, unless they are MDs)	Use a translator, define your jargon, explain sx they should look for
	Overreporters of symptoms	
	Anxiety, PTSD, or recent severe illness	Treat anxiety with meds or CBT, schedule routine short follow-ups
	Lonely or seek sympathy	Do not tie your attention to the number of their complaints
	Skilled observers (e.g., chronically ill, MD, or nurse pts)	Stress need for big picture; tell them which sx they can ignore
Pt.'s relation to rx	**Med-fearing patients**	
	Fear side effects; nocebo effect from previous rx failures	Slow drug loads; novel rx modality—"This one may be better"
	Fear dependence on meds or MD	Stress pt.'s ability to stop rx; query subst. abuse hx
	Med-seeking patients	
	Borderline or histrionic personalities, substance abuse	Meds with low abuse potential (e.g., long acting)
Pt.'s relation to authority	**Erratic or self-treating patients**	
	MDs, PhDs, schizotypal personality, alternative med pts	Guide rather than try to veto self-experimentation.
	Dementia, psychosis	Simple regimens, have others dispense, consider depot meds
	Pts. from other cultures	Ask the pt., assimilated family, or translator about pt.'s goals and fears
	Over-docile patients	
	Dependent, passive, or fearful of authority	Encourage their (or family members') report of sx
	Manipulative, ingratiating, or borderline pts.	Prepare for sudden changes in their behavior; do not overpraise

Table 30. Strategies for specific compliance problems.

1. **Indications:** Best for lesions 3 cm or less such as AVMs, vestibular schwannomas, pituitary adenomas, craniopharyngiomas, pineal tumors, metastases, small primary tumors. Cavernous malformations are controversial.
2. **Methods:** Gamma knife (gamma rays), LINAC (requires a linear accelerator to produce x-rays), or proton beam (requires a cyclotron to produce a beam of charged particles).
3. **Post-op care:** ACDs, analgesics, antiemetics. Complications are similar to regular XRT but with more frequent radiation necrosis.

SEIZURES

A. **Status epilepticus:** A seizure that lasts for more than 30 minutes, or seizures that recur for more than 30 minutes without regaining consciousness in between. <u>This is an emergency.</u>
  1. **Initial assessment:** ABCs (airway, breathing, cardiac), O_2 sats, coma exam (see Coma and Brain Death, p. 29), EKG, IV access, and draw labs. Coma exam can almost always be done before intubation and sedation.
  2. **Initial rx:**
      a. **Thiamine, glucose:** 100 mg IV, 50% dextrose 50 cc, naloxone.
      b. **Lorazepam** (Ativan): 2 mg IV q2min × 5, or diazepam (Valium) 5 mg IV q3min × 4 while starting DPH load.
          1) **Pediatric dosing:** Diazepam 0.2 mg/kg IV at 1 mg/min, to max. of 10 mg. Or lorazepam 0.1 mg/kg IV under age 12, 0.07 mg/kg over age 12.
      c. **IV ACD:** Avoid IV phenytoin if possible. Options:
          1) **Fosphenytoin:** See p. 162. Load 1000 mg PE (PE = phenytoin equivalent doses) IV/IM, at <150 mg/min. Cardiac monitor; check BP q min. Pediatric dose = 20 mg/kg IV at 0.5 mg/kg/min.
          2) **Valproate:** Load 1 g over 15-20 min (20 mg/kg). No immediate SEs to follow; check ammonia/LFTs in follow-up. Therapeutic level = 50-100.
  3. **Full assessment:** H&P (see below), intubate if necessary, check labs, stat head CT. Consider lumbar puncture + Abx if pt. is febrile or has never seized before. Consider emergent EEG if pt. is comatose to rule out nonconvulsive status.
  4. **Second-line rx:** Usually require intubation and arterial line (see p. 222) for BP monitoring.
      a. **Phenobarbital** (Luminal): 20 mg/kg IV (100 mg/min) if still seizing after 40 min despite DPH and lorazepam.
      b. **Pentobarbital** (Nembutal): 5 mg/kg IV load if still seizing after phenobarbital. Titrate dose (0.3-9 mg/kg/h) to obtain 3- to 15-sec periods of burst suppression on EEG.
      c. **Midazolam** (Versed): 0.2 mg/kg IV loading dose as alternative to phenobarbital or pentobarbital. Titrate dose (0.1-0.4 mg/kg/h) to get burst on EEG.
      d. **Supportive care:** Pressors if necessary. Cool pt. if febrile. Stop ACD drip once a day to see underlying EEG rhythm.
  5. **Special cases:**
      a. **Partial status epilepticus:** May be confused with tremor.

      b. Nonconvulsive status epilepticus: Usually there is some focal motor activity such as rhythmic blinking; rarely is there merely altered mental status. Nearly all pts. in nonconvulsive status are known epileptics. A test of 1-4 mg lorazepam IV/SL/PO should cause improvement (but may also improve catatonia).

      c. Pyridoxine (B_6) deficiency: Consider giving pyridoxine 1 g IV or more if pt. is on isoniazid.

B. Seizure H&P: Aura, behavior during seizure, postictal period, h/o previous seizures or status epilepticus, drugs tried, nocturnal tongue biting or incontinence, febrile seizures as child, head injury, recent alcohol or other drugs, illness, sleep deprivation, relation to menstruation.

C. DDx of seizures: Syncope, myoclonus, tremor, pontine rigors, pseudoseizure, narcolepsy.

  1. Nonepileptic seizures: See Table 27, p. 104.

D. Management of first seizure:

  1. Causes of new-onset seizures: Cerebral ischemia, bleed, trauma, mass, hydrocephalus, infection, toxin, metabolic, withdrawal (alcohol, benzodiazepine), overdose (cocaine, TCA, isoniazid), amyloid angiopathy, anoxia (usually does not respond to ACDs), idiopathic.

  2. Tests: Consider head CT or MRI, LP, electrolytes (vigorous seizure alone can cause acidosis and hyperkalemia), Ca/Mg/Phos, CBC (vigorous seizure alone can cause WBC), screen urine and blood for toxins, EEG (best with sleep deprivation, photic stimulation, and hyperventilation), CXR to rule out lung primary tumor. Prolactin level elevation is unreliable evidence of a seizure.

  3. Uncomplicated first seizure: Do LP if any suspicion of SAH or infection. If pt. is young, healthy, with normal exam and head CT, no need to admit. Get an outpt EEG and MRI + gadolinium, with thin cuts through hippocampus. Hold ACD unless seizure was prolonged. If workup negative, chance of recurrence is about 30%.

  4. Hospital admission: Consider admitting pts with nonresolving change in their neuro exam, elderly pts with first seizure (for more rapid tumor workup), and alcoholics with active withdrawal.

  5. Acute seizure rx:

      a. Benzodiazepines: For alcohol withdrawal seizures or if pt seizes repeatedly. Lorazepam 2-4 mg IV/IM or diazepam 5-10 mg IV. Use only lorazepam in liver failure. Lorazepam has a slower onset but lasts longer (1 h vs. 20 min) because it is less fat soluble. This is the opposite time course of its sedative effects.

      b. DPH: Not for alcohol withdrawal seizures. Do not need to load it IV if pt not seizing.

         1) Oral: 300 mg PO q3h × 3; then 300 mg qhs. Warn pt. of SEs: double vision, vertigo, fatigue.

         2) 1g DPH over 45 min on cardiac monitor; if pt. is in status epilepticus, give it in 20 min. Painful.

      c. Transition to chronic drugs: Consider immediately starting a switch to another agent if you think it would be a better long-term choice.

E. Seizure classification by clinical type:

  1. Generalized:

      a. Tonic-clonic ("grand mal"): LOC with bilateral jerking, often preceded by aura. Often tongue biting or incontinence, postictal con-

fusion. A focal onset or Todd's (transient focal postictal) paralysis suggests the seizure is secondarily generalized from a partial seizure.
  b. **Atonic** ("drop attacks").
  c. **Absence** ("petit mal"): Usually in children; see p. 150.
  d. **Myoclonic epilepsy:** Usually in children; see p. 149.
2. **Partial** (focal, local): May become secondarily generalized.
  a. **Simple** (no impairment of consciousness): May be motor, sensory, or ANS, depending on site of focus.
  b. **Complex** (impairment of consciousness): Often preceded by psychosensory aura. Seizure has confusion ± automatisms. Often from mesial temporal or frontal lesion.
F. **Management of chronic seizures:**
  1. **Causes of chronic seizure disorder (epilepsy):**
    a. **Underlying defect:** Structural damage, genetic, metabolic.
    b. **Precipitants of seizure:** Fever; low ACDs, Ca, Na, or blood sugar; sleep deprivation; or the acute causes listed above.
  2. **Typical seizure, known epilepsy:** Pts. can leave emergency room as soon as they are back to baseline. They do not need a head CT unless they have head injury and nonresolving change in their neuro exam.
  3. **Rx of seizure disorder:**

Indication	Try	AVOID
Seizure Type		
Partial or secondary generalized	Levetiracetam, carbamazepine > valproate	
Primary generalized	Valproate, carbamazepine	Ethosuximide
Absence	Ethosuximide, valproate	DPH
Myoclonic	Valproic acid, clonazepam	DPH, carbamazepine
Centrotemporal	DPH, phenobarbital	
Other Factors		
Young woman	Lamotrigine, carbamazepine	DPH
Depression	Lamotrigine	
HIV	Valproate, lamotrigine	DPH, phenobarbital
Labile, impulsive	Valproate, carbamazepine	
Liver disease	Levetiracetam, lamotrigine	
Overweight	Topiramate, oxcarbazepine	DPH, phenobarbital
Pain	Valproate, carbamazepine, gabapentin	DPH, phenobarbital

Table 31. Choice of anticonvulsant by type and comorbid condition.

  a. **ACD choice:** Lower doses of two agents are sometimes more tolerated than high doses of one agent. For dosing, side effects, and mechanisms, see Anticonvulsants, p. 161.

   b. **Avoid precipitants:** Alcohol, sleep deprivation. Oral contraceptives may help perimenstrual seizures.
   c. **Avoid driving:** Laws vary; it is typically illegal for pt to drive for 6 mo after a seizure.
   d. **In pregnancy:** See p. 97.
   e. **Discontinuing ACDs:** Typically considered if pt has not had a seizure in 2 years. May want to check EEG; chance of recurrence is higher if EEG is abnormal. See also p. 161, for taper regimens.
   f. **Epilepsy surgery:** To treat poorly controlled, disabling seizures after more than a year of failed aggressive medical management.
G. **Seizure prophylaxis:** Pts. should sometimes be on ACDs even if they have never seized, e.g., in:
   1. **Brain tumor:** See p. 120. Usually not necessary, unless there is danger of herniation or it is a melanoma.
   2. **Post head injury:** See Trauma, p. 119.
   3. **Intracranial hemorrhage:** Q.v. p. 61. All pts. with spontaneous subarachnoid hemorrhage should get an ACD; subdural and parenchymal bleeds are controversial; probably do not need prophylaxis.
   4. **Routine craniotomy:** Consider 2 wk of ACD.
H. **Proconvulsant drugs:** The following may lower seizure thresholds in some pts.: some Abx (amphotericin B, β-lactams, fluconazole, isoniazid, metronidazole, praziquantel, zidovudine), anticholinergics, antihistamines, glucocorticoids, lithium, naloxone, narcotics (especially meperidine), neuroleptics, oxytocin, all stimulants, TCAs, x-ray contrast agents.

SENSORY LOSS

A. **H&P:** Pts. use "numbness" to mean everything from tingling to paralysis. Ask about pain, paresthesias, hyperpathia. Look for dermatomal or individual nerve distributions, distal vs. proximal differences, spinal cord level, spared modalities, graphesthesia, stereognosis, neglect to bilateral simultaneous stimulation. Associated signs: weakness, skin changes, cranial nerve abnormalities. For hysterical numbness, see p. 104.
B. **DDx:**
   1. **Mononeuropathies and monoradiculopathies:** Usually trauma or compression; sometimes vasculopathy (e.g., in DM), zoster, leprosy.
   2. **Symmetric distal sensory loss** ("stocking glove"): Usually polyneuropathy from chronic illness or toxin.
   3. **Hemianesthesia:** Damage to sensory cortex, thalamus, white matter.
   4. **Dissociated or crossed sensory deficits:** Often from brainstem or spinal cord lesions; generally with other neurological deficits.
      a. **Brainstem syndromes:** See brainstem stroke syndromes, p. 28.
      b. **Posterior column:** Ipsilateral decreased position, vibration, stereognosis (but often bilateral involvement).
      c. **Hemisection** (Brown-Sequard syndrome): Ipsilateral decreased position and vibration; contralateral decreased pain and temperature. Little change in fine touch. Upper motor neuron signs beneath level of lesion.
      d. **Central cord syndrome:** Usually from syringomyelia: cavity near the central canal. Often begins cervically, with cape-like loss of

pain and temperature sensation; then gradual spasticity and loss of light touch, sometimes facial or tongue weakness.

  e. Suspended sensory loss: Isolated numb band on thorax. Specific for spinal cord lesions.

5. **Paresthesias:** Peripheral neuropathy or compression; peripheral vascular dz; spinal cord dz; metabolic disturbance, e.g., hypocalcemia or respiratory alkalosis; postherpetic neuralgia. . . .

SLEEP DISORDERS AND FATIGUE

A. See also: Table 28, p. 105.

B. H&P: Distinguish sleepiness that stems from insomnia or sleep deprivation from fatigue from meds or illness. Ask about sleep latency, daytime sleeping, medications, snoring, scratchy throat in AM, cataplexy, sleep paralysis, trouble with initiating vs. maintaining sleep, movements in bed.

C. Insomnia:

1. **DDx:** Pain, anxiety, depression, bad sleep hygiene, alcohol or tranquilizer dependence, medications (steroids, β-blockers, etc.), nocturnal movement disorders, occasionally sleep apnea or midbrain damage.

2. **Acute rx:** In the elderly, use the lowest, shortest acting dose.

   a. Nonbenzodiazepine GABA receptor drugs: E.g., zolpidem 5-10 mg. Little addiction, short half-life.

   b. Benzodiazepines: Good for comorbid anxiety, but rapid tolerance. Avoid these, esp. in elderly pts.

   c. Melatonin agonists: Melatonin itself soon habituates. Ramelteon 8 mg is nonaddictive; effects last ~8 h.

   d. Sedating antidepressants: Trazodone: 25-50 mg PO qhs; doxepin: 25-50 mg PO qhs.

   e. Sedating antihistamines: E.g., diphenhydramine 25-50 mg. Rapid habituation.

3. **Chronic rx:** Stop caffeine, alcohol, offending meds; retire and rise at same time every day; no reading in bed. Consider zolpidem or ramelteon, but cognitive-behavioral therapy may work better than medications.

D. Shift work syndrome and sleep deprivation:

1. **H&P:** Flight attendant? Hospital resident? etc.

2. **R/o mood disorder:** Depression and mania can be both cause and effect of odd sleep cycles.

3. **Rx:**

   a. Maintain constant wake time: Sleep time is less important. This means waking early on weekends to avoid Monday "jet lag."

   b. Light box therapy: 10,000 lux for ≥30 min, as early in AM as possible. Small boxes are fine (e.g., SunLight Jr., sunbox.com); they fit better beside the computer or box of Cheerios (generalmills.com), and user need not stare at light.

   c. Drugs:

   1) **Avoid:** Alcohol, stimulants. Caffeine, dexedrine, methylphenidate can cause rebound hypersomnolence that leaves pt. more tired.

   2) **Consider:** Modafinil. More helpful at noon than in AM. Not a substitute for sleep. Do not self-prescribe.

E. Excessive sleepiness:
  1. **DDx:** Sleep deprivation, depression, drugs, metabolic disorder.
  2. **Tests:** Overnight sleep-EEG study.
  3. **Sleep apnea:** Cessation of breathing during sleep.
     a. **Obstructive apnea:** If severe, can cause pulmonary hypertension, arrhythmia. Treat with d/c of sedatives, weight loss, AM/noon modafinil 100-200 mg, nightly CPAP.
     b. **Central apnea:** From brainstem lesions, dysautonomias, neuromuscular dz. May require tracheostomy.
  4. **Narcolepsy:** Lifelong disorder of REM sleep architecture.
     a. **Sx:** Frequent daytime sleep attacks, episodes of cataplexy (hypotonia), and more nonspecific signs of sleep deprivation, e.g., sleep paralysis, hypnagogic hallucinations.
     b. **Rx:** For sleepiness, modafinil 200 mg q AM/noon has less habituation than methylphenidate 5 mg q AM and noon. For cataplexy: TCAs, e.g., imipramine 25 mg tid.

F. Nocturnal movement disorders:
  1. **DDx:** Hypnagogic jerks (benign, single), nocturnal seizures (often at REM transitions), akathisia....
  2. **Restless leg syndrome (RLS):** While resting but still awake, pt feels an urge to move legs to remove "creepy feeling" (not really pain). Rx: DA agonists, e.g., ropinirole (raise slowly to ~2 mg qhs).
  3. **Nocturnal myoclonus:** While sleeping, pt has rhythmic leg jerking that may awaken him. May occur in combination with restless leg syndrome. Try clonazepam.
  4. **Periodic limb movements of sleep (PLMS):** Rhythmic leg jerk, may awaken pt. Often with RLS. Try clonazepam, ropinirole.

G. Parasomnias:
  1. **REM behavior disorder:** Loss of normal REM atonia; pt acts out his dreams. Associated with alcohol. Treat with safety precautions, clonazepam 0.5-2 mg.
  2. **Sleep walking:** Occurs during non-REM sleep. Try clonazepam.

SPINAL CORD DISORDERS

A. Acute cord compression is an emergency: Consider this in any pt with rapidly progressive spinal cord sx, especially of bladder or bowel.
  1. **Exams:** Rectal sensory and motor exam, emergent spinal MRI. Do whole spine if cancer suspected.
  2. **Rx:** Consider dexamethasone 100 mg IV push or the methylprednisolone protocol available in most ERs, stat neurosurgery consult, or XRT. Goal is to prevent progression, although deficit can sometimes reverse if it is of recent onset.
  3. **Blood pressure:** Very labile with cord lesions, especially during pain. Overtreating BP (e.g., with nifedipine) can cause hypotension.
  4. **Cervical cord contusion:** High-dose steroids, hard collar unless cervical instability already ruled out with C-spine x-ray (but do not flex/extend if there is a known cord contusion).

B. Pts with back pain and known cancer: Assume cord compression until proven otherwise. See p. 117 for workup.

C. Terminology:
1. **Bone problems:** Spondylosis = degeneration. "Cervical spondylosis" sometimes used as synonym for "stenosis." Spondylolisthesis = anterior subluxation. Spondylolysis = isthmic spondylolisthesis.
2. **Cord problems:** Myelopathy and myelitis are spinal cord damage and inflammation, respectively. Cf. myopathy and myositis, which are muscle conditions.

D. History: Radiation of pain, triggers, numbness, weakness, incontinence, weight loss, IVDA, DM, previous surgery, trauma, litigation, degree of disability, assoc. depression. With neck pain, ask about chest pain, shortness of breath, radiation to jaw.
1. **Location:** Thoracic level suggests metastases.
2. **Character:** Burning, electric, aching.
3. **Precipitants:** Walking, sitting, squatting, leaning forward, coughing, time of day.
4. **Bladder changes:** Frequency, urgency, sensation during voiding, sexual function.
   a. **UMN lesion:** Bladder stretch reflex is disinhibited and spastic, so small bladder and frequent voids.
   b. **LMN lesion:** Retention, sometimes with retention overflow.

E. Exam: Document exam carefully, especially if pt. going to OR, to record presurgical deficit.
1. **Reflexes:** Spread, finger flexors, Hoffman's, crossed adductors, clonus, Babinski, abdominals.

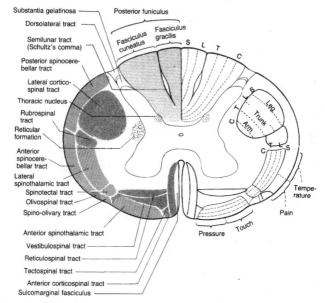

Figure 12. The spinal cord in cross-section. (Reprinted with permission from Duus P. *Topical Diagnosis in Neurology.* New York: Thieme; 1983: 49.)

2. **Straight leg raise (SLR):** For L5, S1 irritation. Pain during reverse SLR (extension) suggests L3 or L4 irritation. Pain on palpation, range of motion, posture (anthropoid in stenosis), abdominal reflexes, clonus, pulses, atrophy, fasciculations, café-au-lait spots, Lhermitte's sign.

3. **FABER** (Flex-ABduct-Extend-Rotate): Put ankle on opposite knee; rotate knee towards exam table. Positive for hip dz and mechanical low back pain, but not for disc dz.

4. **Hysterical back pain:** If pain on simulated axial loading (push top of head), or if cannot tolerate straight leg raise, but can sit/put socks on.

5. **Bowel/bladder:** Prostate, bulbocavernosus (finger in rectum, pull on penis or bladder catheter), cremaster, anal wink, percuss bladder, measure postvoid residual (if residual >100 cc, leave catheter in). Any abnormality may be indication for emergent MRI.

6. **Sensory lesions:** Look for sensory level, dissociation of sensory modalities. Pinprick is lost first (vs. peripheral nerve injury, where light touch is lost first). See Sensory Loss, p. 111.

F. **DDx:**

1. **Conus medullaris vs. cauda equina compression:** The former is a cord lesion, the latter peripheral nerve. However, prognosis is similar, and sx often overlap.

	Conus Medullaris	**Cauda Equina**
Onset	Sudden, bilateral	Gradual, unilateral
Pain	Mild, bilateral	Severe, radicular
Bladder/bowel	Severe, early	Late
Sensory loss	Symmetric, saddle distribution.	Asymmetric
Touch vs. pain	Touch/pain dissociation	No dissociation
Motor loss	Mild, symmetric	Marked asymmetric atrophy
Fasciculations	Common	Rare
Reflexes	Lose ankle but not knee jerk	May lose knee jerk too

Table 32. Distinguishing conus and cauda syndromes.

2. **Cortical vs. spinal or peripheral lesion:** Former has slow mvts., latter has fast but weak mvts.

3. **Disc herniation vs. spinal stenosis:**
   a. **Provocation:** Both worse with coughing, Valsalva. Stenosis worse with walking, better with leaning forward (→ anthropoid posture).
   b. **Reflexes:** Stenosis causes brisk reflexes, toes can be up. Disc herniation causes dropped reflexes.

4. **Central cord syndrome:** Arms weaker than legs, pain and temperature sensation worse than dorsal column modalities—vibration and proprioception. LMN signs in some segments. Later, UMN signs below the lesion. Anterior spinal artery infarct can do this. (Relative preservation of dorsal column modalities of vibration and proprioception.)

5. **Cervical cord contusion:** Usually after hyperextension with underlying stenosis or instability.

6. **Paraparesis:** Consider spinal stenosis or mass, falx meningioma, spinal ischemia, thyrotoxic paralysis. Check orthostatic BPs.
7. **Onc:** Pain worse lying/at night. Weakness usually legs first; not clear why there is usually sacral sparing. Position/vibration sense very sensitive for compression. Occasionally ataxia. Consider leptomeningeal metastases, q.v. p. 124; lumbosacral plexopathy in pelvic cancer. Most spine tumors compress rather than invade.
   a. **Leptomeningeal tumors:** See Tumors of Brain p. 120.
   b. **Extradural** (55%):
      1) **Metastases:** Common. Consider lung, breast, prostate, lymphoma, kidney.
      2) **Primary:** Rare. Chordomas, neurofibromas, osteoid osteomas, osteoblastomas, aneurysmal bone cysts, vertebral hemangiomas.
   c. **Intradural extramedullary** (40%): Schwannomas, meningiomas, neurofibromas, lipomas.
   d. **Intramedullary** (5%): Astrocytomas (30%), ependymomas (30%), miscellaneous.
8. **Ortho:** Compression fracture, ankylosing spondylitis (get plain films of sacral joint; HLA B-27 Ag), Paget's dz.
9. **Other:** Epidural abscess, osteomyelitis, vasculitis, transverse myelitis, spondylitis, aortic dissection, cord embolus, bleed, Guillain-Barré, CIPD, schistosomiasis....

G. **Tests:**
   1. **Spine MR:** Useless if metal in back (e.g., previous surgery), but hip replacements are usually okay. Consider pain premedication. 24% of <u>asymptomatic</u> pts have bulging disc; 4% have stenosis.
      a. **Screening sagittal view of whole spine:** If you suspect metastasis (30% have second met).
      b. **Contrast:** If you suspect leptomeningeal dz or myelitis or if there was previous surgery and you need to tell scar from disc.
   2. **X-rays:** Get C-spine if recent neck trauma. Consider flexion-extension C-spine films, especially if transient quadriparesis after a neck injury or if there is A-P pain. Lumbosacral x-rays are usually useless except if spine may be unstable; then get flexion-extension films.
   3. **CT myelogram:** If MRI contraindicated, previous back surgery, suspected dural AV fistula, CSF leak or obstruction.
   4. **LP:** Can show high prot. below cord comp, because of pooling.
   5. **Bone scan:** Not useful except as screen for infection or metastases all over. Rarely positive if plain films and ESR nl. Does not show myeloma.
   6. **Blood:** Consider ESR, UBJ, SIEP, PSA, CA125, CEA.
   7. **CSF:** Avoid LPs, as risk of deterioration in...
   8. **EMG:** If need to distinguish radiculopathy (nl nerve conduction velocity, but F-wave abnormal) from peripheral neurop. Denervation changes after disc occur 1-2 wk in paraspinous muscles; 2-5 wk in leg. Polyphasic renervation potentials start ~10 wk.

H. **Rx of noncancer spinal pain:** NSAIDS, gabapentin, duloxetine, nortriptyline, soft collar or back brace, physical therapy; consider surgery if myelopathy. Bed rest rarely helps.

1. **Disc herniation:**
   a. **Home neck traction:** Kit available in surgical supply stores. 10-20 min qd, facing door, 6-8 lb in sandbag. Head should be pulled 15 degrees forwards, not back. Pressure on both occiput and mandible. Should not hurt.
2. **Spinal stenosis:** NSAIDS, physical therapy, surgery. Pt may tolerate bicycling more than other forms of exercise.

I. **Rx of spine pain in a pt with cancer:** Assume spinal cord compression until proven otherwise.
   1. **Neurological deficit on exam:**
      a. **Dexamethasone:** 100 mg IV bolus.
      b. **Emergent MRI** or myelogram: Multiple lesions are common, so request longitudinal scout of entire spine. For MRI appearance of spinal cord tumors, see p. 189.
         1) **Tumor and >80% stenosis:** Give emergent XRT, consider surgery. Continue dexamethasone 96 mg qd; taper as tolerated.
         2) **Tumor and <80% stenosis:** Nonemergent XRT ± surgery.
         3) **No tumor:** Symptomatic rx.
   2. **No neuro deficit:** Get plain spine films.
      a. **If abnormal x-ray** with >50% collapse of a vertebral body or pedicle erosion, get emergent MRI and proceed as above.
      b. **If normal x-ray:** Get nonemergent MRI.
   3. **Acute cord compression rx in cancer:**
      a. **Dexamethasone:** 100 mg bolus, then 24 mg q6h. In breast cancer and lymphoma, steroids kill tumor, as well as decrease edema and pain.
      b. **Neurosurgery consult:** Emergent.
         1) **Indications:** Decompression, tissue diagnosis, displaced bone or ligament, unstable spine, or relapse at previously irradiated site. May reverse paraplegia.
         2) **Relative contraindications:** Very radiosensitive tumor (myeloma, lymphoma), total paralysis >24 h. Laminectomy no better than radiation. Anterior decompression and stabilization beneficial, but most pts are poor surgical candidates.
      c. **Radiation therapy** within 12 h: See below. After XRT, 80% of pts. who could walk before can still walk, <50% if paraparetic before, <10% if paraplegic before.
   4. **Nonemergent cord compression rx in cancer:**
      a. **Dexamethasone:** 10 mg q6h.
      b. **Radiation therapy:**
         1) **Dose limit:** 300 rad fractions × 10, i.e., 3000 rads. Higher dose causes transverse myelitis. Need to simulate and plan field carefully if window may overlap previous radiation therapy area.
         2) **Contraindications:**
            a) **Bone compression:** If bone, not tumor, is compressing cord, pt needs surgery, not radiation therapy.
            b) **Radio-resistant tumor:** E.g., thyroid cancer, renal cancer, sarcoma.
            c) **Previous XRT in same region:** Unless pts have only a few months to live, XRT twice in same field will cause paralysis.

c. **Chemotherapy:**
   1) **Prostate metastases:** Start flutamide several days before Lupron; latter has temporary agonist effect and can cause swelling with acute cord compression.
   2) **Lymphoma.**

SYNCOPE

A. H&P: Try to find a witness who can describe the event.
   1. **Precipitants:** Exertion, stress, meals, alcohol, drug, cough, swallowing, urination, postural change, head movements, poor POs.
   2. **Sequelae:** Tonic/clonic movements, drowsiness, confusion, neuro changes, nausea, sweating, cold, incontinence, tongue biting, injury from fall, amnesia.
   3. **Exam:** Orthostatic BP and HR (immediate and delayed), BP in both arms, bruits (carotid, subclavian, supraorbital, temporal), heart exam. Look for trauma from fall. Stool guaiac.
B. Causes:
   1. **Cardiac:**
      a. **Arrhythmic:** AV block, sick sinus syndrome, long QT interval, pacer malfunction.
      b. **Obstructive:** MI, global ischemia, valve stenosis or dysfunction, PE, pulmonary HTN, aortic dissection, tamponade, left atrial myxoma....
   2. **Vascular reflex:**
      a. **Vasovagal:** From fear, urination, Valsalva maneuver.
      b. **Orthostatic:**
         1) **Hyperadrenergic:** Volume depletion, varicose venous pooling, supine hypotension of late pregnancy (pressure on aorta).
         2) **ANS dysfunction:** Vasoactive or antidepressant drugs, neuropathies, spinal cord dz, paraneoplastic dz, parkinsonian syndromes.
      c. **Carotid sinus hypersensitivity:** A diagnosis of exclusion; can be elicited in 1/3 of normal old men.
         1) **Cardioinhibitory:** Common. Carotid sinus massage (see p. 206) causes sinus pause; blocked by atropine.
         2) **Vasodepressor:** Rare. Carotid sinus massage causes low SBP; blocked by epinephrine, not atropine.
   3. **Neurological:** Vertebrobasilar TIA (carotid TIAs almost never cause syncope), seizure, subclavian steal, NPH.
   4. **Metabolic:** Hypoxia, hypoglycemia, hyperventilation.
   5. **Psychiatric.**
C. Tests: Rule out risk of sudden death; reserve further testing for recurrent syncope only.
   1. **Cardiovascular:** EKG for MI, LV hypertrophy, arrhythmia. Consider echocardiogram, Holter monitor, ETT; perhaps signal averaged EKG, tilt test, cardiac electrophysiology study.
   2. **Blood:** CBC, electrolytes, toxin screen, CPK.
   3. **CXR:** If suspect PE ($\pm$ ABG, V/Q scan), CHF, pericardial effusion, mitral stenosis.

4. **Neuro tests** (low yield unless focal deficit or bruits): CTA or MRA, carotid and cranial ultrasound, EEG.
5. **Carotid sinus massage:** See Arrhythmia, p. 205. Cardiac pause of >3 sec or SBP drop >30 points with sx or >50 points without sx is abnormal. Abnormal response confirms cause only if it reproduces sx and other causes are excluded.

D. Orders: VS q shift with orthostatic BPs, guaiac all stools, cardiac monitor, IV fluids slowly, keep BP >140. For ANS insufficiency, see Hypotension, p. 211.

TRAUMA

A. Indications for head CT: Focal deficit, anticoagulation, significant LOC, drug intoxication. Usually do not need (but highly recommended) to get a CT in pts with very brief LOC and no focal neurological signs.

B. Exam: Note exact time of exam and amount and time of last sedation.
1. **General:** Vital signs and pattern of respiration. Palpate head for skull fractures, facial fractures. Look for lacerations, raccoon eyes, battle sign (bruise behind ear). Fundi (papilledema, hemorrhage, retinal detachment). Blood in nose/ears; CSF leak (q.v., p. 20). Listen for bruits over eyes, carotids. Look for evidence of spine trauma.
2. **Neuro:**
   a. **Quick:** Assess alertness; coma exam (see p. 30), cerebellar exam if cooperative.
3. **R/o spine injury:**
   a. **Rectal:** Including anal wink and bulbocavernosus.
   b. **Sensory:** Pinprick all four limbs and trunk; touch major dermatomes C4, C6-8, T4, T6, T10, L2, L4-S2. Vibration and proprioception for posterior columns.
   c. **Motor:** In more detail than just noting "moving all extremities."

C. Types of head injury: See p. 182 for CT appearance of head trauma.
1. **Concussion:** Any altered consciousness after minor head injury, including confusion, N/V, dizziness. LOC is not required.
   a. **Hx:** Cause of injury, h/o previous concussions.
   b. **PE:** Orientation, attention, memory, CN, coordination, sensation. Symptoms should not be present even after significant exertion, e.g., sprinting 40 meters.
   c. **Complications:**
      1) **Postconcussive syndrome:** Weeks to months of fatigue, HA, attention. Try nortriptyline, load to 75 mg qhs.
      2) **Cerebral edema:** Head reinjury before complete symptom resolution can cause life-threatening cerebral swelling. Concussion grade, determined by presence of LOC and length of other symptoms, predicts risk of returning to contact sports:

Concussion Grade	Symptom Length	Time Until Contact Sports Safe	
		1st Concussion?	>1 Concussion?
1	<15 min, no LOC	That day	1 wk
2	>15 min, no LOC	1 wk	2 wk
3	LOC <1 min	1 wk	>4 wk
3	LOC >1 min	2 wk	>4 wk

Table 33. Contact sport restrictions after concussion.

   2. **Contusion:** Gray matter injury after head trauma.
   3. **Diffuse axonal injury:** AKA shear injury. Seen especially after deceleration injury.
   4. **Contrecoup injury:** Seen when the brain is thrust against the skull opposite from the primary blow.
   5. **Skull fracture:** May not be visible on head CT for several days.
   6. **Intracranial hemorrhage:** Q.v., p. 61.
   7. **Dissection** of carotid or vertebral artery.
D. **Rx:** Consider neurosurgery consult.
   1. **Spinal cord trauma:**
      a. **Methylprednisolone:** Must be given within 8 h of injury. 30 mg/kg initial IV bolus over 15 min; then wait 45 min, then 5.4 mg/kg/h for 23 h.
      b. **Blood pressure and temperature control:** May be very labile.
      c. **Nasogastric tube:** For paralytic ileus.
      d. **Bladder catheter:** To avoid bladder distension.
   2. **Head trauma:**
      a. **Indications for seizure prophylaxis:** Intracranial blood, Glasgow Coma Scale <10, significant alcohol history. Give ACD × 1 wk. If pt. needs craniotomy, give × 3-6 mo (may discontinue at 3 mo if no h/o seizure).
      b. **Indications for mannitol:** Evidence of herniation (e.g., dilated pupils) or local mass effect (e.g., hemiparesis) or sudden deterioration. Hypotension is a relative contraindication.
      c. **Indications for intubation:** Glasgow Coma Scale (GCS) <7, inability to protect airway (e.g., from maxillofacial trauma or when heavy secretions), recurrent seizures, high ICP.
      d. **Admission orders for moderate head injury:** GCS 9-13.
         1) **Neuro checks:** q 1-2 h.
         2) **Activity:** HOB up 30-45 degrees.
         3) **Diet:** NPO until alert or no risk of surgery; then clear liquids. NS + 20 mEq KCl/L at 75 cc/h.
         4) **Meds:** Mild analgesics and antiemetics. Have naltrexone handy. Avoid phenothiazines, which lower seizure threshold.

TUMORS OF BRAIN

A. **See also:** Spinal Cord Disorders, p. 113.
B. **H&P:**
   1. **Generalized sx:** Papilledema, GI sx, fatigue, confusion.

2. **Focal sx:** Reflect tumor. N/V suggests post. fossa or location.
3. **HA:** Worse in AM, lying flat, or with Valsalva suggests high ICP.
4. **Seizures:** In about 1/3 of pts; more common if low-grade tumor or cortical location.

C. DDx of brain tumor: Abscess, bleed, infarct, demyelination, radiation necrosis....

D. Tests: MRI + contrast, or CT + contrast if pt unstable or question of hemorrhage. See imaging of tumor, p. 182. Brain biopsy vs. resection. Consider workup for unknown primary tumor (usually CXR, mammogram, chest/abdominal CT), LP to rule out leptomeningeal spread.

E. Rx of brain tumor: See also specific tumor types, below.

1. **Treat edema:** Consider one or more of the following:
   a. **Dexamethasone:** Bolus 10 mg IV, then 4 mg q6h. Taper after radiation therapy. If you suspect CNS lymphoma, try to withhold steroids until biopsy.
   b. **Fluid restrict:** 1200 cc qd, no free water.
   c. **Mannitol:** 50-100 g IV, then 25-50 g q6h to keep osmolality 305-310.

2. **Neurosurgery:**
   a. **Resection:** Unless inaccessible, multiple foci, or very radiosensitive. Consider surgery for all posterior fossa tumors >3 cm even if there are other metastases.
   b. **Biopsy:** In situations where full resection is inadvisable but a tissue diagnosis is necessary.
   c. **CSF access procedures:** See p. 85. E.g., EVD or VP shunt for hydrocephalus, Ommaya reservoir for intraventricular chemotherapy.

3. **Radiation therapy:** Consider 2-3 d of steroids before beginning XRT to decrease swelling, especially in posterior fossa lesions.

4. **Chemotherapy:** Regimens vary. See p. 166 for side effects.

5. **Seizure prophylaxis:** No need to provide prophylaxis to pts who have never seized, except if there is a risk of herniation. Metastases in the cerebellum or deep subcortical areas rarely cause seizures.

F. Prevalence:

1. **Metastases:** 30%-50% of all brain tumors. Presenting complaint is from a brain met in 15% of all cancer pts. 10% present with seizures.

2. **Primary intracranial tumors:** Astrocytomas (including GBM) 38%, meningiomas 18%, acoustic schwannomas 8%, oligodendrogliomas 4%, lymphomas 4%, craniopharyngiomas 1%.

G. Metastases to CNS:

1. **Most common source:** Usually carcinoma ≫ sarcoma or lymphoma.
   a. **Intracranial metastases:** Lung > breast > melanoma > renal, colorectal, lymphoma, and unknown primary. Prostate is very rare.
   b. **Dural, epidural, skull metastases:** Breast, prostate.
   c. **Leptomeningeal metastases:** See p. 124.

2. **Tumors most likely to have brain metastases:** Melanoma (40%).

3. **Metastases likely to bleed:** Renal, papillary thyroid, melanoma, choriocarcinoma, lung.

4. **Number:** On MRI, only 20%-30% of mets are solitary.
   a. **Solitary metastases:** Resection is usually offered. If cannot resect, consider biopsy because 10% turn out *not* to be mets even if the pt has another known primary.
   b. **Multiple metastases:** Consider resection of the dominant, symptomatic lesion. Stereotactic radiosurgery may help small lesions.
5. **Location:** 80% are supratentorial, 15% cerebellar (50% of cerebellar metastases are pelvic/GI).
6. **Prognosis for brain metastases:**
   a. **No rx:** 4-wk survival.
   b. **Steroids alone:** 8 wk.
   c. **Steroids + XRT:** 3-6 mo (most die of other cause).
   d. **Surgery + XRT:** 10-16 mo.

H. **Gliomas:** Include astrocytomas, oligodendrogliomas, oligoastrocytomas, ependymomas.
   1. **Brainstem gliomas, cerebellar astrocytomas, ependymomas:** Mostly pediatric; see p. 151.
   2. **Astrocytomas:**
      a. **World Health Organization (WHO) grading:**

Grade	Scan of Mass	Survival	Usual Pathol.	Treatment
I	Post. fossa mass	Excellent	Pilocytic astro.	Surgery
II	Nonenhanced	7-10 yr	Diffuse astro.	Surg+XRT ±chemo
III	Enhanced	~2 yr	Anaplastic astro.	Surg+chemo+XRT
IV	Enhanced	<1 yr	GBM: necrosis, vasc. prolif.	Surg+chemo+XRT

Table 34. Astrocytoma grading.

      b. **Recurrence:** ~90% near original site. Some white matter spread (e.g., "butterfly" glioma across callosum). Metastases rare.
      c. **Rx of astrocytoma:** Surgery, XRT (q.v. p. 125), alkylating agents. No longer standard to use procarbazine, CCNU, vincristine.
   3. **Oligodendrogliomas:** May be grade II (low grade) or grade III (anaplastic). Often present with seizures. Often calcified. More chemosensitive than astrocytomas. 50%-70% of anaplastic lesions have loss of chromosomes 1p and 19q, which suggests increased chemosensitivity, good prognosis.
   4. **Meningiomas** (20% of intracranial primaries): Arise from the arachnoid. Mostly indolent, often asymptomatic incidentalomas. Sx relate to tumor location; seizures and HA occur rarely. 8% are multiple, higher in type 1 neurofibromatosis.
      a. **DDx:** Includes prostate or breast metastasis to bone.

     b. Scans: "Light bulb" enhancement, attached to meninges ("dural tail" on post-gado MRI), usually extra-axial, may show peritumoral edema. Often calcified, with adjacent hyperostosis or bone erosion.

     c. Rx: Surgery usually curative, often bloody. Often need re-op angio ($\pm$ embolization) to define vascular involvement and assess venous sinus invasion or occlusion. XRT (and, increasingly, stereotactic radiosurgery for small lesions) is effective for incompletely resected tumors.

I. Pituitary tumors:
1. **H&P:**
   a. **Secretory tumors:** Sx of hormonal excess: Cushing's syndrome, acromegaly, or galactorrhea.
   b. **Nonsecretory tumors:** Sx of mass effect: bitemporal field cuts, headache, hypopituitarism, invasion of cavernous sinus.
   c. **Pituitary apoplexy:** An emergency. See sudden headache, visual deterioration, diplopia, and drowsiness. From bleed into tumor. Requires immediate surgery to preserve vision.
2. **DDx:** Suprasellar mass, pituitary infarct or apoplexy, inflammation.
3. **Tests:** MRI with gadolinium and thin cuts through sella (see p. 190), adrenal function (see p. 199), thyroid function (see p. 201), prolactin, follicle-stimulating and luteinizing hormones, estradiol in women, testosterone in men, growth hormone if there is acromegaly.
4. **Rx:**
   a. **Surgery:** Usually transsphenoidal or pterional (see p. 85). Indications include apoplexy, acromegaly, Cushing's syndrome, macroadenomas, prolactinomas with PRL <500 ng/mL (chance of normalizing PRL >500 is low), or unresponsive to meds.
   b. **Medical:**
      1) **Bromocriptine:**
         a) **Prolactinomas:** Start 1.25-2.5 mg qd; add additional 2.5 mg qd every 3-7 d as necessary. Usual dose 5-7.5 mg qd.
         b) **Growth hormone tumors:** may need more. Max. dose is 100 mg qd.
         c) **SEs:** Include nausea, orthostasis, cognitive complaints, psychosis. Minimize these by giving qhs with food.
      2) **Cabergoline:** At least as effective as bromocriptine in lowering prolactin levels and shrinking tumor, with substantially fewer side effects. Long half-life allows twice-weekly dosing. Start 0.25 mg 2×/wk, incr. monthly by 0.25 mg 2×/wk based on prolactin levels. Max. dose is 1 mg 2×/wk.
      3) **Octreotide:** For growth hormone–secreting tumors. Very expensive. SEs include GI disturbance, gallstones. Dosing varies with GH levels.
      4) **Hormone replacement therapy:** Adrenal, thyroid, or sex hormones when necessary.
   c. **XRT:** Not routinely used. Side effects include hypopituitarism, optic nerve damage, lethargy, diplopia, and pituitary apoplexy.

J. Vestibular schwannomas: Formerly inaccurately called acoustic neuromas and acoustic neurinomas. Benign, cerebellopontine angle tumors.
1. **H&P:** First symptom is usually gradual unilateral hearing loss. Also common are tinnitus, vertigo, imbalance; later headache, facial numbness, weakness, or diplopia. Look for signs of

neurofibromatosis. Bilateral vestibular schwannomas are pathognomonic for NF2.

2. **DDx:** Meningioma (often nerve V involvement before VII, calcification on CT) or other tumor.

3. **Tests:** MRI with thin cuts through internal auditory meatus, or CT with contrast. MRI usually shows a round or ovoid enhancing mass in the IAM. Audiological testing may help establish a baseline for postsurgical comparison.

4. **Rx:** Goal is to prevent complications (esp. hearing loss). Surgery, stereotactic radiosurgery, and fractionated stereotactic radiotherapy appear equally safe and effective.
    a. **CSF leak rx:** 3-5 d of lumbar drainage to allow healing.
    b. **Facial nerve dysfunction rx:** Gold weight (to maintain eye closure) or hypoglossal-facial anastomosis (to restore facial tone).

Tumor	Good Surgical Candidate	Poor Surgical Candidate
<3 cm	If good hearing, surgery If no hearing, observation[1]	Observation[1]
>3 cm	Surgery	Surgery or radiosurgery

Table 35. Management of vestibular schwannomas.

[1] Observation = repeat neuro exam and imaging q 6 mo × 2 yr, then annually if stable. If exam deteriorates or growth is >2 mm/yr, consider surgery or radiosurgery.

K. **Primary CNS lymphomas:** Rare, but much more common in AIDS. Sx relate to location.

1. **DDx:** In HIV, toxo is primary concern. If there are multiple lesions, give 2 wk of empiric toxo therapy and look for response before bx. In immunocompetent host, biopsy is necessary for dx.

2. **Tests:** MRI with gado.
    a. **Immunocompetent:** A homogeneously enhancing mass in white matter or basal ganglia. 20%-40% multifocal.
    b. **AIDS:** Often rim enhanced. Up to 70% multifocal.

3. **Rx/prognosis:** Months if untreated. Chemo regimens are mostly methotrexate based, with 5-year median survival. XRT may be provided after chemo. No role for surgery. Steroids cause temporary (sometimes dramatic) regression.

L. **Leptomeningeal metastases:** Can be the presenting problem. Most common in leukemia, lymphoma, breast cancer, lung cancer.

1. **H&P:** Synchronous signs or sx at multiple sites in brain, cranial nerves, or spinal cord. Often back pain or postural headache.

2. **Tests:**
    a. **CT or MRI:** To r/o mass before LP. Communicating hydrocephalus suggests leptomeningeal dz. Contrast may show meningeal enhancement.
    b. **LP:** Do cytology for malignant cells (80% sensitive after 3 LPs). Send at least 3 cc. Cells degrade quickly; do not let them sit.

3. **Rx:** Depends on primary tumor. Most breast cancers and lymphomas respond, as do about 30% of lung cancers and 20% of melanomas. Untreated pts. usually die within weeks.

    a. XRT: Irradiate symptomatic areas. Often given with
    dexamethasone.
    b. Chemotherapy: Usually intrathecal methotrexate. Consider
    Ommaya reservoir.
    c. Ventriculoperitoneal shunt: For symptomatic hydrocephalus.

URO-NEUROLOGY

A. Bladder detrusor and internal sphincter:
    1. Parasympathetic: Acetylcholine from S2-4 via pelvic nerve constricts bladder via muscarinic receptors.
    2. Sympathetic: Norepinephrine from L2-4 via hypogastric nerve constricts sphincter via α-receptors. The bladder has β-receptors.

B. External sphincter: Voluntary control via S2-4

C. H&P: Often a poor correlation between sx and urodynamic findings.
    1. Autonomic dysreflexia: <u>Urgent problem.</u> In pts with spine injury
    (usually above T5/6). Pain, bladder distension or catheterization,
    bowel distension, or other stimuli can trigger acute hypertension,
    bradycardia, anxiety, and headache. Sit the pt. up, and treat BP
    promptly, e.g., with nifedipine 10 mg SL.
    2. Frequency or urgency: From high fluid intake, urinary tract infection, partial outlet obstruction (prostate, diaphragm), upper or lower
    motor neuron lesion, psychosomatic.
    3. Urinary retention: From drugs (anticholinergics, opiates, anesthetics), pain, prostate, lower motor neuron lesion, bladder-sphincter
    dyssynergia, obstruction.
    4. Incontinence:
        a. Stress: Often a bladder suspension defect or sphincter damage.
        b. Overflow: Dribbling, small volumes, big painful bladder. Causes
        are those of urinary retention, above.
        c. Confusional: Varying volumes, usually shameless.

D. Upper vs. lower motor neuron lesions:

	Upper Motor Neuron	**Lower Motor Neuron**
Bladder	Small, spastic, low PVR	Large, flaccid, high PVR
History	Urgency, trouble starting, wet at night	Strains to empty fully, wet or dry at night.
Bulbocavernosus	Present	Absent
Causes	Bilat. frontal lesion, cord lesion above T12	Anesthetics, neuropathy, ALS, cauda equina lesion
Treatment	Decrease bladder tone with anticholinergics or adrenergics	Increase bladder tone with cholinergics or antiadrenergics; self-catheterization

Table 36. Distinguishing upper and lower motor neuron lesions.

E. Rx by urodynamic finding:
  1. **Flaccid bladder:** Detrusor hyporeflexia, poor voiding.
     Catheterization helps. Try cholinergics, e.g., bethanechol (Urecholine)
     10-50 mg bid-tid. Avoid cholinergics in COPD, PUD, CAD,
     hyperthyroidism.
  2. **Spastic bladder:** Detrusor hyperreflexia, poor storage. Try anti-
     cholinergics, e.g., tolterodine (Detrol) 1 mg bid, oxybutynin
     (Ditropan) 5 mg bid-tid, implanted stimulator.
  3. **Detrusor-sphincter dyssynergia:** Spinal cord lesions above the
     sacral level can leave just the sphincter spastic. The bladder
     eventually dilates, but secondarily. Treat with catheterization,
     anticholinergics, prazosin (an anti-α_1-adrenergic, 1 mg bid-tid),
     Botox.

VENOUS SINUS THROMBOSIS, CNS

A. Sx: "Great mimic" in stroke; HA 80%, papilledema 50%, seizure 40%,
   variable confusion, cranial nerve deficits, uni- or bilateral cortical signs.
   Variable time course. Can look like pseudotumor cerebri.
G. Tests:
  1. **MR or CT venogram:** The test of choice—true angiogram usually
     not necessary. Sinuses need to be traced out. Note that dural venous
     sinuses asymmetry is common; follow contrast flow through to
     bilateral IJ veins to verify flow difference between the dominant
     and hypoplastic sinuses.
  2. **CT** (not sensitive): Focal hypodensity or petechial blood; can
     look like metastases. Small ventricles. Without contrast, the
     triangular "delta" of the sagittal sinus looks dense. If contrast
     given, can sometimes see empty delta sign or gyral and falx
     enhancement.
  3. **MRI** (not sensitive): After day 5, standard MRI may show increased
     T1 and T2 signal along sinus. Iron susceptibility scan may show hem-
     orrhagic transformation of thrombosis-related strokes.
  4. **CSF:** Usually normal; sometimes see decreased protein or
     increased RBCs; may have high opening pressures if significant
     clot burden.
C. Causes of thrombosis: Hypercoagulable state, pregnancy, estrogenic
   meds; septic thrombosis); inflammatory disorders (SLE, GCA, Behçet's
   disease); malignancy (visceral carcinoma, primary CNS tumors,
   Trousseau's syndrome); and idiopathic (15%-20%).
D. Rx of venous thrombosis: Heparin, even if hemorrhagic infarct
   (rationale: the only way to prevent hemorrhage expansion is to
   prevent further clot formation and consequent increase in venous
   congestion/formation of venous infarcts). When therapeutic on
   heparin, start warfarin $\times$ 2-3 mo. Consider thrombolysis, mechanical
   clot retrieval (thrombectomy). Mannitol and steroids. ACD only if
   seizure.
E. Prognosis: Good; 75% have complete recovery.

VERTIGO

A. Dx:
  1. **"Dizziness":** Ask if the feeling is of spinning, and in the feet vs. the head, may distinguish between vertigo (illusion of movement), light-headedness (a feeling that one might faint), and poor balance—all of which pts may call "dizziness."
  2. **Other:** Sudden onset, HA, tinnitus, hearing decrease, other cranial nerves, gait, trouble controlling limbs, length of episode, LOC, change in vision, N/V, worse when lay down/stand/stoop/turn neck, h/o trauma, anxiety, hypo- or hyperglycemia, or hypertension. Orthostatic BPs, bruits, hearing (q.v. p. 54), eye exam, tympanic membranes; consider Romberg, postural reflexes, hyperventilation × 3 minutes, calorics (q.v. p. 222).
  3. **Bárány's test:** On a stretcher, bring pt suddenly back from a seated position to supine with pt's head turned fully to the right and eyes open. Watch for nystagmus and vertigo for at least 1 min. Repeat with head to the left. Have a bucket handy in case of vomit.

B. DDx: R/o dizziness from cardiac problem, bleed, panic, hypoglycemia; poor balance from movement disorder, sensory deficits, or weakness.
  1. **Central vertigo:**
     a. **H&P:** Usually less sudden onset (or if sudden, with HA), less nausea, continuous sx indep. of posture, usually no hearing loss.
        1) **Nystagmus:** All varieties of nystagmus including vertical.
        2) **Side of sx:** Falling and nystagmus are to same side, that of the lesion (vs. peripheral nystagmus, which is to opposite side).
        3) **Bárány's test:** No latency to nystagmus, it lasts >30 sec, no habituation. Nystagmus can go in different directions from same head position.
     b. **Causes of central vertigo:** Brainstem lesion, cerebellar lesion (especially AICA territory), acoustic schwannoma. DPH or barbiturates. Can see central vertigo in migraine or complex partial seizures. Multiple sclerosis may cause poor balance; rarely true vertigo. Vertebral dissection.

C. Peripheral (vestibular) vertigo:
  1. **H&P:** Often sudden, positional, with severe nausea, tinnitus, or decreased hearing.
     a. **Nystagmus:** Horizontal or rotatory, in only one direction.
     b. **Side of sx:** Sx are usually worse with bad ear facing down. Falling and dysmetria are to side of bad ear. Nystagmus (fast phase) is complicated.

D. Excitatory lesion: E.g., positional vertigo. Nystagmus (fast phase) is toward the affected ear.
  1. **Inhibitory lesion:** E.g., vestibular neuronitis, otitis. Nystagmus away from the affected ear.
  2. **Ménière's:** Unreliable.
     a. **Bárány's test:** 2-20 sec latency to nystagmus; habituates in ~30 sec and on repeated testing.
  3. **Causes of peripheral vertigo:**
     a. **Drug-induced:** Alcohol, Abx, furosemide, quinidine, quinine, aspirin. DPH or barbiturates cause central vertigo, not peripheral.

b. Ménière's dz: Usually with decreased hearing, ear fullness, tinnitus. Attacks of vertigo last minutes to hours, recur weeks to years. Try clonazepam 0.5 mg bid, meclizine 25 mg q6h, diuretics, or strict salt restriction.

c. Benign positional vertigo: From loose otoliths. Drugs work poorly. Better to move otoliths back out of posterior canal.

    1) Epley maneuver: See Figure 13.

        a) Briskly lie pt on back with their head tilted 45 degrees towards the symptomatic side until vertigo stops.

        b) Rotate their head the other way until vertigo stops.

        c) Have pt roll body towards that side, carrying the head along until it points down 45 degrees, until vertigo stops.

        d) Sit pt up, with head slightly down. Repeat two more times.

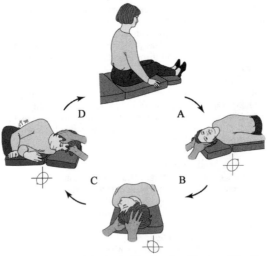

Figure 13. The Epley maneuver in benign positional vertigo. (Courtesy of Timothy Hain, MD.)

    2) Brandt-Daroff desensitization exercises: If Epley fails. Do each step for 30 sec (or until vertigo stops). Sit on edge of bed. Lie on R side of body with head turned 45 degrees up toward ceiling. Sit up. Lie on L side with head turned 45 degrees up. Repeat this cycle five times per session, three sessions per day.

E. Vestibular neuronitis: Usually young, sudden onset, not recurrent, postviral, normal hearing, and no tinnitus.

    a. Vestibular neuronitis: Usually young, sudden, not recurrent, postviral. No decreased hearing or tinnitus.

    b. Other infections: Chronic otitis media, herpes zoster oticus, syphilis (usually bilateral)....

F. Psychosomatic vertigo and dizziness: Fluoxetine may help both this and true peripheral vertigo. See "Psychosomatic Neurology", p. 102.

WEAKNESS

A. See also: Neuromuscular Disorders, p. 80.
B. Terminology: Paresis is partial; plegia or paralysis is complete.
C. H&P: Numbness, pain, distal vs. proximal, bowel and bladder function, injuries, diurnal or exercise-induced fluctuation, tone, reflexes, atrophy, fasciculations, etc.

Muscle strength grading:

0 : No contraction
1 : Flicker of contraction
2 : Active movement; can't resist gravity
3 : Active movement against gravity
4 : Active movement against resistance
5 : Normal strength

Figure 14. Muscle strength grading.

D. Upper motor neuron (UMN) vs. lower motor neuron (LMN) weakness: Both may be flaccid initially, but UMN lesion (corticospinal, pyramidal) usually develops spasticity and hyperreflexia; reflexes should be depressed in LMN lesion. May see fasciculations in LMN lesion; EMG will show fibrillations only after a few weeks. Dexterity is preferentially affected by upper motor neuron corticospinal lesion.
  1. Spasticity: An exaggeration of stretch reflexes, causing velocity-dependent, "clasp-knife" rigidity, flexion dystonia, and flexor spasms, hyperreflexia.
    a. DDx: Extrapyramidal rigidity, muscle spasms,
    b. Rx: Muscle relaxants, see p. 173. Physical therapy. Orthopedic procedures to release contractions.
E. Bulbar vs. pseudobulbar palsy:
  1. Bulbar palsy: Lower motor neuron flaccid lesion of lower cranial nerves. Decreased gag.
  2. Pseudobulbar palsy: Spastic, upper motor neuron lesion. Hyperactive gag. Causes include ALS, MS, and bilateral cerebral strokes. In the latter two, there is often "pseudobulbar affect": excessive, inappropriate laughing and crying.
F. Hemiparesis: Ipsilateral arm and leg. Typically from corticospinal damage. Look for other signs (e.g., neglect, cranial nerve abnormalities) to localize further.
G. Monoparesis: Single limb. May have peripheral or central cause.
H. Paraparesis: Both legs. Usually spinal cord; look for sensory level. But consider falx meningioma or bilateral ACA infarcts.
I. Proximal, distal, or generalized weakness:
  1. Severe or quickly progressive quadriparesis: Consider high cervical or brainstem lesion, Guillain-Barré syndrome, botulism.

2. **Slowly progressive:** Consider neuropathies, neuromuscular dz.
3. **Fluctuating weakness:** Consider myasthenic syndromes, TIAs, hyper- or hypokalemic periodic paralysis.
4. **Generalized weakness in the ICU:** Mnemonic for DDx is <u>MUSCLES</u>: <u>M</u>edication, <u>U</u>ndiagnosed neuromuscular disorder, <u>S</u>pinal cord damage, <u>C</u>ritical illness polyneuropathy, <u>L</u>oss of muscle mass, <u>E</u>lectrolyte disorders, <u>S</u>ystemic illness.

CHILD NEUROLOGY

DEVELOPMENT

A. **History:** Problems or drug use in pregnancy, weeks gestation, Apgars, birth weight, postnatal problems, developmental milestones (see Table 37), school performance. For adolescents, try to ask about drugs and sexual activity with parents out of the room.

B. **General exam:** Head circumference (see Figure 17, p. 139), eye exam, face and limb morphology, skin (café-au-lait, ashleaf, palmar creases), and cardiovascular exam. In infants, fontanelles (see p. 137), skull, and base of the spine.

C. **Neurological exam:** See primitive reflexes and developmental milestones, below.

1. **Infants:** Alertness, posture, spontaneous movements, cry pitch and volume, pupil responses, ability to track a face, orientation towards noise, reflexes (see Table 36), response to pinch. Assess tone (premature infants are normally hypotonic).

   a. **Supine:**
      1) **Hypertonic:** Arched back, more than a few beats of clonus, asymmetric tonic neck reflex that is obligate or present after age 6 mo, and inability to dorsiflex the foot to the shin in infants <6 mo.
      2) **Hypotonic:** Frog-legged, little spontaneous movement.

   b. **Traction response:** Pull the infant from supine to sitting.
      1) **Hypertonic:** Persistent leg extension.
      2) **Hypotonic:** Head lag, no compensatory leg flexion.

   c. **Horizontal suspension:**
      1) **Hypertonic:** Back extension.
      2) **Hypotonic:** Infant drapes over your hands.

   d. **Vertical suspension:** Hold baby under armpits.
      1) **Hypertonic:** Scissoring of legs with plantar ankle flexion.
      2) **Hypotonic:** Head droops; baby slips through your fingers.

2. **Older children:** Toddlers may be examined better on a parent's lap. Use toys to engage them; watch movement during spontaneous play.

D. **Normal patterns of myelination:** In general, myelination progresses caudal to rostral, central to peripheral, and dorsal to ventral. Because there is no gray-white differentiation in infants, it is easy to miss small amounts of edema.

1. **Imaging:** Use T1 MRI for the first 4 mo of life, T2 thereafter.

2. **At birth:** Central cerebellar white matter, superior and inferior cerebellar peduncles, brainstem, and thalamus.

3. **By 1 month:** Corticospinal tracts, pre- and postcentral gyri, optic nerves and tracts.

4. **By 3 months:** Middle cerebellar peduncles, optic radiations, and posterior limb of the internal capsule.

5. **By 8 months:** Anterior limb of the internal capsule, corpus callosum, centrum semiovale, and subcortical U-fibers.

6. **By 18 months:** Nearly adult appearance except for the peritrigonal region posterior to the occipital horns.

7. **By 20 years:** Peritrigonal region is myelinated.

E. Normal reflexes and milestones:

Reflex	Appears By	Gone By
Gag	32 wk gest	Persists
Suck	34 wk gest	4 mo
Palmar grasp	34 wk gest	6 mo
Plantar grasp	34 wk gest	10 mo
Tonic neck–incomplete (asymmetric)	34 wk gest	4 mo
Moro (arms, legs extend when head falls supine)	34 wk gest	3 mo
Automatic stepping when upright on table	35 wk gest	2 mo
Crossed adductor	35 wk	7 mo
Extensor plantar response (Babinski)	Birth	10 mo
Placing (when baby upright and foot brushes table)	1 day	2 mo
Asymmetric tonic neck reflex (ATNR)[1]	2-3 wk	4-6 mo
Landau (head, trunk, leg extension while prone)	3 mo	24 mo

[1] ATNR: Turn and hold baby's head laterally. Ipsilateral arm extends, contralateral arm flexes briefly. Lasting >3 sec is not nl at any age.

Table 37. Primitive reflexes.

Age	Gross Motor	Fine Motor	Language	Social
2 mo	Lifts chest off table	Follows object past midline	Responsive smile	Recognizes parent
4 mo	Rolls over	Moves arms in unison to grasp	Orients to voice	Enjoys looking around
6 mo	Sits unsupported	Grasps with either hand, transfers	Babbles	Recognizes strangers
9 mo	Crawls, pulls to stand	Pincer grasp, holds bottle	Understands no	Explores, plays pat-a-cake
12 mo	Walks alone	Throws objects	Uses two words besides dada/mama	Imitates, comes when called
18 mo	Runs	Feeds self with spoon	Knows body parts	Copies tasks, plays w/others
24 mo	Walks stairs alone	Turns single pages, removes clothes	Uses two-word sentences, follows two-step commands	Parallel play
3 yr	Pedals tricycle	Dresses partially, draws a circle	Uses three-word sentences, plurals	Group play, shares toys
4 yr	Hops, skips	Can button, catches ball	Knows colors, asks questions	Tells "tall tales"
5 yr	Jumps over low barriers	Ties shoes, spreads with knife	Prints name, asks word meanings	Competitive play, obeys rules

Table 38. Developmental milestones.

F. Progressive developmental delay or regression:

1. **H&P:** Ask about progression ("Are there things your child could do before but can't do now?"), CNS trauma, family history, consanguinity, child abuse or neglect. Perform a good general exam as well as neurological exam and head circumference.

G. Intelligence quotient (IQ): Average = 100; with 15 points for each standard deviation from the mean.

Degree of Retardation	IQ	Mental Age as Adult
Dull normal	80-90	—
Borderline	70-79	—
Mild	55-69	9-11
Moderate	40-54	5-8
Severe	25-39	3-5
Profound	<25	<3

Table 39. Degrees of mental retardation.

1. **Causes:** Consider hydrocephalus, tumors, autism, epilepsy, infections, toxins, abuse, and metabolic disorders.
   a. **Gray matter dz:** Cerebral cortex dz → cognitive loss, seizures. Basal ganglia dz → movement disorders, cerebellar dz → ataxia. Causes include tumors, severe epilepsy, lysosomal disorders, ceroid lipofuscinosis, autism spectrum, aminoacidopathy.
   b. **White matter dz:** Corticospinal sx, blindness, and other focal deficits, but seizures rare. Causes include progressive hydrocephalus, childhood multiple sclerosis, leukodystrophies, Alexander's dz, Canavan's dz, galactosemia, Pelizaeus-Merzbacher dz.
   c. **Peripheral as well as central nervous system dz?** Suggests lysosomal storage disorders; mitochondrial disorders.
   d. **Other organs involved besides nervous system?** Look especially at skin, eyes, viscera (murmurs, hepatomegaly), dysmorphic features, growth failure. Suggests aminoacidurias (p. 143), neurocutaneous syndromes (p. 146), chronic infections, e.g., TORCH (see p. 142), hypothyroidism, chronic toxin exposure.
2. **Tests:**
   a. **Blood:** Electrolytes, CBC, lactate, liver function tests, lead level.
   b. **Neuroimaging:** Look for hydrocephalus, focal lesions, atrophy, diffuse white matter change. Compare with normal progression of myelination, above.
   c. **Other:** Consider metabolic screen (p. 142), LP (p. 224).
H. Static developmental delay:
1. **Tests:** First, MRI. Evaluate structural lesions; if none are found, consider further metabolic workup. Pts with global developmental delay should have tests for fragile X, Rett syndrome, and others if appropriate. Any patient with language delay should always have hearing formally tested.
2. **DDx:** Slowly progressive congenital disorders.

3. **Cerebral palsy:** Generic name for static encephalopathy, usually from prenatal rather than perinatal factors. Classified by motor findings.

   a. **Spastic hemiplegia** (arm and leg): Usually from developmental malformation or stroke. Usually normal intelligence, sometimes seizures.

   b. **Spastic diplegia** (legs ≫ arms): Usually from prematurity. Intelligence may be near normal; seizures rare. May need orthopedic rx of spasticity.

   c. **Spastic quadriplegia:** Usually from severe diffuse brain injury. Severe seizures and mental retardation are common.

   d. **Athetoid:** From hypoxia, cerebellar or basal ganglia lesions, kernicterus (severe neonatal jaundice).

4. **Perinatal events:**

   a. **H&P:** Maternal risk factors and delivery. Poor alertness, periodic breathing, hypotonia, seizures. Bulging fontanelles and signs of high ICP in severe hemorrhage.

   b. **Term newborns:**

      1) **Hypoxic-ischemic encephalopathy (HIE):** Defined as cord blood gas pH <7, Apgar 0-3 at >5 min, neuro sx (seizures, coma, hypotonia), and other organ involvement.

         a) **Acute total asphyxia:** Injures thalamus and brainstem more.

         b) **Prolonged partial asphyxia:** Injures cerebral cortex and white matter more.

         c) **Prognosis:** Alertness may improve between 12-24 h of age, then worsen over the next 72 h. Severe HIE causes mental retardation, spastic quadriparesis, and seizures, but mild HIE resolves within 2 d without sequelae.

      2) **Other:** Stroke, CNS bleed, etc.

   c. **Premature infants:**

      1) **Periventricular leukomalacia** (PVL): Presumed to be from HIE. In premature newborns, this mostly affects subcortical white matter, causing spastic diplegia, quadriplegia, or visual impairment. Severe HIE also causes mental retardation and microcephaly. PVL can be shown, after 1-2 wk, with CT or MRI.

      2) **Periventricular-intraventricular hemorrhage** (PIVH): A germinal matrix hemorrhage, probably the effect of transient hypertension on vessels previously weakened by ischemia. Occurs in about 25% of newborns weighing <2 kg, within the first 4 d.

         a) **Tests:** Head ultrasound. Should be performed as a screen in all newborns <32 wk gestation and in symptomatic newborns >32 wk. Follow PIVH with serial US; 10% will develop hydrocephalus.

         b) **Prevention:** Avoid premature birth. Avoid blood pressure fluctuations with therapeutic paralysis of vented newborns, rapid volume expansion.

         c) **Management:** Continue BP control; treat hydrocephalus with drugs that decrease CSF production (e.g., mannitol, acetazolamide), EVD, or ventriculoperitoneal shunt.

5. **Structural malformations:**
   a. **Neurulation disorders:** E.g., encephaloceles, myelomeningoceles: when spinal, AKA spina bifida. The defect should be surgically closed within the first week or two of life. Hydrocephalus requiring VP shunt usually develops because of associated aqueductal stenosis.
   b. **Midline malformations:** E.g., holoprosencephaly (undivided anterior brain), septo-optic dysplasia.
   c. **Migration disorders:** E.g., schizencephaly (brain cleft from partial defect in neuronal germinative zone), lissencephaly (agyria), pachygyria (few gyri), polymicrogyria.
   d. **Differentiation disorders:** E.g., microcephaly, megalencephaly, neurocutaneous disorders, corpus callosum aplasia, Aicardi's syndrome (callosal agenesis with chorioretinal lacunae, vertebral defects, and infantile spasms in a girl), colpocephaly (enlarged occipital ventricular horns), congenital vascular malformations and tumors, porencephaly (cerebral cavity), hydranencephaly (severe bilateral porencephaly).
   e. **Cerebellar malformations:**
      1) **Chiari malformation:** See also p. 181 for radiologic appearance of tonsillar herniation. Sx range from headache to sx of cerebellar and brainstem compression.
         a) **Type I:** Cerebellar tonsils herniate below the foramen magnum.
         b) **Type II:** Cerebellar vermis, fourth ventricle, and medulla are below the foramen magnum. Usually with myelodysplasia and lumbar myelomeningocele.
         c) **Type III:** Brain displaced into a myelomeningocele. Rare.
      2) **Dandy-Walker malformation:** Vermis hypoplasia with fourth ventricle cyst and hydrocephalus, from blocked foramen of Magendie. Both the fourth and lateral ventricles must be shunted.
   f. **Myelination disorders.**
   g. **Arachnoid cysts:** Seen in 4% of normals; only 20% are symptomatic, usually from secondary hydrocephalus.
6. **Chromosomal defects:** E.g., trisomies, translocations, deletions, mosaicism.
   a. **Down syndrome** (trisomy 21): 1/1,000 live births.
      1) **General features:** Short, dysmorphic, simian crease; cardiac, thyroid, GI problems; increased risk of leukemia.
      2) **Neurological features:** Hypotonia, mental retardation, early Alzheimer's dz, cervical narrowing and risk for atlantoaxial subluxation, seizures in 10%, nystagmus and sluggish pupils, hearing loss.
   b. **Fragile X syndrome:** See p. 151.
7. **Gene disorders:** May be static or progressive (see p. 132).
8. **Maternal diseases and toxins:**
   a. **Fetal alcohol syndrome:** Dx requires sx in each of three categories:
      1) **Growth retardation:** Weight, length, or head circumference <10th percentile (corrected for gestational age).
      2) **CNS involvement:** Neurological abnormality, developmental delay, or cognitive impairment.

3) **Facial abnormalities:** ≥2 of the following: head circumference <3rd percentile; narrow eye slits; flat and long upper lip; underdeveloped midface; flat nose bridge.
  b. **Other:** TORCH infections (p. 142), prenatal cocaine.
9. **Postnatal insults:** E.g., infections, malnutrition, toxins, cerebrovascular events, trauma, neglect.

EYES AND VISION

A. **See also:** Adult Eyes and Vision, p. 44.
B. **Nystagmus:**
  1. **Congenital nystagmus:** Begins at age 2-3 mo, not at birth. Pts. do not feel spinning vertigo but sometimes have poor acuity.
  2. **Spasmus nutans:** Nystagmus with head nodding and abnormal head position. Onset 6-12 mo, lasts 1-2 yr, improves spontaneously.
C. **Oculomotor palsy:**
  1. **H&P:** Babies >3 mo old should have conjugate gaze and good fixation. See adult eye movements, p. 46, for exam (although you will probably need something more interesting than your finger to get a 2-year-old to track).
  2. **Causes:** Causes also seen in adults include raised ICP, tumor, aneurysm, thrombosis, myasthenia, trauma, orbital entrapment, mitochondrial dz, etc. Additional pediatric causes include:
    a. **Infantile botulism:** Hypotonia with big, sluggish pupils, ANS dysfunction. May see ptosis without ophthalmoplegia. Associated with eating honey. Unlike adult form, spores colonize gut. Antitoxin and antibiotics do not help.
    b. **Congenital palsies:** Duane's syndrome (poor ab- or adduction with globe retraction), Möbius syndrome (bilateral 6th and 7th palsies), Brown syndrome (congenitally short superior oblique muscle), congenital myasthenia.
    c. **Infection:** E.g., meningitis, Gradenigo's syndrome (petrous inflammation).
    d. **Ophthalmoplegic migraine:** Sx begin during or just before a migraine but may last up to 1 mo. Oculomotor nerve is affected in 80%.
D. **Strabismus:** Nonparalytic ocular misalignment. If constant and persistent, child will often fixate only with one eye, develop amblyopia (loss of acuity) in the other, and have no complaint of diplopia.
  1. **H&P:** If misalignment is fixed, test EOM monocularly to r/o paralysis. If it is intermittent, perform alternating cover test, p. 48. Test acuity, fundus exam.
  2. **Rx:** Alternate patching of the eyes. Corrective surgery. Botulinum toxin has recently been tried.
E. **Visual loss:**
  1. **H&P:** In babies, test pupillary, red, and blink reflex. By 6 wk, babies should make and maintain eye contact. Babies under 3 mo should only be expected to fix and follow. Babies over 3 mo should have conjugate gaze and a visual grasp, but the latter is hard to test before 6 mo. Look

for abnormal eye movements, structural abnormalities such as cataracts, fundal lesions, microphthalmia.

2. **Tests:** Visual evoked responses should be present by 30 wk gestation and mature at 3 mo.
3. **Causes:** See causes also seen in adults (retinal ischemia, optic nerve or cortical lesions, etc.), p. 44.
   a. **Acute:** Carotid dissection, ICH, hysteria, migraine, optic neuropathy (demyelinating, ischemic, toxic), pseudotumor cerebri, trauma.
   b. **Subacute or chronic:**
      1) **Compression:** Tumor, aneurysm, AVM, inflammatory mass.
      2) **Cataracts:** Genetic, intrauterine drug exposure (chlorpromazine, steroids, sulfonamides) or infection (mumps, rubella, syphilis), prematurity, endocrine abnormalities, trauma, postnatal varicella. Remove cataracts before 3 mo to prevent amblyopia.
      3) **Hereditary optic atrophies:** Sometimes isolated. Multisystem involvement is most often mitochondrial dz.
      4) **Tapetoretinal degeneration:** Usually disorders of carbohydrate or lipid metabolism, and associated with dementia, neuropathy, and ataxia.
   c. **Other:** Congenital optic nerve hypoplasia, coloboma (an embryonic retinal defect), Leber's congenital amaurosis (unrelated to the mitochondrial disorder of Leber's hereditary optic neuropathy), dislocated lens, corneal clouding (e.g., in mucopolysaccharidosis and Fabry's dz).

HEAD CIRCUMFERENCE DISORDERS

A. **H&P:** Maternal history (toxins, infections, hypoxia), family head sizes. Get pt's prior head sizes. Rule of thumb for normal growth rate is premature infants: 1 cm/wk; 1-3 mo: 2 cm/mo; 3-6 mo: 1 cm/mo; 6-12 mo: 0.5 cm/mo.
   1. **Ophthalmoscopic exam:** Look for papilledema, retinal bleed.
   2. **Head shape:** Frontal bossing suggests hydrocephalus; lateral bulging suggests SDH.
   3. **Fontanelles:** Posterior and sphenoid fontanelles closes by 2-3 mo, mastoid fontanelle by 1 yr, anterior fontanelle by 1.5-2.5 years.
   4. **Head circumference:** Largest measurement around forehead and occiput excluding ears. For a normal baby, it is approximately the crown-rump length. Abnormal = more than 2 SD above mean, circumference out of proportion to height and weight, or upward deviation of growth curve over time (crossing curves).
B. **Tests:** CT, MRI, or ultrasound. Genetic and metabolic evaluation if microcephaly.
C. **Causes of microcephaly:** Genetic, intrauterine infections (CMV, toxoplasmosis, rubella), toxins (alcohol, ACDs), asphyxia, metabolic disorders, radiation (especially 4-20 wk gestation).
D. **Causes of macrocephaly:** Hydrocephalus, SDH, hydranencephaly, megalencephaly.

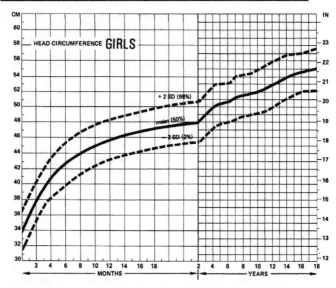

Figure 15. Head circumference, girls. (Reproduced with permission from Neilhaus G. *Pediatrics.* 1968;41:106.)

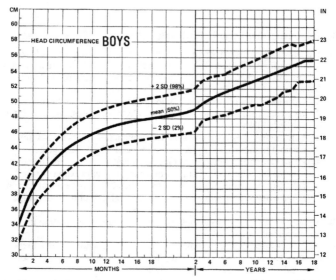

Figure 16. Head circumference, boys. (Reproduced with permission from Neilhaus G. *Pediatrics.* 1968;41:106.)

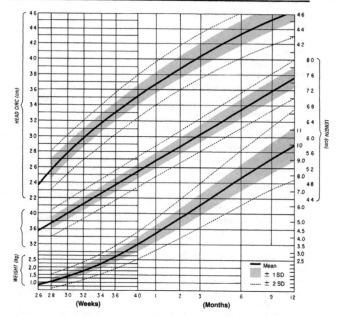

Figure 17. Fetal and infant head circumference, weight, and length. (From Babson SG, Benda GI. *J Pediatrics.* 1976;89:814.)

E. **Craniosynostosis:**
1. **H&P:** Deformed skull, firm pressure on either side of affected suture fails to cause movement. Look for other facial or body dysmorphisms; developmental delay.
2. **Causes:** Premature fusion of sutures, failure of brain growth. Little evidence that it can be caused by shunting for hydrocephalus.
   a. **Sagittal synostosis:** Most common type, has long, boat-shaped skull with keel-like ridge.
   b. **Coronal synostosis:** If unilateral, affected forehead is flat or concave, and normal eye falsely appears to bulge. Can cause amblyopia.
      1) **Crouzon's syndrome:** Coronal synostosis plus midface hypoplasia. Hydrocephalus is rare.
      2) **Apert's syndrome:** Coronal synostosis plus syndactyly. Hydrocephalus is common.
   c. **Metopic synostosis:** Pointed forehead with midline ridge. Often with 19p chromosome abnormality and mental retardation.
   d. **Lambdoid synostosis:** Flattened occiput. If unilateral, causes rhomboid skull with bulging ipsilateral forehead.

3. **DDx:** "Lazy lambdoid syndrome" (positional flattening from decreased mobility), congenital torticollis (causing baby to always lie on same side).
4. **Rx:** Surgery.

F. **Hydrocephalus:**
   1. **H&P of active hydrocephalus:**
      a. **Hydrocephalus before cranial sutures close:** Cranium grows faster than face does, bulging fontanelles, irritability, N/V, poor head control, engorged scalp veins, Macewen's sign (cracked pot sound when percussing over dilated ventricles), 6th nerve palsy, upgaze palsy (see Dorsal midbrain lesion, p. 48), hyperactive reflexes, apneic spells.
      b. **Hydrocephalus after cranial sutures close:** Headache, papilledema, N/V, ataxia, 6th nerve palsy, upgaze palsy.
      c. **Entrapped 4th ventricle:** Sometimes seen with chronic shunting of lateral ventricles after infections. Headache, lower cranial nerve palsies, decreased alertness, ataxia, N/V.
   2. **Differential diagnosis of hydrocephalus:** Macrocrania (from rickets, chronic hemolysis, osteopetrosis), megalencephaly, hydranencephaly, benign external hydrocephalus (asymptomatic enlargement of subarachnoid space, with large head size).
   3. **Causes of hydrocephalus:** Either noncommunicating (obstructive) or communicating (decreased absorption or, rarely, increased production of CSF). Hemorrhage may cause hydrocephalus by either mechanism.
      a. **Congenital** (70%): Chiari II malformation, aqueductal stenosis, Dandy-Walker malformation, X-linked hydrocephalus.
      b. **Hemorrhagic** (15%): Postintraventricular, postsubarachnoid. Common in premature infants.
      c. **Mass lesion** (11%): Often tumors around the aqueduct, e.g., medulloblastoma. Colloid cyst can intermittently block foramen of Monro. Because there is no gray-white differentiation in infants, it is easy to miss small amounts of edema.
      d. **Postinfectious** (8%): Purulent or basilar meningitis, cysticercosis.

HEADACHE

A. **See also:** Adult Headache, p. 52; Concussion, p. 119; Ophthalmoplegic migraine, p. 136.
B. **H&P:** How much school is missed? Does the HA stop pt from playing or watching TV? Visual changes? Very young children may have only paroxysmal vomiting with or without paroxysmal vertigo. Check for stiff neck, papilledema, head circumference, tooth and ear infection, cerebral bruits (common, but should not be asymmetric), heart murmur.
C. **Causes:** See p. 52. In very young children, consider also occipital seizures (rare).
D. **Tests:** No need for MRI in pts with stable recurrent HA >6 mo and normal neuro exam including fundi.

E. Rx of migraine: Similar to adults.

  1. Acute rx: Consider an NSAID + promethazine (Phenergan) 1 mg/kg PO. Sumatriptan has been safely used in school-aged children; divide the dose in half for smaller ones.

  2. Prophylaxis: For children with >2-3 significant HAs/mo. Try propranolol 0.5-1.0 mg/kg bid (asthma, DM, and depression are contraindications) or cyproheptadine 2-4 mg PO bid-tid. Consider also nortriptyline (monitor serum level and QT interval) or valproate 15-45 mg/kg/d age 7-16; 500-1,000 mg/d age 9-17.

INFECTIONS, CNS

A. Meningitis: See also meningitis in adults, p. 56.

  1. H&P: Irritability or somnolence, fever, cyanosis, high-pitched cry, poor feeding, sometimes a bulging fontanelle or seizures. Before 1 yr of age, there is usually no meningismus; after that, you may see HA, stiff neck, Kernig's or Brudzinski's sign. Look for rash, mouth or ear lesions.

  2. DDx: Mass lesion, including abscess, toxic exposure. . .

  3. Tests: CBC, electrolytes, blood cultures. LP, usually with prior head CT. See Table 3, p. 19, for CSF findings. Never delay empiric Abx; LP can be done up to 2 h after first dose without destroying culture results.

  4. Rx:

   a. Empiric Abx: These suggestions are heavily influenced by vaccine use and do not apply outside the United States. Adjust on basis of culture and sensitivities.

Patient	Likely Pathogen	Antibiotic
<1 mo	*S. agalactiae, E. coli, L. monocytogenes, Klebsiella*	Ampicillin + (cefotaxime or aminoglycoside)
1 mo-2 yr[1]	*S. pneumo., H. influenzae, E. coli, N. meningitides, L. monocytogenes*	Vancomycin + (ceftriaxone or cefotaxime)
2–50 yr[1]	*N. meningitidis, S. pneumo.*	Vancomycin + (ceftriaxone or cefotaxime)
Head trauma, surgery, shunt	*Staph*, gram-neg. bacilli, or pneumococcus	Vancomycin + (cefepime, ceftazidime, or meropenem)

[1] Most infants and children need only vancomycin unless gram stain has gram-negative bacilli.

Table 40. Empiric antibiotics for pediatric meningitis. (Adapted from Tunkel AR, et al. *Clin Infect Dis.* 2004;39:1267–1284.)

   b. Respiratory precautions if you suspect *N. meningitidis*.

   c. Dexamethasone: 20 min before, or at least with, the first Abx dose, at 0.15 mg/kg every 6 h for 2-4 d, or until pathogen determined. Helps *H. influenzae* primarily. No point in starting it after the first dose of Abx.

B. TORCH infections: Acronym for the major nonbacterial infections of neonates: <u>T</u>oxoplasmosis, <u>O</u>thers (especially syphilis), <u>R</u>ubella, <u>C</u>ytomegalovirus, and <u>H</u>erpes simplex. All are acquired transplacentally except herpes, which the fetus catches in the birth canal.

  1. Toxoplasmosis:
    a. H&P: Signs of diffuse cortical and subcortical lesions. Cataracts, microphthalmia. Sometimes liver, marrow, lung, muscle, and heart problems.
    b. Tests: Cerebral cortex and periventricular necrosis and calcification on CT; watch for hydrocephalus. *Toxoplasma*-specific IgM is often negative. CSF may show lymphocytosis, high protein, and trophozoites.
    c. Rx: Spiramycin, pyrimethamine, and sulfadiazine to infected mother and baby during the first year. Infected infants are highly infectious.

  2. Rubella: Congenital rubella syndrome occurs when the fetus is infected <20 wk gestation.
    a. Mild cases: Normal at birth, then show CNS and ocular deficits, deafness, and heart dz.
    b. Severe cases: Low birth weight, liver failure, petechiae, cataracts, deafness, heart dz, microcephaly, bone lesions, and low platelets.
    c. Tests: Viral culture of throat and urine. Serum rubella IgM.
    d. Rx: Symptomatic.

  3. Cytomegalovirus:
    a. H&P: Only 10% of infected newborns are symptomatic at birth (liver failure, petechiae, microcephaly, periventricular calcifications, chorioretinitis). Of the 90% who are asymptomatic, 10% will later get deafness or microcephaly.
    b. Tests: Urine culture.

  4. Herpes simplex: Maternal hx may be absent for newborns since mother sheds virus before lesions are visible.
    a. H&P: Local oral or ophthalmic lesions (both may be <u>absent</u>), meningitis, or disseminated HSV with hepatosplenomegaly, DIC, renal failure, and encephalitis.
    b. Tests: CSF is consistent with viral meningitis, and CSF HSV PCR+. Throat, urine, and stool cultures.
    c. Rx: 14 days of acyclovir, 60 mg/kg/d, div tid for neonates. Do not wait for culture results to start.

METABOLIC DISEASES

A. See also: Progressive developmental delay, p. 132.

B. H&P: Progressive neurological deterioration with recurrent unexplained ataxia, spasticity, altered consciousness, vomiting, acidosis; or mental retardation in the absence of major congenital brain abnormalities.

C. Tests: Electrolytes, glucose, ABG, ammonia, lactate, urine ketones, urine colorimetric tests (ferric chloride, DNPH, reducing substances, nitroprusside, CTAB Berry spot). Consider carnitine, serum and urine amino acids, urine organic acids, ferritin glycosylation, full ophthalmologic exam, CT or MRI, skeletal films for bone age and defects, lysosomal enzyme studies, tissue biopsy.

1. **Isolated ketosis:** Suggests maple syrup urine dz.
2. **Ketosis and acidosis:** Organic acidopathy, lactate/pyruvate disorders.
3. **Lactic acidosis:** Lactate/pyruvate or mitochondrial disorders; hypoxia, sepsis, liver or renal failure, DM.
4. **Hyperammonemia:** Urea cycle disorders (without ketosis), organic acidopathies, Reye's syndrome, liver failure.
5. **No ketosis, acidosis, or hyperammonemia:** Nonketotic hyperglycinemia, sulfite oxidase deficiency; peroxisomal, lysosomal, or fatty acid disorders.

D. **Causes:** The entries below focus on disorders for which prompt rx is essential.

E. **Abetalipoproteinemia** (Bassen-Kornzweig dz): Infants have steatorrhea, ataxia, retardation, retinitis pigmentosa, low cholesterol, acanthocytes. Responds to vitamin E and special diet.

F. **Aminoacidurias:**
   1. **Homocystinuria:** Autosomal recessive defect in cystathionine synthase causes accumulation of sulfur metabolites.
      a. **H&P:** Normal at birth. The neurological sx are from strokes. Frequently mentally retarded, with psychiatric disorders. Also see skin and eye problems. Adult heterozygotes are also at risk for strokes.
      b. **Rx:** Pyridoxine (B_6) 250-1,000 mg qd, and a methionine-restricted diet supplemented with cystine and betaine.
   2. **Maple syrup urine dz:** Autosomal recessive defect in branched-chain amino acid metabolism (valine, leucine, isoleucine).
      a. **H&P:** Normal at birth; sweet-smelling urine. Within a week, get opisthotonos, intermittent increased muscle tone, irregular breathing. If untreated, severe retardation and spasticity; may die in infancy.
      b. **Tests:** Ferric chloride test on urine; serum amino acids.
      c. **Rx:** Diet restricted in branched-chain amino acids. If started in first 2 wk of life, most children develop normally. However, they are vulnerable to sepsis.
   3. **Phenylketonuria:** Autosomal recessive defect of phenylalanine hydroxylase (converts phenylalanine to tyrosine)
      a. **H&P:** Normal at birth, vomiting and irritability by 2 mo, mental retardation by 4-9 mo; later seizures and imperfect hair pigmentation.
      b. **Rx:** Phenylalanine-restricted diet. If started early, children develop normally.
   4. **Nonketotic hyperglycinemia:** Autosomal recessive defect in glycine processing.
      a. **H&P:** Severe early seizures sometimes associated with gyral abnormalities, agenesis of corpus callosum, cerebellar hypoplasia.
      b. **Tests:** CSF to plasma glycine ratios.
      c. **Rx:** Benzoate and dextromethorphan.

G. **Hyperammonemias:** Major causes include neonatal asphyxia, severe liver dz, drugs (e.g., valproic acid), urea cycle disorders, organic acidurias, lactic acidoses, and dibasic aminoacidurias.
   1. **Rx:** Arginine, sodium benzoate, phenylacetate, dialysis, and low-protein diet.

H. Leukodystrophies: Defects in myelin metabolism, usually lysosomal or peroxisomal, causing white matter dz and peripheral neuropathy. See below.

I. Lysosomal enzyme disorders: Glycoprotein degradation disorders, mucolipidoses, mucopolysaccharidoses, sphingolipidoses.

   1. Krabbe's leukodystrophy (globoid cell): Galactocerebrosidase deficiency. Onset in infancy, with irritability, hypertonia and opisthotonos, vision and hearing loss, seizures, $\pm$ peripheral neuropathy. Death in 2-3 yr.

   2. Metachromatic leukodystrophy: Arylsulfatase A deficiency. Infant to adult onset. May be spastic or flaccid. Severe peripheral neuropathy and CSF protein elevation. Also dementia, ataxia, optic atrophy.

   3. Others: Niemann-Pick's, Gaucher's, Tay-Sachs, GM1 gangliosidosis, Fabry's, Hurler's. . . .

J. Peroxisomal disorders:

   1. Zellweger's syndrome (cerebrohepatorenal syndrome): Reduced or absent peroxisomes. Severe hypotonia, seizures, developmental delay, liver failure, and early death.

   2. Adrenoleukodystrophy (ALD):

      a. Neonatal ALD and infantile Refsum's dz are milder variants of Zellweger's syndrome, above. N-ALD pts benefit from docosahexaenoic acid.

      b. X-linked ALD: Buildup of very long–chain fatty acids. Childhood onset form starts with ADHD, progresses to seizures, dementia, ataxia, death. Adult onset form (adrenomyeloneuropathy) causes progressive spastic paraparesis, sphincter trouble, and adrenal insufficiency.

K. Others: E.g., metabolism of carbohydrate, glycoprotein, lipid, or purine; mucopolysaccharidoses, mucolipidoses; mitochondrial defects; endocrine defects.

   1. Galactosemia: Autosomal recessive defect in galactose-1-uridyltransferase.

      a. H&P: Usually normal at birth. First week: listlessness, jaundice, vomiting, diarrhea, no weight gain. Second week: hypotonia, cataracts, hepatosplenomegaly. Untreated infants get mental retardation and die of cirrhosis.

      b. Tests: Reducing substances in the urine; erythrocyte transferase activity.

      c. Rx: Lactose-free diet. Most treated infants have a normal IQ but visual-perceptual defects.

   2. Hypothyroidism:

      a. H&P: Postterm, macrosomy, jaundiced, large fontanelles, skin mottling, listless, big belly, umbilical hernia. By age 2 mo: hypotonic, grunting cry, wide-open sutures. Later: mental retardation, deafness, and spasticity.

      b. Rx: Thyroid replacement. Even with early rx, pts usually have learning and cerebellar disorders.

   3. Mitochondrial disorders: See p. 72.

   4. Neuronal ceroid lipofuscinosis:

      a. Sx: Myoclonic seizures, ataxia/extrapyramidal abnormalities, visual loss (except in adult onset).

    b. Cause: Encoded by different gene with variable ages of onset.
    c. Dx: Skin biopsy and/or genetics.
  5. Congenital disorders of glycosylation.
  6. Pyridoxine (B_6) dependency: Can cause neonatal seizures that respond only to pyridoxine.

MOVEMENT DISORDERS AND ATAXIA

A. See also: Adult Movement Disorders and Ataxia, p. 74.
B. Ataxia:
  1. Acute or intermittent:
    a. Cerebellitis: Usually postviral, especially varicella and EBV. CSF shows mild lymphocytosis. Usually resolves completely.
    b. Intoxication: DPH, lead, alcohol, thallium. . . .
    c. Occult neuroblastoma: Usually with opsoclonus-myoclonus. Thought to be paraneoplastic.
    d. Metabolic disorders: Including maple syrup urine dz, Hartnup's dz, pyruvate decarboxylase deficiency, arginosuccinic aciduria, hypothyroidism.
    e. Paroxysmal disorders: Seizure, migraine, benign positional vertigo, familial episodic ataxia.
    f. Other: Guillain-Barré syndrome, posterior fossa hemorrhage or stroke, multiple sclerosis.
  2. Progressive ataxia:
    a. Congenital malformations: Aplasias, Dandy-Walker, Chiari.
    b. Hereditary degeneration:
      1) Spinocerebellar ataxias: Besides ataxia, there are often neuropathies, absent DTRs, weakness, and other organ system involvement, depending on the syndrome; See Table 18.
      2) Ataxia-telangiectasia syndrome: A defect in DNA repair causing ataxia, telangiectasias, infections, and tumors.
      3) Abetalipoproteinemia (Bassen-Kornzweig syndrome): Treat with vitamin E.
      4) Other: Leukodystrophy, mitochondrial dz. . . .
    c. Posterior fossa tumors: See HA, vomiting (especially if early AM, not preceded by nausea), cranial nerve abnormalities, papilledema, meningismus.
    d. Vitamin deficiencies: E.g., E, B_{12}.
C. Chorea: Causes include Sydenham's dz, Wilson's dz, Huntington's dz, hyperthyroidism, vasculitis, basal ganglia tumors or strokes, estrogens, pregnancy, kernicterus, pantothenate kinase–associated neurodegeneration (PKAN, née Hallervorden-Spatz dz; see eponym rant, p. 28.)
  1. Sydenham's chorea: Poststreptococcal, in association with rheumatic fever, often after other sx have resolved. Often with emotional lability and OCD. Check antistreptolysin O titer. Pt should get prophylactic penicillin until adulthood because 1/3 will develop valvular dz.
  2. Wilson's dz: Autosomal recessive, copper builds up in liver and basal ganglia.
    a. H&P: Usually childhood onset. Cirrhosis, corneal Kayser-Fleischer rings, personality changes, and extrapyramidal sx including tremor, ataxia, dysarthria, and dystonia.

    b. Tests: Low serum ceruloplasmin, high urine copper, abnormal LFTs, subcortical and brainstem changes on CT or MRI.

    c. Rx: D-penicillamine 250–500 mg PO qid. Pyridoxine supplements. Side effects include transient decline of neurological function, allergic sensitivity, nephrotic syndrome, a lupus-like syndrome, low platelets, myasthenia, and Goodpasture's syndrome.

D. Dystonia: See also causes of chorea, above, and adult dystonia, p. 76.

    1. Drug effect: E.g., from neuroleptic or antiemetic.

    2. Idiopathic torsion dystonia (dystonia musculorum deformans): Onset usually age 5-15, with action dystonia of one foot that then spreads. Often mistaken for hysteria. Often autosomal dominant, from the DYT-1 gene. Rx: high-dose anticholinergics or deep brain stimulation.

    3. Dopa-responsive dystonia: Autosomal dominant, incomplete penetrance. Worsens throughout day, improves with sleep. Responds to levodopa.

E. Tics: Common in normal 6- to 9-year-olds. Tourette's syndrome is motor and vocal tics for more than 1 yr without interruption; often with ADHD, OCD, echolalia, coprolalia (uncommon, strong family history). For motor tics, consider clonidine or pimozide. For OCD, use high-dose fluoxetine.

NEUROCUTANEOUS SYNDROMES

	Neurofibromatosis Type I	Neurofibromatosis Type II
Incidence	1/3000	1/30,000
Onset of sx	Early childhood	Adolescence or adulthood
First sx	Café-au-lait spots, freckling	8th nerve problems
Acoustic tumors	Almost never bilateral	Hallmark of NF2
Typical tumors	Neurofibromas, astrocytomas	Schwannomas, meningiomas
Nontumor sx	Macrocephaly, low IQ, bone dz	Retinal dz, juvenile cataracts
Typical spine sx	Scoliosis, syringomyelia	Intradural tumors, syringomyelia
Screening MRIs?	Less useful	To catch schwannomas early
Malignancy risk	NFS, leukemia, pheo	No
Inheritance	Chromosome 17, dominant	Chromosome 22, dominant
Severity	Wide variation within a family	Consistent within a family

Table 41. Distinguishing NF1 and NF2.

A. Neurofibromatosis Type I (von Recklinghausen's dz):

    1. H&P: Family history of NF1; café-au-lait spots, neurofibromas, axillary or inguinal freckling, optic glioma, iris (Lisch) nodules, typical osseous lesion (thoracic scoliosis, anterolateral tibia bowing, pseudoarthrosis, sphenoid wing dysplasia).

    2. Tests: MRIs for symptoms; screening MRIs less useful.

    3. Rx: Surgery for symptomatic lesions.

B. Neurofibromatosis Type II:

    1. H&P: Acoustic schwannomas (usually bilateral, and before age 30), café-au-lait spots, posterior lens opacities, family history of NF2.

No Lisch nodules; not associated with seizures, mental retardation, or macrocephaly.

    2. Tests: Screening MRI can detect acoustic tumors early.

    3. Rx: Resect acoustic schwannomas before they cause deafness.

C. Tuberous sclerosis: Autosomal dominant gene on either chromosome 9 or 11, very variable expression. Many spontaneous mutations.

    1. H&P: Characteristic triad of seizures, retardation, and facial adenofibromas (misnamed adenoma sebaceum). See also hypomelanotic macules, shagreen patches (connective tissue hamartomas). Family history. Heart, pulmonary, and kidney tumors are often silent.

    2. Tests: MRI of head shows focal cortical dysplasias (tubers) and subependymal nodules. Renal, cardiac, and pulmonary screening.

    3. Rx: Steroids or vigabatrin for infantile spasms, ACDs for seizures; resect intraventricular tumors causing hydrocephalus.

D. Sturge-Weber syndrome (encephalotrigeminal angiomatosis): Chromosome 3 defect, causes vascular port-wine nevus on face (usually in V1 distribution), contralateral hemiparesis and field cut, ipsilateral glaucoma, seizures, retardation.

E. Incontinentia pigmenti (Bloch-Sulzberger syndrome) and hypomelanosis of Ito: Erythema/bolus lesions only in girl (X-linked dominant) and hypopigmented lesions, respectively. Both in dermatome distribution and associated with seizures, microcephaly, and mental retardation.

F. Von Hippel-Lindau dz: Dominant gene defect on chromosome 3. Not really a neurocutaneous disorder, but we had to stick it somewhere.

    1. H&P: Sx of hemangioblastomas, usually in posterior fossa, in second to fourth decade. Also see retinal hemangiomas, renal cell carcinomas, pheochromocytomas.

    2. Rx: Early surgery for cerebral or spinal cord tumors, laser or cryosurgery for retinal tumors, frequent screening exams.

SEIZURES

A. See also: Adult Seizures, p. 108.

B. Status epilepticus: A medical emergency. See p. 108.

C. H&P: Ask about birth history, maternal illnesses, precipitating factors, fever, skin color changes, movements, family history. Try to get parents to videotape an episode. Thorough skin and physical exam.

D. Tests:

    1. EEG: Baseline rhythms change dramatically with age. Many pts with epilepsy have normal EEGs. Sleep EEGs help; if necessary, give chloral hydrate 50 mg/kg PO, max. 1,000 mg. Consider continuous video-EEG monitoring.

    2. Tests: Glucose, electrolytes, Ca, Mg, UA. In newborns and infants, consider ammonia, lactate, pH, metabolic screens.

    3. Head scans: Intracranial ultrasound in newborns to rule out hemorrhage. CT in acute workups. MRI for structural detail.

E. Neonatal seizures:
1. **Sx during seizures:** Seizures in newborns are poorly organized and multifocal. Look for eye deviations, repetitive movements, tonic stiffening, apnea.
   a. **Premature infants:** Apnea and bradycardia may be the only sign.
   b. **Intubated, chemically paralyzed infants:** Sudden blood pressure changes may be the only sign.
2. **DDx:** Benign jitteriness, benign sleep myoclonus, nonconvulsive apnea, normal movement, opisthotonos (back arching from meningitis or brain injury), hyperekplexia (genetically exaggerated startle reflex causes transient stiffness).
3. **Causes of neonatal seizures:** The time frames are approximate.
   a. **First 72 h of life:** Hypoxic-ischemic encephalopathy, cerebral hemorrhage, bacterial meningitis, TORCH infection, cerebral dysgenesis, drug withdrawal, hyperammonemia, hypoglycemia, hypocalcemia, effect of local anesthetic, pyridoxine dependency. Rarely from inborn errors of metabolism.
   b. **After 72 h:** Cerebral hemorrhage, infection, hypocalcemia, inborn errors of metabolism, herpes simplex encephalitis, stroke, cerebral dysgenesis, kernicterus, benign familial neonatal seizures. Rarely from hypoxic injury.
4. **Rx of neonatal seizures:** Correct electrolyte abnormalities. If no hypoglycemia (<30mg/ml), give:
   a. **Phenobarbital** Load 15 mg/kg IV; may repeat to a total load of 40 mg/kg. Monitor SBP and breathing. Maintenance is 3-5 mg/kg qd IV or PO.
   b. **DPH:** A second-line agent. Poorly absorbed PO in infants. Load 10 mg/kg IV $\times$ 2. Monitor cardiac rhythm. Maintenance 5 mg/kg qd.
   c. **Pyridoxine?** Severe, refractory seizures in infancy may be pyridoxine dependent. Test with pyridoxine 100 mg IV $\times$ 2; EEG usually improves within minutes. Can become apneic during test. Rx pyridoxine 10-30 mg/kg/d.
F. Infantile seizures (1 mo-2 yr):
1. **DDx:** Apnea, migraine (can present as paroxysmal vertigo), paroxysmal dystonia, benign myoclonus, cyanotic syncope (usually triggered by anger or fear), pallid syncope (usually triggered by sudden pain). Both types of syncope can be associated with tonic/clonic movements.
2. **Simple febrile seizures:** Seizure lasts <15 min, single occurrences in 24 h, febrile illness, nonfocal seizure and exam.
   a. **Relation to nonfebrile seizures:** Febrile seizures are seen in 4% of children; only 2% of those will have epilepsy. Features that suggest epilepsy: neurodevelopmental abnormality, focal seizure, family history.
   b. **Tests and rx:** Unnecessary unless the seizure is focal, prolonged, or leaves residual deficits. Prophylactic acetaminophen and prn rectal diazepam may help.
3. **Nonfebrile seizures:** Causes are similar in infants and children; *see next section. The following are types of seizures that present between 1 mo and 2 yr.

- **a. Infantile spasms:** AKA West's syndrome.
  - **1) H&P:** Onset is always before 1 yr. See brief myoclonic extensor or flexor spasms (salaam movements), sometimes mistaken for colic. "Symptomatic" spasms are those with known cause; "cryptogenic" spasms are idiopathic.
  - **2) EEG:** Usually shows interictal hypsarrhythmia (chaotic, very high–voltage slow waves and spikes) or ictal burst-suppression pattern. If high suspicion and normal interictal EEG, do long-term monitoring.
  - **3) Rx:** ACTH, especially in cryptogenic cases (in which the ACTH toxicity is justified because the prognosis is slightly better). In symptomatic cases, where prognosis is poor, consider clonazepam.
- **b. Myoclonic epilepsy:** May be benign or severe.
  - **1) H&P:** Brief seizures, no LOC, vary from head nodding to sudden leg flexion and fall (with arms flung up and out). In severe myoclonic epilepsy, there is developmental delay and progressive ataxia and hyperreflexia.
  - **2) EEG:** 3-Hz spike-wave in benign myoclonic epilepsy; >3-Hz polyspike-wave in severe myoclonic epilepsy.
  - **3) Rx:** Valproic acid 15 mg/kg qd divided bid. Watch closely for hepatotoxicity. Avoid carbamazepine, lamotrigine.
- **c. Biotinidase deficiency.**

G. Childhood seizures:

1. **DDx:** Migraine, syncope, hyperventilation, narcolepsy-cataplexy, night terrors, startle dz (hyperekplexia), pseudoseizures, daydreaming.
2. **Generalized tonic-clonic seizures:** The most common type.
   - **a. H&P:** See p. 109.
   - **b. Causes:** Traumatic hypoxic or ischemic brain injury, CNS infection, cerebral dysgenesis, metabolic abnormality, drug or toxin effect, drug withdrawal.
   - **c. Rx:** No need to start ACDs after a single seizure in an otherwise normal child. Phenobarbital (5 mg/kg qd), DPH (5 mg/kg qd; poorly absorbed in infants), and carbamazepine (load slowly to 15 mg/kg qd) are equally effective for recurrent seizures.
3. **Simple partial seizures:**
   - **a. H&P:** Focal movement or dysfunction, often with subsequent secondary generalization.
   - **b. Causes:** Benign centrotemporal or occipital epilepsy is the most common cause; see below. Any focal lesion, most often a neuronal migration disorder, mass, neurocysticercosis.
   - **c. Benign centrotemporal (rolandic) epilepsy:** Genetic.
     - **1) H&P:** Onset usually age 5-10; stop before age 14. Seizure usually occurs during sleep and wakes the child with mouth paresthesias and twitching for 1-2 min. Usually no LOC. Seizures sometimes spread to the arm or generalize.
     - **2) EEG:** Interictal uni- or bilateral centrotemporal spikes, enhanced in sleep.
     - **3) Rx:** Usually unnecessary.
   - **d. Benign occipital epilepsy:** Probably genetic.

     1) **H&P:** Onset usually age 4-8; stop before age 12. Seizure usually has visual changes, often followed by migraine-like headache or nausea. Often induced by sleep-wake transition, photic stimulation, or video games.

     2) **EEG:** Interictal 2-Hz uni- or bilateral occipital spike-wave, inhibited by eye opening.

     3) **Rx:** Standard ACDs are usually successful.

4. **Complex partial seizures:** See p. 110.

5. **Myoclonic seizures:** See p. 149.

6. **Absence seizures:**

    a. H&P: Onset 3-12 yr. Attacks last 5-10 sec, up to $100 \times$ qd. The child stares vacantly, sometimes with rhythmic eyelid movement; some have automatisms. No aura or postical confusion. Absence status can cause confusion. 50% of pts. with absence will also have at least one generalized seizure.

    b. Cause: Autosomal dominant gene, age-dependent penetrance.

    c. EEG: Bilateral synchronous 3-Hz spike-wave during the seizure. Can be triggered by hyperventilation.

    d. Rx: Ethosuximide, initial dose 20 mg/kg qd divided tid. Or valproate.

7. **Landau-Kleffner syndrome:**

    a. H&P: Onset age 2-11 yr. Usually starts with selective word deafness or seizures (partial or generalized), followed by autistic personality changes.

    b. Cause: Unknown, except in rare cases of temporal lobe tumor. Hard to tell from autism, which may also have abnormal EEG.

    c. EEG: Multifocal parietal and temporal spikes. Sometimes associated with electrical status epilepticus of sleep (ESES), with seizures during >80% of sleep.

    d. Rx: ACDs help the seizures but not aphasia. Early steroids may cause remission of aphasia and seizures. Some use high-dose oral diazepam for ESES.

8. **Lennox-Gastaut syndrome:**

    a. H&P: Seizures (atypical absence, atonic, and myoclonic) and mental retardation. Onset usually at age 1–5 yr. May follow infantile spasms.

    b. Causes: Usually from neurocutaneous disorder, peri- or postnatal brain injury.

    c. EEG: Slow (1-2.5 Hz) spike-wave complexes.

    d. Rx: Valproate, benzodiazepines, felbamate.

SOCIAL AND LANGUAGE DISORDERS

A. Autism: One of the pervasive developmental disorders.

    1. **H&P:** Usually normal early milestones, early language development followed by regression at age 1-2 yr. The classic triad is poor language, poor social interaction, and restricted or repetitive behavior and interests (abnormal imitative play, stereotyped movements such as whirling, rocking). Motor skills and memory may be normal.

    2. **Tests:** Audiology, EEG. Imaging usually not indicated.

    3. **Rx:** Behavioral therapy.

4. **Syndromes with prominent autistic features:**
   a. **Fragile X syndrome:** Most common cause of mental retardation. See also dysmorphic facies, macro-orchidism after puberty, hyperactivity. 1/3 of female heterozygotes are also mildly retarded.
   b. **Angelman syndrome** ("happy puppet" syndrome): Same 15q gene deletion as Prader-Willi syndrome, but of the maternal, not paternal, chromosome. Infant feeding problems, severe retardation, autism, microcephaly, jerky puppet-like ataxia, paroxysmal laughter, protruding tongue. By contrast, Prader-Willi syndrome has severe floppiness at birth; dysmorphic, mental retardation, later hyperphagia, hypogonadism, Pickwickian syndrome.
   c. **Rett syndrome:** Idiopathic syndrome seen only in girls, in which autism is associated with progressive microcephaly, ataxia, breathing irregularities, seizures, scoliosis, spasticity, and dystonia.
   d. **Others:** Tuberous sclerosis, TORCH infections, phenylketonuria.
B. **Attention-deficit/hyperactivity disorder:**
   1. **H&P:** Birth history, milestones. School performance: get detailed records. Are behavior problems limited to one domain? Staring spells? Family history of learning disability, stress, or substance abuse?
   2. **Tests:** Use DSM-IV criteria or Conners' Motor Overactivity Scale.
   3. **Rx:** Methylphenidate 5 mg PO qAM, titrate up. Alternatives are dextroamphetamine and pemoline (watch LFTs on the latter). All can cause nausea, anorexia, insomnia, rebound hyperactivity. Tics may worsen.
C. **Dyslexia:**
   1. **H&P:** Family history of dyslexia or left-handedness. Selective difficulty reading and writing with intact visuospatial, mathematical, and memory abilities.
   2. **Rx:** Individualized educational intervention. Experimental rx targets the visual and auditory processing defects.

TUMORS

A. **See also adult sections:** Tumors of Brain, p. 120, and Spinal Cord Disorders, p. 113.
B. **XRT in children:** Causes IQ loss and is usually avoided in pts <3 yrs.
C. **Infratentorial tumors:** The most common pediatric location.
   1. **H&P:** Ataxia, signs of high ICP or hydrocephalus, corticospinal and cranial nerve signs, head tilt.
   2. **Brainstem gliomas:** Malignant. Usually no hydrocephalus until late. Peak incidence age 2-12 yr. Rx: XRT, dexamethasone.
   3. **Cerebellar astrocytoma:** Benign, usually cystic. Rx: Surgery, usually do not need XRT.
   4. **Ependymoma:** Malignant, often on floor of 4th ventricle. Peak incidence 0-4 yr. Early vomiting. Can seed spinal cord. Rx: surgery; high-grade tumors need XRT of head and spine.
   5. **Medulloblastoma:** Malignant, often in vermis, neuronal origin. Peak incidence age 3-6 yr. Can seed spinal cord. Rx: surgery, head and spine XRT, ± chemotherapy.
D. **Supratentorial tumors:** Seizures and hemiparesis are common (vs. infratentorial tumors).

1. **Craniopharyngiomas:** Suprasellar tumor, presents with signs of high ICP, pituitary dysfunction, or visual field deficits. Rx: surgery and XRT; prognosis relatively good.
2. **Gliomas:** Rx of cerebral gliomas depends on the grade of the tumor. Rarely, children age 0-4 yr present with weight loss despite a voracious appetite caused by a hypothalamic glioma.
3. **Optic gliomas** present with poor vision, strabismus, exophthalmos, optic atrophy, or papilledema. Surgery vs. XRT is controversial; rx is sometimes conservative. Often associated with neurofibromatosis.
4. **Primitive neuroectodermal tumors (PNETs):** Pathology similar to medulloblastoma. Often presents in pts <3 yr. Rx: XRT of head and spine ± chemotherapy.

E. **Intracranial metastases:** Rare in children, except from leukemia or lymphoma.
   1. **Leukemic infiltration of the meninges:** Pts present with headache, papilledema, diplopia. To prevent this, methotrexate and XRT of head and spine are usually given during hematological remission; this can cause an encephalopathy.
   2. **Intracranial hemorrhage:** From low platelets; not seen in lymphoma.
   3. **CNS infection:** If peripheral white counts are low, CSF may not show lymphocytosis.

WEAKNESS

A. **See also:** Adult Neuromuscular Disorders, p. 80, Adult Weakness, p. 129. The following focuses on static or progressive weakness. Acute weakness suggests vascular event or trauma. Subacute weakness suggests tumor, infection. If onset was prenatal, there is often arthrogryposis, dislocated hips.

B. **Hypertonia vs. hypotonia:**
   1. **Hypertonic infants:** From CNS damage. May be hypotonic first.
      a. **Static hypertonia:** Usually cerebral palsy or a perinatal event.
      b. **Progressive hypertonia:** Can be a mass lesion or metabolic dz.
   2. **Hypotonic infants:** From CNS trauma or vascular lesions, genetic dz, mitochondrial dz, congenital hypomyelination syndrome, myasthenia, benign central hypotonia, spinal muscular atrophy, congenital myopathies and dystrophies. Specific causes discussed below.

C. **Upper motor neuron hypotonia:** See Developmental delay, p. 132. CNS hypotonia in infants usually has decreased tone with relatively preserved strength, in contrast to peripheral causes. CNS hypotonia progresses to hypertonia and spasticity.

D. **Lower motor neuron dz:**
   1. **H&P:** Weakness, hypotonia, areflexia, fasciculations.
   2. **Tests:** CPK, NCS, EMG; consider genetic tests, e.g., for spinal muscular atrophy.
   3. **DDx:**
      a. **NCS normal:**
         1) **Acute:** Polio, Coxsackie, echoviruses.

  2) **Chronic:** Pure anterior horn cell sx suggest spinal muscular atrophies. Additional lethargy suggests organic acidurias. Glycogen on muscle biopsy suggests Pompe's dz.
  b. **NCS very slow:** Do sural nerve biopsy; consider congenital hypomyelinating neuropathy, neuroaxonal dystrophy, infantile neuronal degeneration.

E. **Spinal cord damage:**
  1. **H&P:** Difficult or breech delivery, sensory level, sphincter disturbance.
  2. **Causes:** Trauma can present with hypotonia in newborns. Also consider tumor, hypoxic myelopathy.
    a. **Atlantoaxial dislocation:** From dislocation of C1-2. Presents as acute or slowly progressive quadriplegia.
    b. **Meningocele or spina bifida:** See p. 135.
    c. **Occult spinal dysraphism:** AKA tethered cord syndrome, spina bifida occulta.
      1) **H&P:** Pts present with back pain, bladder trouble, distal weakness or numbness, hemiatrophy, or scoliosis. Look for sacral dimple or lipoma, brisk leg reflexes.
      2) **Tests:** MRI shows a low-lying conus. A conus below L2-3 is always abnormal in children over 5.
      3) **Rx:** Surgery (controversial).
    d. **Syringomyelia:** See Sensory Loss, p. 111.

F. **Peripheral weakness:** Pts. are hyporeflexic with normal mental status.
  1. **Peripheral neuropathy:** Toxic, metabolic, traumatic (e.g., brachial plexus injuries, p. 94), Guillain-Barré syndrome, infectious, congenital hypomyelination syndrome, Charot-Marie-Tooth dz (types 1, 2, 4).
  2. **Neuromuscular junction (NMJ) dz:**
    a. **Botulism:** Infants can get botulism from honey.
    b. **Myasthenia:** Two types:
      1) **Neonatal:** Via transplacental IgG; resolves with time.
      2) **Congenital:** Genetic dz of NMJ; does not resolve with time.
  3. **Myopathy:**
    a. **H&P:** Proximal > distal weakness, reflex loss proportional to weakness, muscle pain, steppage gait, waddle, trouble rising from floor, Gower's sign ("walking" hands up thighs to help straighten torso), atrophy, contractures, sometimes myotonia, family history.
    b. **Tests:** CPK, EMG/NCS, muscle biopsy.
    c. **DDx:**
      1) **CPK markedly high:**
        a) **Inflammatory changes on biopsy:** Dermatomyositis or polymyositis. Gradual onset of weakness, malaise, muscle pain, fever, rash, edema. May cause GI ulcers or infarcts. Treat with high-dose steroids.
        b) **Muscle biopsy dystrophic:** Muscular dystrophy.
          i. **Duchenne's:** Most common. X-linked dystrophin deletion, with onset < age 5, proximal weakness, cardiac and GI involvement.
          ii. **Becker's:** Dystrophin alteration, onset > age 5, milder. Early rx with steroids can slow progression.

        iii. Merosin: Congenital dystrophies have merosin-positive, primary merosin-deficient, and secondary merosin-deficient forms.

  2) CPK normal or mildly high:
    a) Myopathy on EMG and biopsy:
      i. Shoulder and hip weakness worst: Endocrine, genetic, or metabolic myopathies, limb-girdle dystrophy.
      ii. Other muscles involved early: Dystrophies (fascioscapulohumeral, Emery-Dreyfuss, oculopharyngeal).
    b) Myotonia present: Myotonic dystrophy (not present in infants), myotonia congenita, paramyotonia.
    c) Congenital myopathies: Central core, central nuclear, and nemaline (rod) myopathies.
    d) Muscle weakness is intermittent: Hypo- or hyperkalemic periodic paralysis, deficiency of phosphorylase, carnitine-palmital transferase, or phosphofructokinase.
    e) Endocrine causes: Myopathy from thyroid, parathyroid, or adrenal abnormalities (either hyper or hypo).
    d) Rx: Treat specific cause; close respiratory and cardiac follow-up, scoliosis screening.

G. Genetic disorders causing, initially, weakness alone:
Adrenoleukodystrophy, familial spastic paraplegia (a variant of spinocerebellar degeneration), spinomuscular atrophies, Charcot-Marie-Tooth dz, muscular dystrophies, metabolic myopathies, Prader-Willi dz.

H. Benign central hypotonia: Usually mild, often with some gross motor delay. Dx of exclusion.

DRUGS

NOTE: In general, mechanisms and side effects are covered in this section. Indications and choice algorithms are typically covered in the relevant section (e.g., Pain).

ADRENERGIC DRUGS

A. **See also:** ICU Drip, p. 172, for indications and dosing.
B. **Alpha-receptor agents:**
1. **Endogenous ligands:** Epinephrine (E) and norepinephrine (NE) have roughly equal binding to α-receptors. Dopamine (DA) at high doses (>10 μg/kg/min) stimulates α-receptors (as well as β-receptors).
2. **Location of receptors:** Mostly postganglionic sympathetic nervous system.
3. **$Alpha_1$-receptors:** Postsynaptic. Cause vasoconstriction, intestinal relaxation and sphincter constriction, increased heart contractile force, arrhythmias, pupillary dilatation.
   a. **Selective agonists:** Phenylephrine, etc.
   b. **Selective antagonists:** Prazosin, etc. Peripherally acting.
4. **$Alpha_2$-receptors:** Presynaptic and nonneuronal. Cause platelet aggregation, lower insulin secretion; lower NE and acetylcholine release, some vasoconstriction.
   a. **Selective agonists:** Clonidine, dexmedetomidine, etc. Centrally acting. Side effects include dry mouth, dizziness, constipation, low BP.
   b. **Selective antagonists:** Yohimbine, etc.
C. **Beta-receptor agents:**
1. **Non-selective agents:** Isoproterenol is an agonist; propranolol an antagonist, for both β_1- and β_2-receptors. DA at midrange doses (>2 μg/kg/min) stimulates β-receptors much more than α-receptors.
2. **$Beta_1$-receptors:** Cardioselective. Cause increased heart contractile force, HR, AV conduction; renin secretion. E and NE are approximately equipotent.
   a. **Selective agonists:** Dobutamine, etc.
   b. **Selective antagonists:** Metoprolol (low dose), etc.
3. **$Beta_2$-receptors:** Cause vasodilation and bronchodilation, intestinal relaxation. E is more potent than NE.
   a. **Selective agonists:** Albuterol, terbutaline.

ANALGESICS

A. **See also:** Pain, p. 86, for choice of meds.
B. **Acetaminophen:** 650 mg PO/PR q4h prn. Avoid in liver dz.
C. **Anticonvulsants:** Q.v. p. 161. Valproate or carbamazepine may be stronger than Neurontin, lamotrigine, topiramate.
D. **Na channel blockers:** Includes local anesthetics and ACDs.
1. **Carbamazepine, valproate, gabapentin:** See Anticonvulsants, p. 161.

    2. Lidocaine: See also ICU Drips, p. 172. When subcutaneous, epinephrine prolongs its action.

    3. Mexiletine: Check EKG first. Start mexiletine slowly to avoid GI side effects: 150 mg PO qd, then increase slowly to 300 mg tid; check level.

E. Nonsteroidal anti-inflammatory drugs (NSAIDS): For most types of pain; particularly bone pain, inflammation.

    1. Dosing: Ketorolac (Toradol) is the only NSAID that can be given IM; it is quick and effective, although expensive. When it is given PO, it has no more effect than ibuprofen. Ibuprofen PO may work more quickly PO than naproxen, although the latter requires less frequent dosing.

    2. Side effects: In one overall toxicity index, from safest to worst is salsalate > ibuprofen > naproxen > sulindac > piroxicam > fenoprofen > ketoprofen > meclofenamate > tolmectin > indomethacin.

        a. Heart: COX-2 NSAIDS increase MI risk 30%-100%; nonselective NSAIDS about 10%.

        b. CNS: Rebound after NSAID is stopped. Tinnitus with high doses. Rare aseptic meningitis.

            1) On the other hand: NSAIDS may lower the risk of Alzheimer's and Parkinson's.

        c. GI: Nausea, bleeding. Consider checking stool guaiacs; GI prophylaxis, NSAIDS with reportedly fewer GI side effects (e.g., Trilisate), or giving in conjunction with misoprostol.

        d. Antiplatelet: Salsalate (Disalcid) may impair platelets the least.

        e. Renal: Fluid retention, decreased GFR. Can cause acute renal failure in high-catecholamine states. Long-term use can cause interstitial nephritis.

F. Norepinephrine reuptake inhibitors: Analgesic effect is duloxetine ≫ venlafaxine > bupropion. Note: SSRIs have no analgesic effect. Duloxetine seems particularly useful for somatization; see Table 28, p. 105.

G. Opiates: Underutilized for acute (e.g., post-op) pain. In chronic pain, do not confuse physical dependency (withdrawal sx when stopped suddenly) with addiction (escalating dose requirements without other evidence of dz progression).

    1. Dosing:

        a. Longest acting opiates: MS Contin, methadone, levorphanol, fentanyl patch. These are less likely to produce euphoria and dependence than short-acting opiates.

        b. IV drip management: When dose is increased, bolus with the difference, or it may take 12-24 h to reach new steady-state level.

    2. Combination therapy: Adding acetaminophen or an NSAID can decrease the need for opiates, even if they were not effective as single agents.

    3. Overdose:

        a. H&P: Dry mouth, dizziness, constipation, low BP. CNS and respiratory depression with small pupils.

        b. Rx: For respiratory depression, naloxone 2 mg IV; if only altered mental status, can try 0.4-0.8 mg. If pt responds, give additional doses, preferably as continuous drip. Beware of severe withdrawal sx in addicted pts.

  4. **Withdrawal:** From abrupt cessation of heavy prolonged use.
     a. **H&P:** Muscle aches, lacrimation or rhinorrhea, pupillary dilation, sweating, diarrhea, yawning, fever, insomnia.
     b. **Rx:** Clonidine 0.15 mg PO bid, methadone 40 mg PO bid.
  5. **Side effects:** Confusion, hypoventilation, constipation, addiction. Differences in side effects may be folk neurology—hard to prove in controlled trials.
     a. **Analgesic rebound:** Can cause headache when opiate is discontinued, leading to a vicious cycle of dependence.
     b. **Sedation:** Try modafinil or methylphenidate. Sedation dissipates with chronic use.
     c. **Constipation:** Does not improve with chronic use. Put everyone on 2 senna tabs tid, metoclopramide 10 mg tid (only in pts at low risk for movement disorders), colace 100 mg tid. Lactulose or polyethylene glycol (Miralax) is a good bail-out. Oral Narcan can treat opiate-induced ileus: give 2-3 amp PO (or as enema) q4h until bowel movement.
     d. **Seizures and myoclonus** when doses high.
H. **TCAs:** See Antidepressants, p. 164. For neuropathic pain. Third-line for pain because of their many SEs.

Opioid	Comparative Side Effect Profiles (rough)
Morphine, MS Contin (slow release)	Smooth muscle relaxation (cardiac, vascular, GI); respiratory and psychiatric depression; more nausea and itching than hydromorphone
Meperidine (Demerol)	Fast acting, blocks shivering, metabolite buildup lowers seizure threshold, risk of hypotension and cardiac arrest; Vistaril does *not* help the nausea; MAOI interaction
Hydromorphone (Dilaudid), Fentanyl	Very addictive; respiratory depression, increased ICPs, hypotension, myoclonus Patch available; used for sedation in ICU; causes spasm of sphincter of Oddi, urinary retention, constipation, high ICPs, bradyarrhythmias
Oxycodone, Oxycontin (slow release)	Pure agonist opioid; causes constipation, depression, can be ground and abused; similar side effect profile to morphine
Methadone	Mu-receptor agonist; delayed onset, no "high" but still dependence potential; used in heroin detox under supervision, useful for severe chronic pain
Codeine	Very weak for pain relief, mostly used for antitussive properties but some dependence and abuse

Table 41. Rough comparison of opioid side effects.

Narcotic	IM/IV	PO	Action	Narcotic	IM/IV	PO	Action
Butorphanol	2	—	3-4 h	Methadone	10	20	4-6 h
Codeine	120	200	4-6 h	Morphine	10	60	3-7 h
Fentanyl	0.1	—	1-2 h	Nalbuphine	10	—	3-6 h
Hydrocodone	1.5	7.5	4-5 h	Oxycodone	15	30	4-6 h
Hydromorphone	1.5	7.5	4-5 h	Oxymorphone	1	6	3-6 h
Levorphanol	2	4	6-8 h	Pentazocine	30	150	2-3 h
Meperidine	75	300	2-4 h	Propoxyphene	—	130	4-6 h

Table 42. Equivalent narcotic doses, in mg.

ANESTHETICS

A. Lidocaine: See Analgesics, p. 155; ICU Drips, p. 172.
B. Thiopental: 50-mg test dose; then 100-200 mg. Onset 30 sec, lasts 5 min; consciousness returns in 30 min.
C. Propofol: Give 10-20 mg (=1-2 cc) q10sec until induction. Effective in refractory status epilepticus.
D. Methohexital: More potent and shorter action than thiopental. Can induce seizures.

ANGIOTENSIN-CONVERTING ENZYME INHIBITORS

A. Indications: To lower BP by decreased peripheral vascular resistance, with little change in cardiac output, HR, or glomerular filtration rate.
B. Side effects: Raises K. Dangerous in bilateral renal stenosis.

ANTIBIOTICS

A. See also: Infection, p. 212.
B. Neurological SEs of:
   1. **Acyclovir:** May see encephalopathy in association with renal failure, methotrexate, or interferon.
   2. **Aminoglycosides:** Vestibular and ototoxicity, neuromuscular blockade (especially in myasthenia).
   3. **Amphotericin B:** Rare headache, tremor, confusion, akinetic mutism.
   4. **Dideoxynucleosides** (stavudine, didanosine, zalcitabine): Distal symmetrical polyneuropathy.
   5. **Isoniazid:** Seizures, altered mental status, optic neuritis.
   6. **Metronidazole:** Distal axonopathy, psychosis, hallucinations.
   7. **Penicillin derivatives:** Rare myoclonus, asterixis, coma.
   8. **Tetracyclines:** Rare pseudotumor cerebri in infants.
   9. **Vancomycin:** Ototoxicity.
   10. **Zidovudine (AZT):** HA, insomnia, sometimes confusion, seizures, myopathy.

Antibiotic	Normal Dose	Max. Dose in Renal Failure			Dialysis Removes?
		GFR >50	GFR 10-50	GFR <10	
Gentamicin	80 mg IV q8h	1.0-1.7 mg/kg q (8 × serum Cr) h			Yes H+P
Tobramycin	80 mg IV q8h	1.0-1.7 mg/kg q (8 × serum Cr) h			Yes H+P
Amikacin	300 mg q8h	5 mg/kg q (8 × serum Cr) h			Yes H+P
Cefazolin	1 g IV q8h	q8h	bid	qd	Yes H, No P
Cefotaxime	1 g IV q6h	NC	NC	1-2 g bid	Yes H, No P
Cefotetan	1 g IV q12h	NC	1-2 g qd	1 g qd	Yes H
Ceftazidime	1 g IV q8h	NC	1-2 g bid	1 g qd	Yes H+P
Ceftriaxone	1 g IV q24h	NC	NC	NC	No H
Cefuroxime	0.75 g IV q6h	NC	1 g q8h	0.75 g qd	Yes H+P
	0.5 g PO bid	NC	NC	0.25 g qd	—
Cephalexin	0.5 g PO qid	NC	NC	NC	Yes H+P
Cephalothin	1 g IV q4h	1 g q6h	1-2 g q6h	1 g q8h	Yes H+P
Amoxicillin	0.5 g PO tid	NC	0.25 g bid	0.25 g bid	Yes H, No P
Amox.-clav.	0.5 g PO tid	NC	0.25 g bid	0.25 g bid	Yes H, No P
Ampicillin	1 g IV q4h	NC	1 g q8h	1-2 g bid	Yes H, No P
Amp.-sulbact.	3 g IV q6h	NC	1 g bid	1.5-3 g qd	—
Dicloxacillin	0.5 g PO qid	NC	NC	NC	No H+P
Imipen.-cilast.	0.5 g IV q6h	NC	0.25 g q8h	0.2 g bid	Yes H
Mezlocillin	4 g IV q4-6h	NC	2-3 g q6h	2-3 g bid	Yes H, No P
Nafcillin	1.5 g IV q4h	NC	NC	NC	No H,P
Oxacillin	1.5 g IV q4h	NC	NC	NC	No H,P
Penicillin G	2 MU IV q4h	NC	NC	1-2 MU q4h	Yes H, No P
Penicillin VK	0.5 g PO qid	NC	NC	NC	Yes H, No P
Piperacillin	4 g IV q6h	NC	2-4 g q8h	2-4 g bid	Yes H, No P
Piper.-tazobact.	4.5 g IV q6h	NC	2.25 g q6h	2.25 g q8h	Yes H
Ticarcillin	3 g IV q4h	NC	2-3 g q6h	2 g bid	Yes H+P
Ticar.-clavulan.	3.1 g IV q6h	NC	3.1 g q6-8h	2 g bid	Yes H
Ciprofloxacin	0.5 g PO bid	NC	0.25 g bid	0.25 g qd	—
	0.4 g IV q12h	NC	0.4 g q12h	0.4 g q24h	—
Levofloxacin	0.5 g PO/IV qd	NC			—
Ofloxacin	0.4 g PO/IV bid	NC	0.4 g q24h	0.2 g q24h	—
Azithromycin	0.5 g qd	?	?	?	—
Clarithromycin	0.5 g PO bid	?	?	?	—
Erythromycin	0.5 g PO q6h	NC	NC	NC	No H,P
Clindamycin	0.6 g IV q8h	NC	NC	NC	No H,P
	0.3 g PO qid	NC	NC	NC	No H,P
Tetracycline	0.5 g PO qid	0.5 g q8h	Avoid	Avoid	No H,P
Doxycycline	100 mg q12h	NC	NC	NC	No H,P
Aztreonam	1 g IV q8h	NC	NC	1 g IV bid	Yes H+P
Chloramphen	1 g IV/PO q6h	NC	NC	NC	Yes H, No P
Metronidazole	0.5 g IV/PO q6h	NC	NC	NC	Yes H, No P
Nitrofurantoin	50-100 mg q6h	NC	Avoid	Avoid	Yes H
TMP-SMX	DS PO bid	NC	2 mg/kg bid	Avoid	Yes H, No P
Vancomycin	0.5 g IV q6h	1 g q1-3d	Follow levels; redose <10		No H,P

GFR = glomerular filtration rate; H = hemodialysis; P = peritoneal dialysis; NC = no change; MU = million units.

Table 43. Commonly used antibiotics.

ANTICOAGULANTS

A. Contraindications to anticoagulation (relative): Large territory brain infarct, brain tumor, cerebral aneurysm, abdominal aortic aneurysm >6 cm, fever/new heart murmur (?septic emboli), thrombocytopenia, SBP >210, recent surgery or trauma, history of cerebral or severe GI bleed, cholesterol emboli.

B. Prevent complications: Consider GI prophylaxis, checking CBCs, stool guaiacs, relevant coagulation parameters (PT, PTT, or anti-Xa).

C. Warfarin (Coumadin): Goal PT/INR = 2-3 for A fib (unless under 65 with no risk factors), DVT, LV thrombus, antiphospholipid syndrome (see p. 192). Goal is 3-4.5 for mechanical valve. Typical load is 10 mg qd × 2 d, then 5 mg qd; decrease this for small or old pts. Overlap with heparin for at least 24 h of therapeutic PT to prevent early paradoxical hypercoagulability. With an INR of 2-3, bleed rate per year is about 2%; 0.6% for cerebral bleed. Concomitant aspirin probably doubles the bleed rate.

   1. Drugs that decrease warfarin clearance, raise PT: Acetaminophen, allopurinol, amiodarone, Bactrim, cimetidine, fluconazole, isoniazid, metronidazole, indomethacin, omeprazole, oral hypoglycemics, phenothiazines, quinidine, salicylates, TCAs.

   2. Drugs that increase warfarin clearance, lower PT: Barbiturates, oral contraceptives, rifampin.

D. Heparin: Goal PTT = 60-80, except as below. Watch for heparin-induced thrombocytopenia (see p. 193).

   1. For prophylaxis of DVT: 5000 U SQ bid.

   2. For rx of stroke, DVT, PE:

      a. Boluses: Avoid them in stroke, unless there is brainstem ischemia or a fluctuating neuro exam. Use boluses in PE, MI. Typically 3,000-5,000 U.

      b. Initial rate: Typically 1,000 U/h; give 600-800 U/h if pt. small, old, or frail; consider 1,300-1,500 U for big young pts.

      c. Sliding scale: For bid PTT:

E. Low molecular weight heparin (LMWH): Enoxaparin (Lovenox), dalteparin (Fragmin). Fragments of unfractionated heparin. QD dosing, greater bioavailability, longer duration, fixed weight–based dosing, no

PTT	Dose Correction
>120	Stop heparin, recheck PTT "superstat" in 2 h
100-119	Hold hep. × 2 h; decrease 200 U/h, recheck in 4 h
90-99	Decrease 200 U/h
80-89	Decrease 100 U/h
60-79	No change
50-59	Increase 100 U/h
40-49	Increase 200 U/h
<40	Bolus 3000 U, increase 200 U/h, recheck stat in 4 h

Table 44. Heparin sliding scale.

need for PTT monitoring or IV. All inactivate factor Xa and have lesser effect on thrombin. Lower risk of HIT. Better than warfarin for DVT prophylaxis in cancer pts and in acute PE.

F. Heparinoids: E.g., danaparoid, fondaparinux (Arixtra). Synthetic heparin-like polysaccharides. They bind antithrombin III and thus inhibit factor Xa. Use instead of IV heparin if pt. has heparin-induced thrombocytopenia (see p. 193).

    1. Danaparoid (Orgaran): A heparinoid. Bolus 1,250-2,000 U, then 400 U/h for 4 h, then 300 U/h for 4 h, then 150 U/h. After a few hours on 150 U/h, draw danaparoid level and anti-Xa level; use these to adjust danaparoid rate. Kidney elimination.

G. Direct thrombin inhibitors: All used as anticoagulants in patients with heparin-induced thrombocytopenia (HIT; see p. 193). They are hard to monitor and have no specific antidotes.

    1. Lepirudin and **hirudin:** Contraindicated in renal failure.

    2. Argatroban: Contraindicated in liver failure. It interferes with INR measurements, so switching to coumadin is complicated.

    3. Ximelagatran: The single oral alternative to warfarin.

H. Reversing anticoagulation:

    1. Contraindications: Prosthetic valve, basilar thrombosis, etc.

    2. Warfarin: Vitamin K 1 mg IV/SQ to lower PT a little. 10 mg qd × 3 d normalizes it but makes anticoagulation hard for the next week.

    3. Heparin: Protamine 10-50 mg IV over 5 min. 1 mg reverses approximately 100 U of heparin.

    4. Others: If active bleeding, consider fresh frozen plasma; DDAVP to boost platelets.

ANTICONVULSANTS

A. See also: Seizure classification, p. 109.

B. Slow release forms: Better compliance, fewer SEs.

C. Drug rash: Stop likely med immediately. Beware progression to Stevens-Johnson syndrome (mucous membranes blister) or toxic epidermal necrolysis (epidermis peels off too).

D. Pregnancy and ACDs: See p. 97.

E. Carbamazepine (Tegretol):

    1. Load: First check CBC, LFTs, iron. Do not start if iron >15 µg%. Carbamazepine autoinduces its metabolism.

        a. Input load: 200 mg qhs × 2 d, 200 bid × 2 d, then 200 tid; check levels after 3 d.

        b. Output load: Consider starting SR (Carbatrol or Tegretol XR) 200 mg qhs × 1 wk, then 200 bid, then dose per level or effect.

    2. Side effects: Rash, leukopenia, hepatitis, low Na, HA, nausea, ataxia. Need to increase oral contraceptive dose. Check Na, CBC, LFTs, level q mo at first.

    3. To taper carbamazepine: Taper 200 mg qd q2wk.

    4. Carbamazepine lowers levels of: Ethosuximide, tiagabine, topiramate, valproic acid, contraceptives (need to increase estrogen from 35-50 µg), steroids, warfarin, antipsychotics, cyclosporine.

    5. Carbamazepine raises levels of: Phenobarbital.

6. Carbamazepine levels raised by: (sometimes to *toxic* levels) cimetidine, erythromycin, Ca channel blockers, propoxyphene, isoniazid, lamotrigine.

7. Lithium and carbamazepine interact without raising level of either drug but can cause confusion, ataxia, tremor, hyperreflexia.

8. Mechanism: Stops high-frequency firing via Na channel.

F. Ethosuximide (Zarontin): Starting dose is 20 mg/kg qd divided tid. For absence seizures. Acts on Ca channels in thalamus; also potentiates dopamine. Lowers carbamazepine levels.

G. Fosphenytoin (Cerebyx): Dosed in mg phenytoin equivalents (PE). Status epilepticus load 1000 mg PE IV/IM, at <150 mg/min. Maintenance 4-6 mg PE/kg/min IV/IM.

H. Gabapentin (Neurontin): Load 300 mg PO qhs &times 2 d, then 300 mg bid × 2 d, then 300 mg tid; max. 3,600 mg qd. Enhances GABA synthesis; may inhibit Ca channels.

I. Lamotrigine (Lamictal): Levels raised significantly by valproic acid. Beware rash. Load slowly—at most 50 mg PO qhs × 2 wk, then 50 mg bid × 2 wk, then 150-250 mg bid. Slower if treating with valproic acid.

J. Levetiracetam (Keppra): Not approved for monotherapy but effective and broad spectrum. Beware rash. Can load quickly (500 mg bid for 1 wk, then 1,000 mg bid). Renally cleared, has few interactions. Well tolerated, can cause drowsiness and behavior disturbances.

K. Oxcarbazepine (Trileptal): Closely related to oxcarbazepine but fewer side effects and less rash. Approved for monotherapy; start at 600 mg/d bid, increase to 300 mg/d every 3 d to dose of 1,200 mg/d. Causes drowsiness.

L. Phenobarbital: A barbiturate.

1. Contraindications: Myasthenia, myxedema, porphyria, attention-deficit/hyperactivity disorder, depression.

2. Side effects: Very sedating, nystagmus, ataxia.

3. Dose: Typically 60 mg bid-tid qd, children 3-6 mg/kg qd.

4. Drug interactions: Decreases levels of carbamazepine, lamotrigine, DPH (variable), tiagabine, valproic acid.

5. Overdose: Similar to alcohol overdose. See ataxia, nystagmus, small reactive pupils, eventually respiratory depression and fixed and dilated pupils.

6. Withdrawal after heavy use: Similar to delirium tremens. Timing varies with the half-life of the barbiturate used, but generally seizures, hallucinations, and fever begin on the second day of withdrawal.

M. Phenytoin (Dilantin, DPH): Overused. Often started because it can be loaded IV, but so can valproate.

1. Contraindications: Secondary or complete AV block, bradycardia, hypotension, low ejection fraction, pregnancy. All pts. on DPH should take folate.

2. Side effects:

a. Short term: Sedation, nystagmus, ataxia, transient dystonias, ophthalmoplegia, rash.

b. Chronic: Coarse features, gingival hyperplasia, ataxia, cerebellar atrophy.

3. Dose: Start 300 mg PO qd; adjust per symptoms. Because of zero-order kinetics, at near-therapeutic doses, a small dose change can cause large level changes. See Table 45.

Present Level	Change to Make
<6 mg/dL	100 mg/d
6-8	50
>8	25

Table 45. Phenytoin dose adjustments for goal level of 10-20 mg/dl.

4. **To discontinue DPH:** Taper 100 mg qd every 2 wk.
5. **DPH lowers levels of:** Carbamazepine, ethosuximide, primidone, topiramate, valproic acid, warfarin, steroids, cyclosporine, doxycycline, estrogen, furosemide, quinidine, rifampin, theophylline, vitamin D.
6. **DPH raises levels of:** Phenobarbital.
7. **DPH levels raised by:** Acute alcohol, Depakote, cimetidine and other H_2 blockers, allopurinol, amiodarone, diazepam, estrogens, ethosuximide, imipramine, isoniazid, phenothiazines, sulfonamides, salicylates, trazodone. . . .
8. **DPH levels lowered by:** Chronic alcohol, carbamazepine, sucralfate, osmolyte, calcium antacids.
9. **Mechanism:** Lowers posttetanic potentiation in Na channel.
10. **Low albumin or renal failure:** Lowers DPH plasma level. The adjusted level should be 10-20 μg/mL (or free level 1-2 μg/mL).
    a. **Low alb:** Adj. level = measured level / [(0.2 × albumin) + 0.1].
    b. **Renal failure:** Adj. = measured level / [(0.1 × albumin) + 0.1].
11. **To raise subtherapeutic level:** Kinetics change from first-order to saturation near-therapeutic dose, so can increase level by 100 mg qd if level <8, but by no more than 50 mg if >8.
    a. **IV dose** (mg/kg) = 0.7 × (desired − observed plasma conc.).
    b. **Oral dose** (mg/kg) = IV dose + 10%.
N. **Topiramate** (Topamax): Approved for monotherapy. Start at 25 mg bid, increased by 50 mg qd every week up to 400 mg qd maintenance. Effective in migraine prophylaxis (not effective after 100 mg qd), causes weight loss but also cognitive dulling.
O. **Valproate** (Depakote): Strictly, Depakote is divalproex. Valproate is Depakene; less well tolerated. They act on chloride channel, GABA receptor.
    1. **Side effects:** Check LFTs. Nausea, weight gain, thin hair, teratogenicity, polycystic ovarian syndrome. Small increased risk of bleeding; pancreatitis, hepatitis.
    2. **Dose:** PO takes several weeks for effect. 1 wk on each dose: 250 mg qd, 250 bid, 250 tid, 250-250-500. IV: 10-15 mg/kg qd divided tid.
    3. **To discontinue valproate:** Taper 250 mg qd q2wk.
    4. **Valproate lowers levels of:** Carbamazepine, DPH (total, but free DPH levels increase), phenobarbital.
    5. **Valproate raises levels of:** Ethosuximide, lamotrigine (lower the dose from tid to bid), phenobarbital, primidone.
    6. **Valproate levels raised by:** Aspirin.

ANTIDEPRESSANTS

A. **See also:** Table 25 (antidepressant choice), p. 100.
B. **Withdrawal syndrome:** Rapid taper of any antidepressant, especially SSRIs, can cause depression and suicidality even in pts with normal mood. Warn your pts.
C. **Selective serotonin reuptake inhibitors (SSRIs):**
   1. **SSRI withdrawal syndrome:** Can cause suicidality even when pt is therapeutic on another antidepressant. The last part of the SSRI taper seems key. Lower the dose ~50% per week to smallest pill, then 2 wk on that, then 1-2 wk on 1 pill qod or ½ pill qd.
   2. **Serotonin syndrome:** Rare, and rarely (though potentially) fatal.
      a. **H&P:** Confusion, HTN, myoclonus, tremor, hyperreflexia and ANS instability, sometimes with hyperthermia. Med list and illicit drug exposures; consumption of tryptophan-rich foods, DIC, rhabdomyolysis.
      b. **Tests:** None. Specifically, blood levels do not help.
      c. **Causes:** Carcinoid; drugs that boost serotonin, esp. when they are of several different mechanisms simultaneously, high tryptophan consumption. MAO-A inhibitors are especially risky. MAO-B inhibitors, e.g., selegiline, rasagiline, are less risky.
      d. **DDx:**
         1) **NMS:** Hyperreflexia is more common in serotonin syndrome; global rigidity and fever more common in NMS. See p. 170.
         2) **Others:** Toxicity syndromes such as anticholinergic excess or sedative withdrawal; heat stroke, viral illness, anxiety.
      e. **Rx:** Usually resolves spontaneously 1-2 d after stopping the offending agent—<u>unless</u> drug is long acting, e.g., MAOI. Benzodiazepines help, and also help NMS. Cyproheptadine and methysergide may help.
   3. **Citalopram** (Celexa): Fewest SEs.
   4. **Fluoxetine** (Prozac): The most stimulating SSRI; can cause short-term anxiety, insomnia. Start 10 mg qAM, max. 80 mg qd, but higher for OCD, e.g., 100-120 mg.
   5. **Sertraline** (Zoloft): Intermediate in anticholinergic effect. Start 50 mg qd; max. 200 mg qd. Has mild dopamine antagonism—bad in Parkinson's, good in psychosis.
   6. **Paroxetine** (Paxil): The most sedating, most anticholinergic common SSRI; SEs include nausea, sedation, dry mouth, urinary hesitancy, constipation, orthostasis. Start 10 mg qhs; max. 50 mg.
D. **Serotonin-norepinephrine reuptake inhibitors (SNRIs):** Good for pain; anxiolysis without sedation.
   1. **Loading syndrome = withdrawal syndrome:** Both starting and stopping the med sometimes cause HA and N/V as well as depression. Warn your pts.
   2. **Venlafaxine** (Effexor): Quite stimulating; makes some pts uncomfortable. Start 37.5 mg in AM and noon, increase dose q4d.
   3. **Duloxetine** (Cymbalta): Best if comorbid pain. Start 20-30 mg qd, increase in a week to 30 mg in AM and noon, or 60 mg qd.

E. Buproprion (Wellbutrin): Less likely to provoke sexual dysfunction, mania. Tolerated in the elderly. Not sedating. Has some dopamine agonist effects.

   1. Dosing: 75 mg qd × 3 d, then 75 mg bid × 1 wk, then 150 mg bid.

   2. Side effects: Lowers seizure threshold; avoid in alcoholics.

F. Mirtazapine: Good for tremor, anxious depression, insomnia, cachexia.

   1. Dosing: Start 15 mg qhs × 1 wk, then 30 mg. Max. 60 mg.

   2. SEs: Sedation and weight gain.

G. Monoamine oxidase inhibitors (MAOIs):

   1. MAO-A inhibitors: E.g., phenelzine, tranylcypromine. Effective but very dangerous antidepressants, with high risk of:

      a. Serotonin syndrome: See p. 164.

      b. Hypertensive crisis/tyramine reactions: Interaction with many different drugs or tyramine-containing food can cause rapidly severe HTN with N/V, HA, MI, death.

   2. MAO-B inhibitors: Selegiline and rasagiline; treat Parkinson's. Much lower risk of MAO-A–like problems.

      a. Em-Sam has mixed effects: This high-dose selegiline antidepressant patch may have MAO-A effects. However, at 6 mg, it does not cause gut tyramine reactions because it is transdermal.

H. Tricyclic antidepressants (TCAs): Side effects make these third-line choices, except when there is also neuropathic pain. Check EKG before prescribing.

   1. Side effects:

      a. Anticholinergic effects: See Cholinergic Drugs, p. 168. Consider adding bethanechol to counteract these side effects.

      b. Alpha$_1$-adrenergic blocking effects: Causes orthostasis, syncope. Check EKG before prescribing TCAs to the elderly.

      c. Antihistaminergic effects: Sedating. High in doxepin.

      d. Rx of overdose: Symptomatic; gastric lavage, monitor ECG, keep blood pH >7.45 with Na bicarbonate rapid IV injection to prevent arrhythmias. Diazepam usually helps CNS effects. Severe anticholinergic sx may require physostigmine 2 mg slowly IV, with repeat of 1-4 mg prn at 20- to 60-min intervals.

   2. Nortriptyline: Less anticholinergic than amitriptyline. Start 10-25 mg PO qhs × 1 wk; gradually increase to 75 mg qhs. Max. 125 mg.

   3. Amitriptyline (Elavil): Very anticholinergic. Consider instead using duloxetine, nortriptyline, or mirtazapine (see Table 25, p. 100). Start 10-25 mg qhs × 1 wk; gradually load to 75 mg.

BENZODIAZEPINES

A. Indications: Anxiolysis, sedation, muscle spasms, seizures.

B. Time course: Diazepam has the shortest onset; oxazepam the shortest duration. Short-acting drugs, e.g., alprazolam, can cause rebound anxiety.

C. Mechanism: Benzodiazepines are GABA-A receptor agonists.

D. Side effects: Respiratory depression, hypotension. Mildly teratogenic during first trimester only. Although shorter acting ones, e.g., alprazolam,

are less sedating, they cause more rebound and withdrawal. Do not use them as analgesics; they can worsen pain.
1. **Withdrawal:** Can occur after prolonged use, so taper slowly. Sx are similar to alcohol withdrawal and can be life threatening.
2. **Overdose:** Flumazenil partly reverses effects but probably <u>not</u> the respiratory depression, and it may trigger seizures. Try 0.2 mg (2 mL) IV over 30 sec, then 0.3 mg q min to effect, max. of 3 mg (10 doses). Since half-life is 15 min-2.5 h, consider IV drip of 1 mg/h.

Generic Name	Brand Name	Half-Life	PO Dose (mg)	Liver Metab?
Alprazolam	Xanax	12 h	0.25-0.5 tid	—
Clonazepam	Klonopin	18-48 h	0.25-2 tid	Yes
Chlordiazepoxide	Librium	24 h	5-25 tid/qid	Yes
Diazepam	Valium	20-80 h	2-10 bid/qid	Yes
Lorazepam	Ativan	8-20 h	0.5-2 q6-8h	—
Oxazepam	Serax	8 h	10-15 tid/qid	—

Table 46. Benzodiazepine half-life and metabolism.

E. **Comorbid dz:**
1. **Liver failure:** In cirrhotics and the elderly, benzodiazepines metabolized in the liver (e.g., diazepam) can linger for weeks. Lorazepam or oxazepam, metabolized primarily in the kidney, are preferred. If pt has hepatic encephalopathy, avoid benzodiazepines completely; use narcotics if sedation is required.
2. **Kidney failure:** Use lorazepam, oxazepam (no active metabolites).
3. **The elderly:** Oxazepam is usually better tolerated than lorazepam.

CALCIUM CHANNEL BLOCKERS

A. **Effects:**
1. **Lower blood pressure:** Nifedipine > diltiazem > verapamil. They lower afterload because they dilate arteries more than veins.
2. **Nodal blockade and negative inotropy:** Verapamil > diltiazem >>> nifedipine.
3. **Migraine prophylaxis?** No net benefit in controlled trials.

CHEMOTHERAPY

A. **Neurological complications of cancer:** Metastases; encephalopathy (metabolic, drug, or radiation induced), paraneoplastic syndromes, CNS infection, infarct or bleed, myopathy (steroid-induced, cachectic), myositis, myasthenic syndromes.
B. **Neurological side effects of chemotherapy by class:**
1. **Alkylating agents:**
   a. **Nitrogen mustards:** Cyclophosphamide, melphalan, chlorambucil. Neuro side effects rare.

   b. **Nitrosoureas:** Lomustine (CCNU), carmustine (BCNU). BCNU causes leukoencephalopathy at high doses. CCNU causes blindness in combination with cranial irradiation.
2. **Antimetabolites:**
   a. **Folate analogs:** Methotrexate:
      1) **Acute transient chemical meningitis:** 4-6 h after intrathecal dose, in ~10% of pts.
      2) **Transient encephalopathy:** 7-10 d after third or fourth intrathecal dose, in ~4% of pts.
      3) **Transverse myelopathy:** After intrathecal dose, uncommon; paraplegia often permanent.
      4) **Leukoencephalopathy:** Weeks or months after brain XRT plus intrathecal or high-dose IV methotrexate.
   b. **Pyrimidine analogs:** 5-Fluorouracil, cytarabine. Occasional transient cerebellar dysfunction. Cytarabine can cause neuropathy.
3. **Purine analogs:** Azathioprine, fludarabine. Avoid allopurinol.

	Neuro	Heart	Liver	GI	Vasc	Lung	Renal	GU
Azathioprine			X	X				
Bleomycin				X		X		
Busulfan						X		
Carboplatin	X							
Carmustine (BCNU)	X		X	X		X	X	
Cisplatin (CDDP)	X						X	X
Cyclophosphamide		X						
Cytarabine (Ara-C)	X			X				
Dacarbazine (DTIC)				X				
Doxorubicin (Adria.)		X		X	X			
Etoposide (VP-16)	X							
Fluorouracil (5-FU)				X				
Ifosfamide		X	X					X
Methotrexate			X	X		X	X	
Mitomycin C				X	X	X		
Taxol	X	X						
Temozolomide				X				
Vinblastine	X				X			
Vincristine	X				X			

Table 47. Antineoplastic agent side effects.

4. **Natural products:**
   a. **Vinca alkaloids:** Vincristine, vinblastine. Especially vincristine: peripheral nerve dysfunction, usually hours to days after dose, usually reversible. Worse if liver dz. See autonomic dysfunction and

ileus (metoclopramide can help), decreased reflexes, toe and finger paresthesias, weak foot and wrist.

b. Abx: Daunorubicin, doxorubicin, bleomycin, mitomycin. Neuro effects rare.

c. Other: Etoposide, L-asparaginase. L-asparaginase causes encephalopathy, usually transient, in ~15% of pts.; also stroke or cerebral bleed in ~2% (drug-induced coagulopathy).

5. Hormonal agents: Tamoxifen, flutamide, leuprolide. Neurological side effects rare.

6. Other: Cisplatin, hydroxyurea, procarbazine, mitotane, aminoglutethimide. Cisplatin (but not carboplatin) causes hearing loss, dose-dependent large-fiber sensory neuropathy; sx can progress even after drug stopped. Sometimes seizures, confusion (but r/o Mg and Ca wasting). Procarbazine can cause encephalopathy and peripheral neuropathy.

7. Antineoplastic agent side effects: See Table 47.

CHOLINERGIC DRUGS

A. Location of receptors: Preganglionic sympathetic nervous system (SNS) + parasympathetic nervous system (PSNS), postganglionic PSNS, postganglionic SNS for sweating and vasodilation.

B. Acetylcholinesterase inhibitors: Inhibit acetylcholine breakdown. E.g., neostigmine (does not penetrate CNS well), physostigmine (does).

C. Muscarinic receptors: Postganglionic. Cause small pupils, high heart rate, secretions, bronchospasm, and bladder tone. Agonists include bethanechol, glycopyrrolate. Antagonists include benztropine, trihexyphenidyl, scopolamine, atropine.

D. Nicotinic receptors: Found in preganglionic ANS (where hexamethonium is an antagonist) and at the NMJ (where curare is an antagonist).

1. Anticholinergic toxicity mnemonic: Mad as a hatter (delirium). Plugged as a pig (stool and urinary retention). Dry as a bone (dry mouth, anhidrosis). Blind as a bat (blurred vision). Hot as a hare (fever). Fast as a fibrillation (tachycardia).

DIGOXIN

A. Elimination: Renal. However, digoxin cannot be dialyzed off.

B. Drug interactions: Cut digoxin dose in half when you start verapamil, quinidine, or amiodarone; check frequent levels.

C. Overdose (Note: digoxin level must be drawn >6 h after dose.):

1. Signs: Vomiting, diarrhea, diplopia, yellow-haloed vision, confusion, low KCl. Long PR interval, heart block, junctional tach., V tach., and V fib. Bidirectional V tach. is pathognomonic for digoxin toxicity.

2. Rx: Cardiac monitor, stop digoxin; replete KCl, Mg, and Ca; lidocaine for V tach./V fib. If heart block, pace. Digibind only if serious arrhythmia.

DIURETICS

A. Acetazolamide (Diamox): A carbonic anhydrase inhibitor that raises extracellular carbon dioxide and decreases CSF formation. It is used in pseudotumor cerebri and sometimes as an adjunct ACD. SEs: rash, agranulocytosis, paresthesias. Follow CBC, electrolytes.

B. Furosemide (Lasix): A loop diuretic. 10-40 mg IV bolus; 20-80 mg PO qd-bid. SEs: low BP, low K, ototoxicity.

C. Mannitol: Osmotic diuretic used to lower intracranial or intraocular pressure. 25% mannitol is 1,375 mOsm/L. Cleared renally in about 3 h, but ICP effect lasts 3-8 h. See p. 68.

DOPAMINERGIC DRUGS

A. Dopamine: Used to increase heart rate, contractility, and SBP. Can cause arrhythmias. See ICU Drips, p. 172.

B. Dopamine (DA) receptors:

    1. D1 receptors: Cause vasodilation.

    2. D2 receptors: Inhibit sympathetic transmission, inhibit prolactin release, cause vomiting.

    3. D3, 4, 5 receptors: Less well characterized; limbic more than motor effects.

C. Agonists: Used mostly for Parkinson's dz.

    1. Levodopa: A precursor to dopamine. Given with carbidopa, which blocks peripheral, but not central, levodopa use.

        a. Start: 25/100 (carbidopa/levodopa) qd, bring to tid. If necessary, give up to total 1000 mg qd of levodopa, dosing q2-4h. Carbidopa dose should be >75 mg/d, but >125 mg/d may itself cause nausea.

        b. Food interactions: Pts. first starting levodopa should take it with meals to minimize nausea. Advanced pts. should take it >30 minutes before or >60 minutes after protein-rich meals because protein blocks CNS levodopa absorption.

        c. Side effects: N/V, low BP, confusion, dyskinesias, hallucinations.

    2. Receptor agonists: Side effects are like levodopa, but agonists are less likely to cause dyskinesias, more likely to cause confusion.

        a. D2 agonists: E.g., bromocriptine (Parlodel), ropinirole (Requip).

        b. D3 agonists: E.g., pramipexole (Mirapex). Start 0.125 mg tid, max. 1.5 mg tid. Or pergolide (Permax). Start 0.05 mg qd, max. 1.5 mg tid.

    3. Inhibitors of DA metabolism:

        a. Monoamine oxidase inhibitors (MAOIs):

            1) Nonspecific MAOIs: Used as antidepressants. <u>Many</u> dietary and drug contraindications, notably meperidine, SSRIs, tyramine-containing foods (red wine, hard cheese).

            2) MAO-B inhibitors: E.g., selegiline (Eldepryl), rasagiline (Azilect). They slow dopamine degradation. Start 2.5 mg bid to 5 bid. SEs are few; sometimes N/V. Avoid opiates, TCAs, and SSRIs (can cause hyperthermia, rigidity, autonomic instability).

        b. Carboxy-o-methyltransferase (COMT) inhibitors: E.g., tolcapone (associated with fulminant liver failure). For end-stage Parkinson's.

    4. Amantadine: DA agonist, mechanism unclear, also anticholinergic and antiviral. Used for Parkinson's dz, fatigue in multiple sclerosis.

        a. Side effects: Rare confusion, depression, edema.

D. Antagonists: Neuroleptics, e.g., haloperidol, Compazine. Used for sedation, psychosis, vomiting. Extrapyramidal side effects are proportional to D2 binding. Clozapine is underused because it requires WBC tests q 1-4 wk. Its risk of aplastic anemia is very low with testing.

Drug	Anti-psych	Extra-pyram	Sedation	Low BP	Weight Gain	Receptor Effect
Typicals						
Haloperidol (Haldol)	+++	++++	+	+	+	D2, high
Pimozide (Orap)	+++	++++	++	+	++	D2, high
Perphenazine (Trilafon)	++	++	+++	++	+++	D2, med
Thioridazine (Mellaril)	++	+	++++	+++	++++	D2, low
Atypicals						
Risperidone (Risperdal)	+++	++	+	+	++	D2 ≅ 5HT
Olanzapine (Zyprexa)	+++	++	+++	+	+++	5HT > D2
Ziprasidone (Geodon)	++	+	+	+	+	5HT > D2
Aripiprazole (Abilify)	++	+	+	+	+	D2 ag/antag
Quetiapine (Seroquel)	+	+	+++	++	++	α_1 > D2
Clozapine (Clozaril)	++++	−	++++	+	++++	5HT > D2

α = noradrenaline; D = dopamine; 5HT = serotonin.

Table 48. Neuroleptic effects.

E. **Neuroleptic-induced movement disorders:**
1. **Neuroleptic malignant syndrome (NMS):** An emergency. Happens in response to a neuroleptic or to sudden withdrawal of an antiparkin-sonian drug. Caused by a sudden release of calcium from sarcoplas-mic reticulum.
   a. **H&P:** Recent drugs. See tachycardia, then acidosis, tachypnea, arrhythmias, muscle stiffness, and fever.
   b. **DDx of NMS:** Malignant hyperthermia, drug interactions with monoamine oxidase inhibitors, central anticholinergic syndromes, catatonia. . . .
   c. **Tests:** ABG, electrolytes, CBC, CPK, EKG.
   d. **Rx of NMS:**
      1) **Transfer to ICU, maintain ventilation**.
      2) **Surface and core cooling.**
      3) **Dantrolene:** Start 1 mg/kg IV, repeat prn to 10 mg/kg qd. Watch for hepatotoxicity, CHF.
      4) **Bromocriptine:** Start 2.5-10 mg IV/pNGT q4-6h.
      5) **Methylprednisolone:** 1 g/d × 3 d may speed recovery.
2. **Acute dystonia:** Within a few days of drug initiation. Rx with diphenhydramine 50 mg IM/PO.
3. **Akathisia:** See Movement Disorders, p. 74.

4. **Subacute parkinsonian sx:** Days to weeks after drug initiation. Add an anticholinergic drug (prophylactic use does not help), switch to clozapine, and use benztropine 0.5-4.0 mg bid—it has better compliance than trihexyphenidyl because bid.
5. **Tardive dyskinesia:** Choreoathetosis, dystonia, orobuccal dyskinesia as late (>6 mo) effect of chronic neuroleptic or antiemetic use. Highest risk in mood disorders, women, children.
   a. **Beware rebound:** TD may greatly worsen if you suddenly stop the neuroleptic. Restart it if necessary and taper slowly.
6. **Rx:** Switch to clozapine. Avoid anticholinergics. Consider tetrabenazine (from England), reserpine.

ICU DRIPS

A. **See also:** Adrenergic Drugs, p. 155; Dopaminergic Drugs, p. 169.
B. **Access:** Most require central line.
C. **Dobutamine:** To treat heart failure. Increases cardiac output while decreasing SVR, so BP often does not change. Does not increase PCWP as much as DA does.
D. **Dopamine (DA):** To treat low BP, low HR, or oliguric renal failure (controversial). You can give low doses by peripheral IV.
   1. **SEs:** Arrhythmia, tachycardia (especially if pt. is hypovolemic).
   2. **Low-dose effects:** 0.5-3 μg/kg/min. Causes renal dilation, Na excretion, via DA receptors.
   3. **Medium-dose effects:** 5-10 μg/kg/min. Causes positive inotropy, via β-receptors.
   4. **High-dose effects:** >15 μg/kg/min. Causes vasoconstriction, via α-receptors. High doses sometimes dilate and even fix pupils.
E. **Epinephrine:** To treat anaphylaxis; to help circulation in cardiac codes.
F. **Lidocaine:** To decrease ectopy. Dangerous in bradycardia or AV block.
G. **Nicardipine:** Calcium channel blocker. Treats high BP in intracranial disease. Can infuse continuously.
H. **Nitroglycerine (TNG, NTG):** To treat cardiac ischemia, coronary or esophageal spasm, CHF if BP not low. Low doses can be given by peripheral IV. It causes venous greater than arterial dilation. May reduce cardiac output. Unlike nitroprusside, it does not cause cerebral steal.
I. **Nitroprusside (NTP):** To treat high BP in stroke, hypertensive crisis, aortic dissection. It causes arterial dilation and venodilation equally. Avoid in ischemic brain; it may cause cerebral steal by dilating peripheral vessels. Low doses can be given by peripheral IV. After 3 days of use, check thiocyanate levels daily.
J. **Norepinephrine (Levophed):** To treat low BP in sepsis. Beta$_1$- and α-receptor effects. Inotropic at 1-2 μg/min; then vasoconstriction and venoconstriction.
K. **Phenylephrine (Neosynephrine):** To treat low BP in stroke; second-line agent for septic shock. Pure α-receptor effects, no β (vasoconstricts without inotropy), so raises afterload without inotropic support.

Category	Target	Dose Per kg	Average Dose	Toxicity
Pressors				
Dopamine (Intropin)	D1, D2	0.5-2 μg/kg/min	50-150 μg/min	↑HR, arrhythmia, big pupils
	β, D	2-10 μg/kg/min	200-500 μg/min	HTN
	α, β, D	>10 μg/kg/min	500-1,000 μg/min	
Norepinephrine (Levophed)	$α_1, α_2 β_1$ >$β_2$		1-16 μg/min	Vasospasm, acute renal failure
Phenylephrine (Neosynephrine)	$α_1$		10-300 μg/min	Vasospasm, acute renal failure
Dobutamine (Dobutrex)	$β_1$	2-20 μg/kg/min	100-1,000 μg/min	Arrhythmia, initial ↓ SVR
Epinephrine (Adrenalin)	$α_1, α_2$ $β_1 β_2$		0.25-4 μg/min	Vasospasm, MI arrhythmia
Isoproterenol (Isuprel)	$β_1, β_2$		0.1-20 μg/min	Arrhythmia, MI hypotension
Amrinone (Inocor)	PDE-III inhibitor	0.75 mg/kg then 5-15 μg/kg/min	40 mg over 3 min then 250-900 μg/min	HR↑, plts↓, hypotension
Cardiac				
Lidocaine	Na channel	1 mg/kg then 1-4 mg/min	bolus 70-100 mg then 1-4 mg/min	Altered MS, seizures, arrhythmia
Procainamide	Na, K channels	15 mg/kg @ 50 mg/min, 1-4 mg/min	1 g over 20 min then 1-4 mg/min	Hypotension, long QT interval
Bretylium	K channel	5 mg/kg then 1-4 mg/min	350-700 mg then 1-4 mg/min	Hypotension, arrhythmia
Amiodarone	K channel	150-300 mg then 0.4-0.8 mg/kg/h	150-300 mg over 5 min then 3-6 mg/h	Hypotension, arrhythmia
Nitroglycerin	Smooth muscle		10-1,000 μg/min	BP↓, hypoxia, methemoglobin
Nitroprusside (Nipride)	Direct vascular	0.1-10 μg/kg/min	5-800 μg/min	Thiocyanate toxicity
Esmolol (Brevibloc)	$β_1 > β_2$ blocker	500 μg/kg then 25-300 μg/kg/min	20-30 mg over 1 min then 2-12 mg/min	CHF, hypotension
Enalapril (Vasotec)	ACE inhibitor	0.625-1.25 mg over 5 min then 0.625-5 mg q6h		K↑, BP↓, acute renal failure
Hydralazine (Apresoline)	Direct vasodilator	5-20 mg q3min up to 400 mg then 5-20 mg q6h		Angina, hypotension
Labetalol (Normodyne)	$α_1, β_1, β_2$ blocker	2.5-10 mg then 10-120 mg/h or 2.5-10 mg q15min		Neg inotrope, BP↓
Verapamil (Calan)	Ca channel	2.5-15 mg then 5-20 mg/h		AV block, BP↓
Diltiazem (Cardizem)	Ca channel	0.25 mg/kg over 2 min, reload 0.35 mg/kg q15min prn, then 10-15 mg/h		AV block, BP↓
Nicardipine (Cardene)	Ca channel	5 mg/h, titrate by 2.5 mg/h q5-15min then ↓ rate by 1-7.5 mg/h when goal BP reached		BP↓

Table 49. ICU drips.

IMMUNOSUPPRESSANTS

A. **Side effects:** Immunosuppressants of all types increase the risk of opportunistic infections and malignancy, especially lymphoma.
B. **Azathioprine:** An antimetabolite. Coadministration with allopurinol will increase its toxicity. Marrow and liver side effects.
C. **Corticosteroids:**
   1. **Indications:** For brain tumors, MS, other autoimmune dz, pre-op neurosurgery.
   2. **Stress-dose steroids:** For pts. on chronic steroids or with adrenal insufficiency, who are exposed to trauma, severe illness, or surgery, give hydrocortisone 100 mg IV q8h × 2-3 d. Unless insult is prolonged, you do not need to taper.
   3. **Adrenal insufficiency after withdrawal:** Taper steroids over several weeks to avoid insufficiency.
   4. **Side effects:**
      a. **Endocrine:** Glucose intolerance, adrenal insufficiency after withdrawal of steroids, hirsutism, growth retardation.
      b. **Electrolytes:** Na and water retention, low K. Give KCl supplements.
      c. **Musculoskeletal:** Osteoporosis, myopathy. Give calcium + vitamin D between steroid courses (risk of kidney stones when given together).
      d. **Connective tissue:** Centripetal obesity, striae, poor wound healing.
      e. **Immune:** Increased infections, decreased allergic reactions, increased WBC count.
      f. **GI:** Ulcers. Give ulcer prophylaxis.
      g. **CNS:** Insomnia, agitation, psychosis. Olanzapine 2.5-10 mg or lithium 300 mg qhs.
D. **Cyclophosphamide (Cytoxan):** An alkylating agent. See Chemotherapy, p. 166.
E. **Cyclosporine:** Inhibits T cells. Major side effects are renal. Some pts. get cyclosporine headaches that are dose dependent; may benefit from propranolol or gabapentin.
F. **FK506 (Tacrolimus):** Inhibits T cells. Major side effects are renal. Some pts. get FK506 encephalopathy, with MRI showing white-matter dz. This is sometimes reversible with stopping FK506.
G. **Interferon:** Cytokines with immunosuppressive and antiviral effects. β-interferon is used in multiple sclerosis. Side effects include a flu-like syndrome, marrow suppression, and rare confusion or seizures.
H. **Methotrexate:** An antimetabolite; see Chemotherapy, p. 166.

MUSCLE RELAXANTS

A. **See also:** Benzodiazepines, p. 165.
B. **Baclofen:** A GABA-B agonist. For spasticity, back pain, trigeminal neuralgia.
   1. **Dosing:** Start 5-10 mg PO bid, to 10-30 tid.
   2. **Side effects:** Sedation, weakness, nausea, depression. If stopped suddenly after several weeks of heavy use, can trigger seizures.
C. **Dantrolene:** A direct muscle relaxant.
   1. **Dosing:** See p. 170 for dosing in neuroleptic malignant syndrome. For spasticity, start 25 mg PO qd, up to 400 mg qd divided bid/qid.

    2. Side effects: Hepatotoxicity, CHF, sedation.
D. Tizanidine (Zanaflex): α_2-adrenergic agonist, used for spasticity.
    1. Dosing: Varies widely across pts., from 2-39 mg PO qd; must titrate over 2-4 wk because it takes about a week to reach max. effect.
    2. Side effects: Sedation, weakness (less than baclofen), dry mouth.
E. Cyclobenzaprine (Flexeril): Central muscle relaxant.
    1. Dosing: 5-10 mg tid; do not use for more than 3 weeks.
    2. Side effects: Sedation, dizziness, dry mouth.
F. Quinine: Not an FDA-approved indication, but helps some pts.
    1. Dosing: Try 300 mg PO qhs.
    2. Side effects: Cinchonism with overdose. Hemolysis with G6PD deficiency.

PARALYTICS

A. Pupils are spared: Large pupils in a pt given paralytics are usually evidence of anxiety from inadequate sedation.
B. Succinylcholine: 1-1.5 mg/kg IV bolus (typically 3.5-5 cc/70 kg of 20 mg/cc solution), onset 60-90 sec, lasts 3-10 min. Infusion 2.5-15 mg/min. A depolarizing blocker that can cause autonomic stimulation and raise intracranial pressure. Blunt this by pretreating with pancuronium (nondepolarizing) 1 mg IV, 5 min before succinylcholine.
C. Vecuronium: 0.07-0.1 mg/kg IV bolus (typically 8-10 mg/70 kg), 2-3 min onset, lasts 15-30 min. Nondepolarizing.

IMAGING

ANGIOGRAPHY

A. **Diagnostic angiogram:** To assess aneurysm, AVM, dural fistula, vessel stenosis, or dissection that is equivocal on CTA/MRA, vessel occlusion before IA thrombolysis, vasculitis, vasospasm, blood flow near a tumor.

B. **Interventional angiogram:** Aneurysm coiling, intra-arterial thrombolysis, balloon angioplasty, cerebrovascular stenting, mechanical clot retrieval, glue embolization of AVM or tumors, severe epistaxis.

C. **Angiographic anatomy:** See also Vascular territories, p. 26.

D. **Consent:** Risk of complication $\cong$ 4%; permanent $\cong$ 1%, death $\cong$ 0.6%. Higher risk with interventional angio, tight stenosis, or h/o migraine.

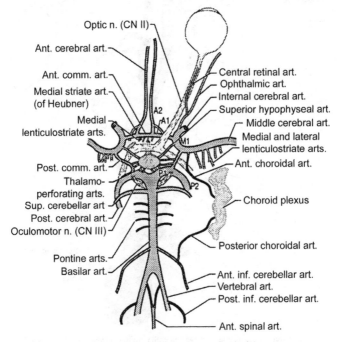

Figure 18. The circle of Willis. (From Greenberg MS. *Handbook of Neurosurgery*. 3rd ed. Lakeland, FL: Greenberg Graphics, 1994, with permission.)

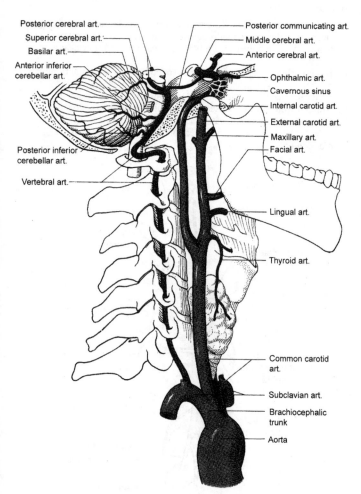

Figure 19. Carotid artery anatomy. (Reprinted with permission from Duus P. *Topical Diagnosis in Neurology*. New York: Thieme, 1983:415.)

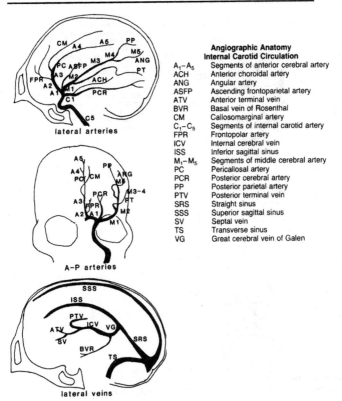

**Angiographic Anatomy
Internal Carotid Circulation**

A_1–A_5	Segments of anterior cerebral artery
ACH	Anterior choroidal artery
ANG	Angular artery
ASFP	Ascending frontoparietal artery
ATV	Anterior terminal vein
BVR	Basal vein of Rosenthal
CM	Callosomarginal artery
C_1–C_5	Segments of internal carotid artery
FPR	Frontopolar artery
ICV	Internal cerebral vein
ISS	Inferior sagittal sinus
M_1–M_5	Segments of middle cerebral artery
PC	Pericallosal artery
PCR	Posterior cerebral artery
PP	Posterior parietal artery
PTV	Posterior terminal vein
SRS	Straight sinus
SSS	Superior sagittal sinus
SV	Septal vein
TS	Transverse sinus
VG	Great cerebral vein of Galen

Figure 20. The carotid circulation. (From Lerner AJ. *The Little Black Book of Neurology.* 3rd ed. St. Louis: Mosby, 1995:20, with permission.)

E. Orders: NPO after midnight, IV fluids, preop labs.

F. Post-angio orders: Keep leg straight for 4 hours; check for groin hematoma and distal leg for pulses (q15min × 4, q30min × 2, q1h × 4). Follow-up noncontrast head CT.

    1. After stenting or mechanical clot retrieval: IIb-IIIa drip, heparin IV, or ASA vs. clopidogrel.

    2. After IA thrombolysis: No anticoagulants or antiplatelets for 24 hrs. Post-tPA precautions, BP control (SBP <180), anticoagulants, or antiplatelets.

    3. After angioplasty or IA treatment of vasospasm etc: IV nicardipine or milrinone.

G. Sheath pull: Usually done at the end of the angiogram; it is sometimes left in longer. Stop anticoagulant drips before pulling sheath. Consider percutaneous closure devices.

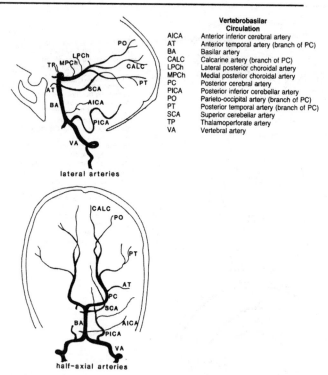

Vertebrobasilar Circulation

AICA	Anterior inferior cerebral artery
AT	Anterior temporal artery (branch of PC)
BA	Basilar artery
CALC	Calcarine artery (branch of PC)
LPCh	Lateral posterior choroidal artery
MPCh	Medial posterior choroidal artery
PC	Posterior cerebral artery
PICA	Posterior inferior cerebellar artery
PO	Parieto-occipital artery (branch of PC)
PT	Posterior temporal artery (branch of PC)
SCA	Superior cerebellar artery
TP	Thalamoperforate artery
VA	Vertebral artery

Figure 21. The vertebrobasilar circulation. (From Lerner AJ. *The Little Black Book of Neurology*. 3rd ed. St. Louis: Mosby, 1995:21, with permission.)

CT AND MRI ANATOMY

A. Opposite of neuropathological conventions: Radiological images are presented with their anatomic left on the right side of the picture. The brainstem on a horizontal scan is upside down compared with pathological or textbook images of the brainstem in coronal section.

B. Sections:
  1. **Axial** (horizontal): Parallel to ground if pt. were standing. The standard section. In the spine, gives a cross-section.
  2. **Coronal:** In plane, not with a crown, but a coronet (or one of those preppy headband things). Good for pituitary, cavernous sinus, skull-base, orbital, and hippocampal lesions.
  3. **Sagittal:** In plane with the interhemispheric fissure. In the spine, gives a longitudinal section.

C. Finding landmarks:
  1. **Ventricles and cisterns:** In horizontal section, the ventricles form a face, with lateral ventricles for eyes, third ventricle for a nose, and a

mouth whose sides are the per-
imesencephalic cisterns and
whose base is the quadrigeminal
cistern below the colliculi. It
should be smiling; flattening of
the quadrigeminal cistern suggests herniation.

2. **Central sulcus:** In horizontal
section, it is most easily seen in
uppermost sections, where it has
a characteristic sickle shape
(look for "omega sign," as in
Greek letter omega, outlining the
motor cortex). The superior
frontal sulcus, running parallel
to the falx,

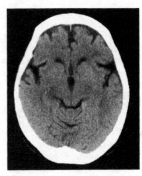

Figure 22. Normal cisterns make a
happy face; herniation makes it sad.

terminates in the precentral
sulcus; the central sulcus is just
posterior.

3. **Orbit:** There is proptosis if more than half the eyeball sticks out past
the line between the zygoma and the nose.

D. **Pediatric neuroimaging:** See p. 131 for patterns of myelination.

COMPUTERIZED TOMOGRAPHY (CT)

A. **Indications for noncontrast study:** STAT scan for ICH, acute stroke, or
altered consciousness after neurosurgery. Good for hydrocephalus, brain
edema, skull fractures, intracranial air, calcifications, metal in head.
Adequate for acute or unstable pt. who cannot have MRI.

B. **Indications for contrast:** ("Contrast head CT" is not a CT angiogram.)
Any process with disrupted blood-brain barrier (e.g., tumor, inflammation, subacute stroke, longstanding hypertensive encephalopathy, etc.).

C. **Indications for CT myelogram:** Spinal cord lesion in pt. with multiple
back surgeries, metal implants causing artifact, or who cannot get an
MRI. Does not show lateral or foraminal herniations.

D. **Indications for CT angiogram:** CTA shows anatomy better; time-of-
flight MRA shows blood flow more accurately. Stroke assessment before
thrombolysis, neck vessel dissection, aortic arch or vessel origin stenoses.
Arterial lesion in pt. who cannot get an MRA.

E. **What CT is bad for:** Posterior fossa and brainstem (much artifact), small
lesions, subacute blood (isodense with brain).

F. **Relative contraindications:**
   1. **Noncontrast:** Limit use in first trimester of pregnancy. Unstable pts.
   should not be sent to the scanner unmonitored.
   2. **Contrast:** Renal failure; creatinine should be <2.0; repeat contrast
   only after 24 h. Previous contrast reaction. Contrast can sometimes
   trigger flash pulmonary edema. See Allergy, p. 191, for prevention
   and rx of contrast allergies.

G. **CT lesions by degree of hyperdensity:** Bone > clotted blood > liquid
blood > subacute (~2 wk) blood ≅ brain tissue > CSF > water > fat.

1. **See also:** DDx by MRI appearance, p. 183, for the DDx of ring-enhancing lesions, etc.
2. **Hyperdense (bright) lesions:** Recent blood, metastases (often), meningioma, calcification, bone.
   a. **Calcifications:** Seen in oligodendroglioma, toxoplasmosis, neuro-cysticercosis, meningioma, Fahr's syndrome, AVM, calcified aneurysms, old infections. Normal in choroid plexus, pineal.
3. **Hypodense (dark) lesions:** Infarct ≥ 3-12 h, brain tumors, inflammation, old blood, edema, posttraumatic changes, fat, cysts, air.
4. **Ventriculomegaly:** Obstruction, atrophy, NPH.

H. **CT of specific lesions:**
   1. **Infarct:**
      a. **Acute:** Infarcts are often hard to see for 12-24 h. Large strokes may show early loss of gray-white differentiation, sulcal definition, and even hypodensity as early as 3 h after sx onset.
      b. **Subacute:** Hypodensity in the distribution of a defined vascular territory, both grey and white matter involved. Look for edema, mass effect, or hemorrhagic conversion. Some tiny lacunar strokes may never be visible by CT. Strokes 2-4 wk old may have ring enhancement with contrast.
      c. **Chronic:** Hypodensity, often with encephalomalacia (tissue loss) that may cause sulcal or ventricular widening.

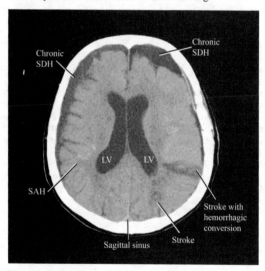

Figure 23. CT appearance of infarcts, SDH, and SAH.

   2. **CT signs of intracranial hemorrhage:** See also Intracranial Hemorrhage, p. 61.
      a. **Epidural hematoma:** High-density biconvex (lens-shaped) area next to skull. Does not cross sutures. Often with skull fracture.

    b. Subdural hematoma (SDH): High-density, crescentic area next to skull. Crosses sutures but not the midline. Look for edema, shift, cortical flattening, associated fracture or scalp bruise. Subacute SDH may be isodense; see only obliteration of sulci and midline shift. There may be no shift if SDH is bilateral.

    c. Subarachnoid hemorrhage (SAH): Serpentine density in sulci, fissures, and basal cisterns, often dissecting into ventricles. Look for associated fracture or scalp bruise, hydrocephalus, hematoma that may need evacuation. Often bleed location predicts aneurysm location. If suspicion of SAH but negative CT, do LP.

    d. Intracerebral hemorrhage: Blood within brain parenchyma. Often surrounded by edema. Location is guide to cause.

        1) Hypertensive bleed: Usually in basal ganglia, thalamus, brainstem, cerebellum, or white matter. Often there is intraventricular blood.

        2) Amyloid bleed: Usually at gray-white junction (lobar), may have subarachnoid component. Get an MRI with iron susceptibility sequence to see additional occult lesions (microhemorrhages) that help confirm the diagnosis.

3. Contusion: Petechial hyperdensity associated with hypodensity, skull fracture or scalp bruise at the site of the blow (the "coup"). Often there is a contrecoup injury in the opposite lobe.

4. Intracranial pressure: <u>The absence of the fourth ventricle is a neurological emergency</u>. It should be visible even if there is much artifact. Look also for sulcal effacement, midline shift, distortion of nearby structures by mass, effacement of cisterns.

5. Herniation: Includes:

    a. Subfalcine herniation: Cingulate gyrus is displaced across the midline under the falx. May have enlargement of contralateral ventricle or ACA territory infarct.

    b. Central transtentorial herniation: Obliteration of the perimesencephalic and quadrigeminal cisterns, sometimes with PCA territory infarcts and small Duret hemorrhages in the brainstem.

    c. Uncal transtentorial herniation:

        1) Early: Loss of the suprasellar cistern's normal smiley face (see Ventricles and cisterns, p. 178).

        2) Mid: Brainstem displacement, compression of contralateral cerebral peduncle, sometimes contralateral hydrocephalus.

        3) Late: Loss of parasellar and interpeduncular cisterns.

    d. Tonsillar herniation: Cerebellar tonsils bulge down into foramen magnum. Best seen sagittally. They should be <5 mm below occipital-clival line.

    e. Upward cerebellar herniation: Vermis is above tentorium; may compress cistern and aqueduct, and cause hydrocephalus.

6. Hydrocephalus: Frontal horns and third ventricles balloon ("Mickey Mouse" ventricles), periventricular low density from transependymal absorption of CSF. In children, plain skull films may show splayed sutures.

a. **Obstructive hydrocephalus:** Large lateral ventricles with effacement of sulci. Third or fourth ventricle may look closed. There is usually a visible compressing lesion.

b. **Communicating hydrocephalus:** All ventricles and the cerebral aqueduct should be large. In hydrocephalus from atrophy, sulci are widened; whereas in hydrocephalus from CSF malabsorption (e.g., after SAH), they may be narrowed.

c. **Ratios that suggest hydrocephalus:** TH ≥2 mm for both temporal horns (see Figure 24) and *either:*

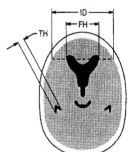

1) **Sulci and fissures are invisible,** *or*
2) **FH/ID >0.5:** where FH = largest width of frontal horns and ID = internal diameter of brain at this level.

d. **Chronic hydrocephalus:** Erosion of the sella turcica with 3rd ventricle herniating downward. Atrophy of corpus callosum on sagittal MRI. In children, macrocephaly.

Figure 24. Ventricular parameters in hydrocephalus. (From Greenberg MS. *Handbook of Neurosurgery.* 3rd ed. Lakeland, FL: Greenberg Graphics, 1994:224, with permission.)

7. **Trauma:**
   a. **Contusion:** Predominantly gray matter hypodensity. See intraparenchymal blood, usually with little mass effect, usually in poles of cerebral hemisphere, next to bone.
   b. **Diffuse axonal injury:** AKA shear injury. Seen especially after deceleration injury. Little change in CT. In severe cases, may see petechial hemorrhages in white matter and brainstem and diffuse cerebral edema. Best seen on MRI.
   c. **Skull fracture:** May be complicated by epidural hemorrhage or CSF leak. Fluid in a sinus or mastoid suggests an occult fracture. May take several days to become visible.

8. **Tumor:** CT is sensitive enough for most cortical tumors that are large enough to be symptomatic. Small metastases, posterior fossa tumors, and some isodense gliomas will require contrast or MRI.
   a. **Mass:** With contrast, most tumors are bright or ring enhancing. Without contrast, they may be dark or isodense, sometimes seen only by distortion of adjacent structures. Look for L-R asymmetries.
   b. **Associated findings:** Look for dark edema surrounding the tissue, midline shift, hydrocephalus, herniation, blood, infarcts.
   c. **In infants,** because there is no gray-white differentiation, it is easy to miss small amounts of edema.
   d. **DDx:** Inflammation, enhancing subacute infarcts.

MAGNETIC RESONANCE IMAGING (MRI)

A. **Indications:** Posterior fossa or small supratentorial lesions, telling new from old strokes, white matter dz, nonacute seizure workup, AVMs. In practice, MRI is privileged as a gold standard, even for unnecessary indications such as NPH. For the indications for specific sequences, see Table 50.

B. **What MRI is bad for:** Unstable pts., fresh blood (except with susceptibility sequence), bone or calcium, cost containment.

C. **Contraindications:**
   1. **Cardiac pacemakers.**
   2. **Old aneurysm clips:** I.e., ferromagnetic ones, e.g., Drake, Heifetz, Mayfield, Scoville. Modern clips are usually MRI compatible, including Olivecrona, Sugita, McFadden, and Yasargil.
   3. **Some cochlear implants:** Verify their compatibility.
   4. **Other ferromagnetic foreign bodies in head:** E.g., bullets.
   5. **Other implants:** Staples, pumps, penile implants, joint prosthetics, spine rods, etc., are usually safe but should be verified.
   6. **Unstable pts.:** This includes pts. who cannot lie flat because of aspiration risk, increased ICP.
   7. **Agitation, claustrophobia, or back pain:** Premedicate with a neuroleptic, benzodiazepine, or opiate, respectively—or combine them. Severe cases may need conscious sedation or intubation.
   8. **Big pts.:** Pts. over 300 lb or girth >50 in. may not fit. "Open MRIs" may help but have worse image quality, especially of spine.
   9. **Contrast allergy?** Rarely a problem. Gadolinium is safe for pts. with renal failure or CT contrast allergies.
   10. **Wrong imaging goal:** E.g., calcium, fresh small bleeds (except with susceptibility sequence), bone or other minerals, cost containment.

D. **MRI findings by appearance:**
   1. **Ring-enhancing lesions:** "MAGIC DR": Metastases, Abscess or aneurysm, Glioblastoma, Inflammation (resolving stroke, infection), Contusion (resolving), Demyelination (active), Radiation necrosis.
   2. **Gray-white junction lesions:** Metastases, septic emboli, thrombosis, vasculitis.
   3. **Periventricular white matter lesions:** MS, hypertensive or diabetic microvascular dz, toxoplasmosis, CNS lymphoma, CMV, lacunar infarcts, glioma.
   4. **Cerebellopontine angle lesions:** "SAME": Schwannoma, Arachnoid cyst, Meningioma, Epidermoid.
   5. **Basal ganglia lesions:** Bleed, stroke, carbon monoxide, lead, methanol, CJD, TORCH infection, glioma, Fahr's dz.

E. **MRI findings by cause:**
   1. **Abscess:** T2/FLAIR hyperintense ring of edema and hypointense capsule, enhances with gadolinium. Bright on DWI and ADC.
   2. **ADEM:** Multiple lesions both supra- and infratentorially, cortical and subcortical, and fluffy in appearance.
   3. **Amyloid angiopathy:** Iron susceptibility sequence shows dark regions at sites of old bleeds (microhemorrhages).
   4. **Arteriovenous malformations:** Serpiginous hyper- and hypodensities on T2/FLAIR MRI; tangle of vessels on MRA.

Sequence	Good For	What's Bright	What's Dark	Comments
T1-weighted	Anatomy	Fat, subacute bleed, protein, calcium, melanomas	CSF, edema, bone, acute bleed; *most T1 lesions are dark*	Most useful when compared with T1-gado
T1 with gadolinium	Highly perfused lesions	Gado and T1-bright structures	T1-dark structures except those with high perfusion	To tell if scan is gado enhanced, look at cerebral veins or nasal mucosa
T2-weighted	Infarcts, inflammation, tumors	CSF, fluid, CVA, edema; *most T2 lesions are bright*	Solids, calcium, intact RBCs, ferritin, hemosiderin, mucinous mets	Good for CSF spaces
FLAIR (fluid attenuated inversion recovery)	Edema, gliosis, small WM lesions, anatomy	Edema, gliosis, old strokes, subacute bleed	CSF, hyperacute bleed	Like T2 but dark CSF; also good for delineating small lesions near CSF spaces
DWI (diffusion weighted)	Acute ischemia (~30 min to 7 days)	Acute stroke, abscess	CSF-filled spaces	Bright artifact at air-bone interface. "T2 shine through": T2-bright signal mimics CVA
ADC (apparent diffusion coefficient)	Acute ischemia	Edema, gliosis (including old strokes), CSF-filled spaces	Acute ischemia (allows to differentiate T2 shine through)	Calculated from DWI maps; ischemia seen from 30 min to 3-7 days

Table 51. Standard MRI sequences. They correspond to images in Figure 25.

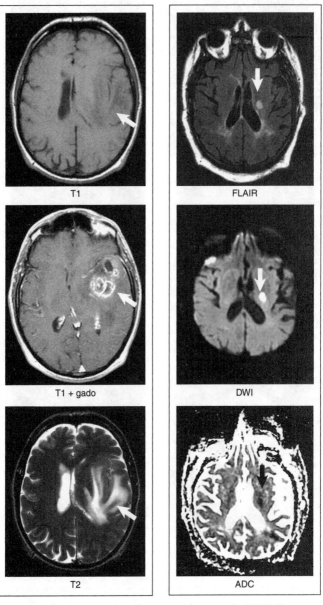

Figure 25. Standard MRI sequences. They correspond to row entries in Table 50; arrows point to pathology. Left: T1, T1+gado, and T2 scans of a tumor. Right: FLAIR, DWI, and ADC of an acute stroke.

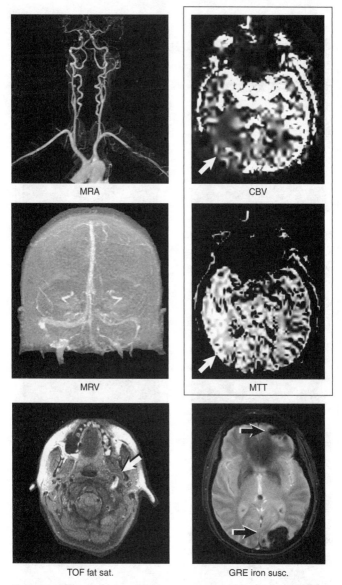

Figure 26. Additional MRI sequences. They correspond to row entries in Table 52. The MRA and MRV are gadolinium enhanced. The arrow in the fat sat sequence points to a carotid dissection. The grouped CBV and MTT sequences are from the same brain, and white arrows point to ischemia. The GRE iron sequence arrows point to hemorrhages.

MRA

CBV

MRV

MTT

TOF fat sat.

GRE iron susc.

Sequence	Good For	What's Bright	What's Dark	Comments
MRA, MRV (either time of flight [TOF] or with gado)	Extra- and intracranial flow	Blood vessels (arteries or veins)	Air, CSF	TOF shows flow but may exaggerate stenosis; gado-enhanced flow gives better view
TOF fat saturation ("fat sats")	Acute blood	Vessel wall clot, e.g., dissection	Fat, CSF (looks like a T1)	Test of choice for carotid/vertebral dissection
Iron susceptibility (gradient echo [GRE])	Iron products, calcium	CSF, gliosis, old strokes	Blood products, calcium	Helps tell blood from CT contrast; vessel cross-sections can look like tiny bleeds
MR perfusion	Diffusion-perfusion mismatch	Ischemia on MTT and TTP maps	Ischemia on CBV or CBF maps	Watch for asymmetry on all maps to identify mismatch
Functional MRI *(not shown)*	Preoperative lesion localization	High blood flow areas	Low blood flow areas	Shows blood flow's focal changes as area's activity changes
MR spectroscopy *(not shown)*	Tumors, metabolic disorders, strokes	N/A	N/A	Spectrum reads R → L: lipid, lactate, NAA, creatinine, choline, myoinositol

Table 52. Additional MRI sequences.

5. **Brainstem lesion:** Request thin cuts through the brainstem.
6. **Carotid or vertebral artery lesion:**
   a. **Stenosis:** MRA of neck and head. Few false negatives but frequent false positives.
   b. **Dissection:** Get TOF fat saturation and MRA. 90% sensitive.
7. **Chiasm/optic nerve/middle fossa problem:** Order gadolinium and fat suppression, with coronal cuts through orbit and middle fossa.
8. **Edema:** Bright T2 and FLAIR.

9. Hemorrhage dating: Complicated. CT is better for fresh blood. Dating uses hemoglobin's oxidation. The clot oxidizes from the outside in, giving a ring appearance at some stages.

Blood Age	Oxidation	T1	T2	Mnemonic
1-3 days	DeoxyHb *(i)*	**I**sodense	**D**ark	***Id****dy*
3-7 days	MetHb *(i)*	**B**right	**D**ark	***Bi****ddy*
7-14 days	MetHb *(e)*	**B**right	**B**right	***BaB****y*
>14 days	Hemosiderin *(e)*	**D**ark	**D**ark	***D****oo****d****oo*

Table 53. Intracerebral hemorrhage dating by MRI: principle, sequences, and the world's most famous mnemonic on MR blood aging.

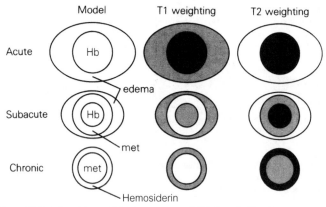

Figure 27. Variation with age of bleed appearance on MRI. (From Berlit P. *Memorix Neurology*. London: Chapman and Hall, 1996, with permission.)

10. Infarct: See also Figure 5, p. 27.
   a. Acute and subacute infarcts: Diffusion-weighted image (DWI) is bright and ADC is dark within 30 min and for 2 wk post stroke. ADC dark signal resolves by 2-7 days. After 4-12 h, see bright T2, bright FLAIR, bright proton density, dark T1. There may be edema or punctate hemorrhage associated with subacute infarcts.
   b. Chronic infarcts: Similar to subacute infarcts except that they are not bright on DWI/or dark on ADC, and may show tissue loss or cavitation rather than edema or hemorrhagic conversion.
11. Multiple sclerosis: T2-bright white matter lesions, usually periventricular, with long axis perpendicular to ventricles (Dawson's fingers). Acute plaques may ring enhance.
12. Spinal vertebral disc herniation: See Figure 28. On T2 images, compressed discs are darker. They bulge into CSF (bright) and sometimes spinal cord (grey). Axial cuts show nerve root impingement best.

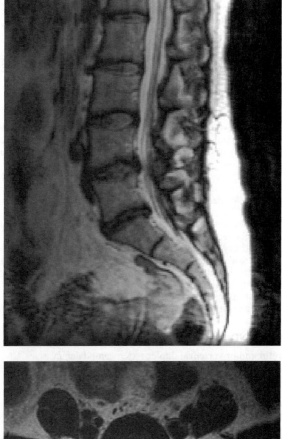

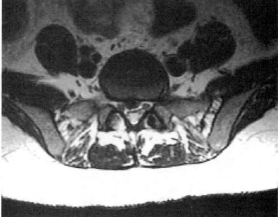

Figure 28. Parasagittal and axial T2-weighted MRI images show a right paracentral disc herniation towards the proximal right S1 nerve root.

13. **Spinal tumor:** Multiple lesions are common, so order a longitudinal scout of entire spine. Consider gadolinium.
   a. **Intramedullary:** Astrocytoma, ependymoma.
   b. **Intradural:** Nerve sheath tumor, meningioma, lymphoma.
   c. **Extradural:** Metastases, bone tumor.
14. **Tumor, brain:** T1 and T2 density will vary with tumor type, presence of hemorrhage, etc. Look for hydrocephalus, shift, necrosis, enhancement, edema. See also Tumors of Brain, p. 120.
   a. **Gray-white junction mass:** Usually metastasis.
   b. **Hemorrhagic mass:** suggests GBM, metastasis (renal cell CA, melanoma, thyroid, choriocarcinoma).
   c. **Calcification:** suggests oligodendroglioma, meningioma, AVM.
   d. **Lymphoma:** Little edema, often subcortical, often travels across corpus callosum ("butterfly appearance"). Enhancement is usually homogeneous, but in AIDS, may ring enhance and look like toxoplasmosis.
   e. **Glioma:** May have heterogeneous appearance, surrounded by significant edema with mass effect. May travel across corpus callosum. Gadolinium enhancing. Rarely multifocal.
   f. **Meningioma:** Extra-axial, usually dark on T2, enhances uniformly ("light bulb sign").
   g. **Pituitary tumor:** Get MRI with thin cuts thru sella. To see microadenoma, scan must be done within 5 min of gadolinium (normal pituitary enhances immediately, but microadenoma takes about 30 min).
   h. **Post-op scans:** Do within 48 h to see residual tumor before inflammation begins. Post-op pituitary scans are rarely helpful.

ULTRASOUND

A. **Carotid and/or vertebral duplex** (AKA carotid noninvasives, CNIs): For stenoses in neck vessels. Uses B-mode and pulsed Doppler imaging.
B. **Transcranial Doppler** (TCD): For stenoses in intracranial vessels. Specify anterior and/or posterior circulation TCDs when ordering. Add TCDs to CNIs if there is greater than 60% carotid stenosis on CNI. Can also help identify vasospasm, AVMs, absence of cerebral blood flow in brain death.
C. **Neonatal brain ultrasound.** For bleeds: periventricular leukomalacia, and congenital malformations in pt. with an open fontanelle.

MEDICINE

ALLERGY

A. Rx of anaphylaxis:
1. **Maintain airway:** Consider intubation.
2. **Epinephrine**:
   a. **Standard:** 0.2-0.5 cc of 1:1,000 IM, or SQ 0.2-0.5 mg q5min.
   b. **Elderly or in shock:** Dilute 0.1 cc of 1:1,000 in 10 cc NS; then give it IV over 5-10 min.
   c. **Stridor:** Racemic epinephrine nebs.
3. **Oxygen:** if slow response to epi or if underlying lung problems.
4. **IVF:** 1-2 L NS initially.
5. **Diphenhydramine + ranitidine:** IM 50 mg + IV 50 mg, respectively, over 5 minutes.
6. **Steroids:** E.g., dexamethasone 10-40 mg IV.
B. Premedication to prevent iodinated contrast reaction: Use nonionic contrast. Give prednisone 50 mg PO 13, 7, and 1 h before; diphenhydramine 50 mg PO 1 h before (but evidence for this is not strong).

BLOOD

A. Anemia:
1. **Neurological complications of anemia:** Lightheadedness, HA; sickle cell anemia can cause strokes, seizures, or extramedullary hematopoiesis in the meninges that mimics masses.
2. **H&P:** H/o ulcers, liver dz, easy bleeding, ecchymoses, stool guaiac, jaundice, adenopathy.
3. **Tests:** CBC, BUN/Cr. Consider reticulocyte count, smear for morphology, iron, TIBC, ferritin, bilirubin, endoscopy or abdominal CT, SIEP, Hb electrophoresis, haptoglobin, Coombs test, bone marrow biopsy.
4. **Causes of anemia:**
   a. **Acute:** Bleeding
   b. **Subacute:**
      1) Normal haptoglobin and bilirubin: Bleeding.
      2) Low haptoglobin, high unconjugated bili: Hemolysis (antibody-mediated, traumatic, toxic, intrinsic cell defect).
   c. **Chronic:**
      1) **Low reticulocyte count** (decreased production):
         a) **Low MCV** (microcytic):
            i. **Iron deficiency:** Fe and ferritin down, TIBC up. Usually from bleeding. Consider endoscopy. Treat with ferrous sulfate 325 mg tid if Fe/TIBC ratio is <20%.
            ii. **Anemia of chronic dz:** Fe down, ferritin up (only if ESR is up), TIBC down.
            iii. **Others:** Thalassemia, sideroblastic anemia.
         b) **Normal MCV** (normocytic): Bone marrow failure (aplastic anemia), either secondary (kidney, liver, or other chronic dz) or primary.

        c) **High MCV** (macrocytic): B_{12} or folate deficiency, drug-induced, liver dz, hypothyroidism.

    2) High reticulocyte count (increased production): Bleeding, hemolysis. See subacute anemia on page 204.

5. Rx of acute or severe anemia: Blood bank sample, type and cross 2 units, guaiac stools, consider transfusion, gastric lavage. For active bleeding, place two 14-gauage IVs, start saline, consider medicine or GI consult.

    a. Bleed on anticoagulants: Reverse anticoagulation. See p. 161.

    b. Transfusions: 1 unit packed red blood cells (PRBC) should raise Hct 3 points.

        1) Typical transfusion order: Transfuse 2 U PRBC over 4 h each; premed before each unit with acetaminophen 650 mg PO and diphenhydramine 50 mg PO.

        2) If severe anemia or danger of CHF: Premedicate with 20 mg furosemide IV before each unit.

        3) If danger of transfusion reaction: E.g., if pt. has received many transfusions, request leukopoor or washed RBCs.

        4) If pt. has suppressed marrow: Use irradiated RBCs.

    c. Transfusion reaction: Call blood bank.

        1) H&P: Sudden fever (most common), sweating, hives, wheezing, tachycardia, hypotension.

        2) Rx: Stop blood product. Diphenhydramine and acetaminophen if mild. If severe, add hydrocortisone 50-100 mg IV. If hemolysis, maintain diuresis with IV fluids and furosemide.

B. Coagulopathy:

1. Neurological complications of coagulopathy: Stroke, hemorrhage, HA, lightheadedness, neuropathy (especially femoral, from retroperitoneal bleed). Paraprotein can cause neuropathy.

2. H&P: Look for hematomas, signs of liver or autoimmune dz, tumor.

3. Tests: Check plts, PT, PTT, fibrinogen, D-dimer, protein C and S (cannot be tested on warfarin), antithrombin III (cannot be tested on heparin), anticardiolipin Ab, lupus anticoagulant, ESR, RF, ANA.

4. Causes of abnormal coagulation:

    a. Long PTT: Heparin, anticardiolipin Ab, lupus anticoagulant, intrinsic pathway defect, hemophilia, DIC.

    b. Long PT: Warfarin, vitamin K deficiency, liver dz, DIC, extrinsic pathway defect.

    c. Long PT and PTT: Very high levels of warfarin; common pathway defect, some lupus anticoagulant.

    d. Hypercoagulable states: DIC, tumors, pancreatitis, vasculitis, oral contraceptives, smoking, DM, nephrotic syndrome, anticardiolipin Ab, lupus anticoagulant, homocystinuria, thrombocytosis, leukostasis. Deficiency of protein C, activated protein C, protein S, or antithrombin III.

5. Anticoagulants: See p. 160.

6. Antibody-mediated coagulation disorders (antiphospholipid syndrome):

    a. Criteria: ≥ 1 each of clinical and laboratory criteria:

      1) Clinical: Stroke or other vascular thrombosis in any location, or complication of pregnancy.

      2) Laboratory: Anticardiolipin IgG or IgM antibodies at moderate-high levels, or lupus anticoagulant antibodies detected on ≥2 occasions ≥6 wk apart.

   b. Other sx: Thrombocytopenia, hemolytic anemia, or livedo reticularis.

   c. Arterial vs. venous clots: Pts. who have had one or the other tend to continue to have that kind. Most common thrombosis is DVT, but most common arterial-side clot is stroke.

   d. PTT: Normal or high, as these antibodies have anticoagulant as well as procoagulant effects.

   e. Cause: Primary or secondary (to autoimmune disease, primarily SLE).

   f. Rx: A thrombotic event is an indication for anticoagulation See Anticoagulants, p. 160, for contraindications. Coumadin goal is INR 2-3. Because these Abs can falsely raise PTT, heparinoids should be measured using anti-factor Xa levels.

C. DIC (disseminated intravascular coagulation): Often post-op, or from sepsis. Platelets and fibrinogen are low; PT, PTT, and D-dimer are high.

   1. Rx of DIC: Treat underlying cause; if necessary, replace with fresh frozen plasma, platelets, cryoprecipitate, blood. Heparin is usually not indicated, unless there is evidence of thrombosis (e.g., stroke, digit ischemia, or oliguria despite good SBP) or in some malignancies. Never give heparin if there has been head trauma.

D. Erythrocyte sedimentation rate (ESR): Nonspecific but useful to rule out temporal arteritis, cancer, chronic infection.

   1. Normal ESR for women = (age)/2 + 10.

   2. Normal ESR for men = (age)/2.

E. Eosinophilia: Mnemonic for causes is "<u>NAACP</u>": <u>N</u>eoplasm, <u>A</u>ddison's dz, <u>A</u>llergy, <u>C</u>ollagen vascular dz, <u>P</u>arasites.

F. Heparin-induced thrombocytopenia (HIT):

   1. H&P: Platelets fall while pt. is receiving heparin; also associated with venous or arterial thrombosis.

   2. Dx: Blood ELISA for heparin bound to platelet factor 4 (HIT test, sensitive but not specific).

   3. Rx: Permanently discontinue heparin (including low molecular weight). Change to argatroban, danaparoid, or hirudin if further anticoagulation is needed. (See Anticoagulants, p. 160.)

G. Platelet disorders:

   1. Neurological complications of platelet problems: See Coagulopathy, p. 192.

   2. H&P: NSAID or heparin use? HIV? Look for petechiae, mucous membrane bleeding.

   3. Tests: Consider bleeding time, von Willebrand's factor test, HIV.

   4. Contraindications: If plts <100: no surgery. Plts <50: no minor procedures. Plts <20: bleed from minor trauma. Plts <10: spontaneous bleeding (except in idiopathic thrombocytopenic purpura, where remaining plts are hyperactive).

5. **Causes:** DIC, drug reaction (e.g., HIT) idiopathic thrombocytopenic purpura (ITP), thrombotic thrombocytopenic purpura (TTP), SLE, HIV.
6. **Rx:** Try Amicar, DDAVP. Autoimmune problem may be helped with steroids, IgG, pheresis. Think twice about platelet transfusion in DIC, ITP, or TTP, where pt. may be hypercoagulable, and in autoimmune or drug-induced platelet dysfunction, where platelet transfusion probably will not help.

H. **Thrombotic thrombocytopenic purpura:**
1. **H&P:** Low platelets, microangiopathic hemolytic anemia, altered mental status (often with seizures); fever, renal problems.
2. **Rx:** Pheresis.

EPIDEMIOLOGY

A. **Sensitivity:** The probability that a test will be positive if the condition it tests for is present: Sens = (true positives)/(true positives + false negatives).
B. **Specificity:** The probability that a test will be negative if the condition it tests for is absent: Spec = (true negatives)/(true negatives + false positives).
C. **Bayes' theorem:** The likelihood of a pt. having a condition given a positive test result (i.e., the positive predictive value, PV^+) depends on the frequency (f) of the condition in the population. PV^+ = (f)(Sens)/[(f)(Sens) + (1 − f)(1 − Spec)]

ELECTROLYTES

A. **Tests:**
1. **Arterial blood gases and serum electrolytes:**
   a. **pH** <7.38 = acidosis; pH >7.42 = alkalosis.
      1) **Respiratory vs. metabolic pH changes:** If pH change is purely respiratory, for every change in pCO_2 of 10 torr, there should be 0.8 pH unit change. Greater or less than this implies superimposed metabolic process.
   b. **Bicarb** <24: Implies metabolic acidosis.
      1) **Anion gap** = Na − Cl − bicarb. Normally is <12 ± 4.
         a) **Correct for low albumin:** Normal anion gap = 2(alb) + 4.
         b) **Correct for alkalosis:** A pH >7.5 causes a high anion gap just by uncovering negative sites on albumin.
      2) **Respiratory compensation?** If 1.5(bicarb) + (8 ± 2) > pCO_2, then there is respiratory compensation for the metabolic alkalosis. But if it is < pCO_2, then there is a superimposed respiratory acidosis.
   c. **Bicarb** >24: Implies metabolic alkalosis. Look at pCO_2 (below) to see if there is a concurrent respiratory alkalosis.
   d. **pCO_2:** If pCO_2 <40, there is an added primary respiratory alkalosis. If pCO_2 >50, there is a primary respiratory acidosis.
      1) **Acute** if for every 10 mm Hg pCO_2 above (or below) normal, the pH is below (above) normal by 0.08.

2) **Chronic** if for every 10 mm Hg pCO_2 above (or below) normal, the pH is below (above) normal by 0.03.

2. **Venous blood gases** can be used to estimate arterial blood gases:
   a. **Venous bicarb + 2** = arterial bicarb.
   b. **Venous pCO_2 − 6** = arterial pCO_2.
   c. **Venous pH + 0.04** = arterial pH.
3. **Urine electrolytes:** Get Na, K, Cr, osms. Get serum Cr and serum osms at same time. Diuretics must have been held for at least 6 h.
   a. **Urine Na <9** is consistent with dehydration (hanging onto salt).
   b. **Urine Na >20** but low serum Na and normal osms might be SIADH or renal failure.
   c. **Urine anion gap:** Useful in hyperchloremic metabolic acidosis. Measure the urine sodium + urine potassium − urine chloride. The remainder is ammonium ion.
      1) **Positive urine anion gap:** Implies renal wasting of bicarb.
      2) **Negative urine anion gap:** Implies GI wasting of bicarb.

B. **Electrolyte abnormalities:**
   1. **Acidosis:**
      a. **Causes of anion gap acidosis:**
         1) **Increased production of acid:**
            a) **Lactate.**
            b) **Ketosis:** DM, alcohol, starvation.
            c) **Ingestion:** Salicylates, methanol, ethylene glycol.
         2) **Decreased excretion of acid:** Renal failure.
      b. **Causes of non–anion gap acidosis:** Diarrhea, dilutional acidosis, carbonic anhydrase inhibitors, renal tubular acidosis. . . .
      c. **Rx:** Treat cause. Respiratory acidosis usually requires intubation. For severe acidosis, pH <7.2, consider 44-88 mEq Na bicarbonate IV, in IV solution appropriate to the pts. fluid status. Do not correct to pH >7.2.
         1) **Complications of bicarbonate rx:** Fluid overload, precipitation of acute tetany in pts. with renal failure, and "relative CSF acidosis" (which can cause coma).
   2. **Metabolic alkalosis:**
      a. **Causes:** Vomiting, NG suction, dehydration, low K, loop diuretics, mineralocorticoids, compensation for chronic respiratory acidosis. . . .
      b. **Rx:** Alkalosis usually resolves with volume correction and KCl—be careful with the latter in renal failure. Correct alkalosis promptly in pts. with neuromuscular or myocardial irritability.
   3. **High sodium:** See Figure 29.
      a. **H&P:** Confusion, thirst, signs of dehydration.
      b. **Rx:** Correct Na slowly to avoid brain edema, CHF. See Dehydration, p. 197.
   4. **Low sodium:** See Figure 30.
      a. **H&P:** Confusion, seizures, signs of dehydration.
      b. **Rx:** Correct Na slowly to avoid central pontine myelinolysis. See p. 197 for correction algorithms.

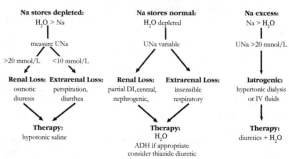

Figure 29. Dx and rx of high serum sodium.

5. **SIADH:**
   a. **Criteria:** Euvolemic hyponatremia from inappropriately concentrated urine, without renal or adrenal dysfunction.
   b. **DDx of SIADH:** Dehydration, overhydration, renal failure, adrenal failure, hypothyroidism, cerebral salt wasting.
   c. **Causes of SIADH:**
      1) **Intracranial processes:** E.g., trauma, infection, tumor. However, you must rule out cerebral salt wasting—see below.
      2) **Lung processes:** E.g., trauma, infection, tumor.
      3) **Other:** Drugs, e.g., carbamazepine; malignancies, anemia, stress, porphyria.

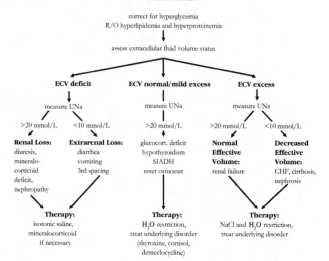

Figure 30. Dx and rx of low serum sodium.

    d. Rx of SIADH:
- **1) Acute:** Free water restriction; if symptomatic hyponatremia, then consider slow correction with hypertonic saline.
- **2) Chronic:** Fluid restriction; high-salt diet. Consider furosemide, demeclocycline 300 mg bid-qid.

6. Cerebral salt wasting (CSW): Hyponatremia from inappropriate excretion of salt in the kidney, via an unknown central mechanism. Unlike SIADH, pts. with CSW are usually hypovolemic. Physical exam, central venous pressure, pulmonary wedge pressure, plasma and urine osms, etc., can help tell if the pt. is hypovolemic. CSW is not uncommon in SAH, and inappropriate fluid restriction for supposed SIADH can worsen SAH vasospasm.

C. Dehydration:

1. H&P: HR, SBP, urine output. Pt. is orthostatic if SBP drops >15 mm Hg or HR increases >20 bpm from lying to sitting after 2 minutes. Look at skin turgor, mucosal hydration.

2. Labs: Electrolytes, BUN, glucose, osms, UA.
- **a. Specific gravity:** <1.015 suggests a renal concentration defect, >1.030 = moderate dehydration, >1.035 = severe.
- **b. Units:** In the following, Na is always measured in mEq/L.

3. Rx of dehydration:
- **a. Discontinue diuretics.**
- **b. Replacement rate** = (deficit/time desired to replete) + maintenance rate.
  - **1) Calculate deficit:**
    - **a) Total deficit** = (old wt − new wt) <u>or</u> = 0.35 (old wt) (1 − old Hct/new Hct). Third-spacing will make these two numbers different; use the Hct estimate.
    - **b) Free water deficit** (in hypernatremia) = TBW (Na − 140)/140, where TBW = total body water = 0.5 (wt) for women, 0.6 (wt) for men.
  - **2) Calculate maintenance** per kg body weight:
    - **a) For 1st 10 kg:** 4 cc/h/kg.
    - **b) For 2nd 10 kg:** 2 cc/h/kg.
    - **c) Above that:** 1 cc/h/kg.
- **c. Type of fluid to use:**
  - **1) For Na 130–150** (isotonic dehydration): Give hypotonic dextrose solution (30–55 mEq Na/L). Give 50% of replacement in 1st 8 h; rest during next 16 h.
  - **2) For Na <130** (hypotonic dehydration): Give isotonic Na.
    - **a) Beware of central pontine myelinolysis**, which may result from overrapid correction of hyponatremia. It presents as mutism, oculobulbar palsies, and quadriparesis. Correct Na slowly, not more than 1 U/h.
    - **b) Beware of seizures** when Na <120.
  - **3) For Na >150** (hypertonic dehydration): Give D5 1/2 NS.
    - **a) Beware of cerebral edema:** Correct Na slowly; it should not fall >10 mEq/24 h.

4. Low potassium:
- **a. H&P:** EKG changes (see Electrocardiogram, p. 207), arrhythmia, muscle twitching, weakness.

    b. Causes: Vomiting, diarrhea, diuretics, alkalosis (intracellular K shift), hyperaldosteronism, familial periodic paralysis. . . .

    c. Complicating conditions: It is important to keep serum K >4.0 in cardiac pts., asthmatics on β_2-agonists, and type 2 DM.

    d. Rx: Be cautious if there is renal failure. With normal pts., KCl 40 mEq PO q4h × 3 doses is usually enough. IV K correction should usually not exceed 10 mEq/h (note: 40 mEq KCl/L at 100 mL/h is 4 mEq KCl/h).

5. High potassium:

    a. H&P: EKG changes (see Electrocardiogram, p. 207), arrhythmia, flaccid paralysis.

    b. Causes: Acidosis, diuretics, renal failure, hemolysis, rhabdomyolysis, Addison's, familial periodic paralysis. . . .

    c. Rx: Stop K supplements. For serum K >5.5 in renal failure, give sodium polystyrene sulfonate (Kayexalate) 30-60 g PO or enema. For emergent rx, consider 1 amp CaCl or Ca gluconate IV, or 2 amps Na bicarbonate with 2 amps D50 given with 10 U regular insulin IV.

6. Low calcium:

    a. H&P: Confusion, papilledema. Ca <7 can cause tetany (Chvostek's and Trousseau's signs), laryngospasm, and seizures.

    b. Correction for low albumin: For every 1 g/dL albumin deficit, lower limit of normal Ca will decrease 0.8 mg/dL. Can also check ionized Ca, which is not influenced by protein, on an ABG. It is normally >1.0.

    c. Rx: Ca carbonate 500 mg PO tid, or Ca gluconate 1-2 amps IV in 250 cc NS, given over 2-4 h. Beware giving Ca to pts. on digoxin.

7. High calcium: Consider medicine consult.

    a. H&P: Abdominal pain, nausea, confusion, muscle weakness.

    b. Causes: Cancer, endocrine, granulomatous dzs, renal failure....

    c. Rx: Emergent if Ca >15. Aggressive hydration, then diuretics; specific drugs such as bisphosphonates, but caution that these effects last up to a month.

8. Low magnesium:

    a. H&P: Nausea, tremor, fasciculations, tetany.

    b. Rx: $MgCl_2$ 10 cc PO × 3 days; or $MgSO_4$ 2 g IV in 250 cc D5 W IV. Be careful in renal failure.

9. Low phosphate: Treat with PO phosphate 2 tabs tid × 3 d, or Na- or K-phosphate 10 mmol over 6-8 h IV. Be careful in renal failure.

10. High phosphate: Treat with PhosLo 1-2 tabs PO tid.

GLANDS

A. Adrenal:

1. Adrenal insufficiency:

    a. Neurological complications of adrenal insufficiency: Lethargy, abdominal pain, neurological signs of low sodium (tremor, aphasia, ataxia, seizures, corticospinal tract signs) and high potassium. All male pts. with Addison's dz should be tested for X-linked adrenoleukodystrophy (see p. 144).

    b. <u>**Adrenal crisis is an emergency:**</u> Besides the above sx, there is dehydration and high BUN. Look for triggers, e.g., infection, MI.

    c. Tests:

        1) Cortisol: May be a better screen for adrenal suppression after prolonged steroid use. Best to do 8 AM cortisol (normal 6-18 μg/dL), but in an emergency, draw a random level before giving steroids.

        2) ACTH stimulation test: Can be done on dexamethasone. For pts. on prednisone, hold it until after cortisol drawn. Give ACTH (Cortrosyn) 0.25 mg IV; measure cortisol then and 60 min later. Nl >18 μg/dL, or >7 μg/dL rise.

    d. Rx: Immediate hydrocortisone 100 mg IV q8h.

  2. Adrenal excess (Cushing's syndrome), or exogenous steroids:

    a. H&P: See Drugs, p. 173, for signs of adrenal excess.

    b. Baseline 8 AM cortisol test: Normal is 6-18 μg/dL.

    c. Low-dose suppression test: Give dexamethasone 1 mg PO at 11 PM, draw serum cortisol at 8 AM. Cortisol <5 μg/dL is normal, 5-10 is indeterminate, and >10 is evidence for Cushing's syndrome.

    d. High-dose suppression test: Helps tell pituitary adrenocorticotropic hormone (ACTH) hypersecretion from adrenal tumor or ectopic ACTH secretion. Give dexamethasone 8 mg PO at 11 PM, draw cortisol at 8 AM. In 95% of pituitary ACTH hypersecretion, but not other causes, cortisol will decrease to <50% of baseline. Phenytoin may interfere with this.

B. Diabetes insipidus (DI): Low antidiuretic hormone (ADH) causes dilute urine, water craving, danger of severely high Na.

  1. Causes: Pituitary damage, e.g., from surgery, head trauma, transtentorial herniation, neurosarcoid, A-comm aneurysm.

  2. DDx: Psychosomatic polydipsia, osmotic diuresis, nephrogenic DI.

  3. Tests: If there is high clinical suspicion, the following four criteria are usually sufficient:

    a. Urine osms: 50-150 mOsm/L or specific gravity <1.005.

    b. Urine output: >250 cc/h (or >3 cc/kg/h).

    c. Serum sodium: Normal or high.

    d. Normal adrenal function: The kidney needs mineralocorticoids to make free water, so steroids may unmask DI by correcting adrenal insufficiency.

  4. Rx: Intranasal desmopressin 10-40 μg bid (typically 20 μg); titrate to urine output.

    a. Post-op transsphenoidal surgery: First try to keep up with fluid loss by IV or PO fluids, as desmopressin sometimes overtreats. Then try desmopressin in above dose range, although you need to give it SQ or IV until nasal packs are out.

C. Diabetes mellitus:

  1. Neurological complications of DM: Glucose-related mental status changes, neuropathy (see p. 93), increased stroke risk.

    a. Hypoglycemia:

        1) H&P: Decreased POs or increased DM medications, with variable tremulousness, fatigue, dysarthria, confusion, seizures (glucose usually <30 mg/dL), coma with pupillary dilatation and extensor posturing (glucose usually <10).

   2) Tests: Low fingerstick glucose.

   3) Rx: Emergent correction of glucose. Hypoglycemic coma can cause permanent neurological damage.

  b. DM ketoacidosis:

   1) H&P: Often type 1 DM with precipitating illness. See subacute polyuria followed by anorexia, confusion (glucose >425 mg/dL), coma (glucose >600).

   2) Tests: Glucose, anion gap, ketones, osmolarity, ABG.

   3) Rx: Correction of glucose, dehydration, potassium. <u>Central pontine myelinolysis</u> can occur when blood osmolarity is lowered more rapidly than brain osmolarity.

  c. Nonketotic hyperglycemic coma:

   1) H&P: Often type 2 DM with infection. Steroids or phenytoin can sometimes be precipitants. Slower onset than DKA. Cerebral dysfunction and seizures are common.

   2) Tests: Glucose, osmolarity, ABG.

   3) Rx: First priority is maintaining blood pressure and cardiac output with IV fluid; correct glucose as needed.

2. Regular insulin (CZI) sliding scale: See Admission Orders, p. 13. All diabetics should be covered with an insulin sliding scale while in house, even if they take only oral hypoglycemics at home. It is best to stop oral agents while pt. is in hospital, as glucose levels will vary from home levels.

3. To convert regular (CZI) to NPH insulin: (2/3)(CZI used qd); give 2/3 of that in AM, 1/3 in PM.

4. Insulin preparations:

Preparation	Onset	Peak	Duration
Lispro (Humalog)	SQ: 5-15 min	0.5-3 h	2-5 h
Aspart (Novolog)	SQ: 5-15 min	0.5-3 h	2-5 h
Regular (CZI)	IV: immediate	15-30 min	2 h
	IM: 5-30 min	30-60 min	2-4 h
	SQ: 30-60 min	2-3 h	6-10 h
NPH, Lente	SQ: 2-4 h	4-10 h	10-16 h
Ultralente	SQ: 6-10 h	No peak	18-20 h
Glargine (Lantus)	SQ: 1.1 h	No peak	24 h

Table 54. Insulin kinetics.

D. Thyroid:

  1. Neurological complications of hyperthyroidism: Tremor, seizures, brisk reflexes, ophthalmopathy, proximal myopathy.

  2. Neurological complications of hypothyroidism: Apathy, "hung-up" reflexes, myopathy, and high CPK. The slow muscle relaxation differs from myotonia in being more painful and worse with exercise. Sometimes see seizures, obstructive sleep apnea, ataxia, hearing loss.

T_3 (triiodothyronine) is better than T_4 (thyroxine) for treating neurological complications.

3. **Tests:** First test TSH. If low, also check T_3, T_4, free T_4, and maybe antithyroid antibodies. If high, check T_4.

E. **Parathyroid:** Psychiatric sx. Hyperparathyroidism can cause myopathy; hypoparathyroidism can cause seizures and other signs of low calcium and magnesium.

GUT

A. **Abdominal pain:**
  1. **Common causes:** Infection, obstruction, ulcer, GI bleed, cholecystitis, pancreatitis, mesenteric ischemia, kidney stone, drug, toxin, urinary tract infection, ectopic pregnancy, ovarian torsion, inferior MI, herpes zoster.
  2. **H&P:** N/V, stool appearance, bowel sounds, rebound.
  3. **Tests:** Consider CBC, electrolytes, β-HCG, LFTs, amylase, UA, guaiac, abdominal x-ray, renal, right upper quadrant, or pelvic US, endoscopy, CT.

B. **Constipation:**
  1. **R/o obstruction in acute-onset constipation.**
  2. **Common neural causes:** Pt. inactivity, medications (e.g., TCAs, opiates), depression, IBS, parkinsonism, spine trauma.
  3. **Rx:** Never give anything from above if pt. may be obstructed, i.e., lower "afterload" before raising "preload" or "inotropy."
    a. **Change offending meds:** E.g., use Comtan rather than Requip, Cymbalta rather than amitriptyline.
    b. **Afterload reducers:** Dulcolax suppositories, Fleets enemas, mineral oil enemas.
    c. **Preload:** MOM 30 cc PO qid prn.
    d. **Inotropy:** Senokot 1-2 tabs bid prn, or Mg citrate 1 bottle, or lactulose 30 cc q2h until pt. stools.
    e. **Stool softeners:** Colace 100 mg tid (<u>not</u> prn).

C. **Diarrhea:** Consider *C. difficile* infection. Symptomatic rx: Lomotil 2 tabs PO qid prn, loperamide 2 mg PO prn (max. 16 qd).

D. **GI bleed (GIB):**
  1. **Upper GIB:** From ulcer, varix, Mallory-Weiss tear.
  2. **Lower GIB:** From ischemia, thrombosis, intussusception, dysentery, colitis, diverticulosis, cancer, polyp, hemorrhoids, anal fissure/ulcer, AVM, angiodysplasia.
  3. **Nasogastric tube** with cold lavage helps both dx and rx.
    a. **Contraindications:** Variceal bleeding.
    b. **False negatives:** Can have upper GIB with negative nasogastric lavage if bleed is duodenal. Look for high BUN.
  4. **Labs:** CBC, blood bank sample, PT, PTT, DIC screen, consider emergent endoscopy.
  5. **Rx of GIB:**
    a. **Orders:** NPO, orthostatic BPs, two large IVs, guaiac all stools, cardiac monitor. GI consult.
    b. **IV fluid or blood.**

    c. Upper GIB: IV ranitidine; consider *H. pylori* Abx. Ranitidine will increase phenytoin and warfarin levels.

    d. Varices: Consider pitressin + nitroglycerine, or octreotide (fewer side effects than vasopressin), or DDAVP (selective splanchnic bed constriction, emergent endoscopy for banding, or sclerotherapy). Pt. should eventually be on long-term beta-blockade.

    e. Catastrophic bleed: Blakemore tube.

    f. Bleed on anticoagulants: Reverse anticoagulation. See p. 161.

E. Hiccups: From diaphragmatic or phrenic irritation; consider brainstem lesion. Treat cause, or:

  1. Hypercarbia: Try repeated breath holding or rebreathing into a paper bag.

  2. Vagal stimulation: Try drinking ice water rapidly, tongue traction, eyeball pressure.

  3. Meds: Sometimes helped by baclofen 5 mg tid, chlorpromazine 25 mg bid, scopolamine, amphetamine, opiates. . . .

F. Liver dz:

  1. Hepatic encephalopathy:

    a. H&P: Confusion, asterixis in pt. with liver failure, usually with precipitating illness.

    b. DDx: Other deliriums, Wernicke's syndrome, aphasia, psychosis.

    c. Tests: Ammonia high, but it may take several days for pt. to recover even after ammonia has returned to baseline. MRI may show T1 signal in basal ganglia, but is not that helpful. EEG will show slowing or triphasic waves.

    d. Rx: Lactulose, low-protein diet, oral neomycin.

  2. Bilirubin: Direct = conjugated. High indirect suggests hemolysis, ineffective erythropoiesis, Gilbert's syndrome.

  3. Alkaline phosphatase up but 5'-nucleotidase normal suggests extra-hepatic source of alk phos, e.g., bone.

  4. Transferases: ALT = SGPT; AST = SGOT.

	Dir/Tot Bili	Alk Phos	Transferases
Hemolysis	+/++	nl	nl
Acute hepatitis	+/+	<3×	SGOT > SGPT, >400
Chronic hepatitis	+/+	<3×	SGPT > SGOT, <300
Acute cholestasis	nl	nl	Ts often > alk phos
Chronic cholestasis	+/+	>4×	<300
Metastasis	nl	>4×	<300
Shock liver	nl	nl	SGPT >> SGOT

Table 55. Enzyme changes in liver disease.

G. Vomiting

  1. H&P: Nausea, color of vomit, diarrhea, fever, precipitating factors, diet, drugs, previous bowel surgery, vertigo, double vision, dysarthria, hearing loss. Neuro and abdominal exam. <u>Always</u> see the pt. walk to rule out ataxia.

2. **DDx:** GI infection, vertigo, drugs, toxins, alcohol, obstruction, gastroparesis, perforated bowel, pregnancy, metabolic disturbance (e.g., uremia and hyperglycemia), brainstem lesion, severe fear or pain.
3. **Complications:** Dehydration and orthostasis, acidosis, low K, gastric or esophageal (Mallory-Weiss) bleed, perforated esophagus.
4. **Tests:** Electrolytes; consider tox screen, MRI for brainstem lesion.
   a. **Abdominal x-ray** is low-yield unless abdomen is severely tender or there is a high suspicion of obstruction.
5. **Rx of vomiting:**
   a. **Orders:** NS + 20 KCl, NG tube, NPO.
   b. **Antidopaminergic drugs** (q.v. p. 169):
      1) **Indications:** GI causes, surgery, radiation, or chemotherapy.
      2) **Contraindications:** Movement disorders, vertigo. In young people, watch for acute dystonia.
      3) **Butyrophenones:** E.g., droperidol 0.0625-2.5 mg q3-6h IV/IM. Sedating. Good for nausea from morphine. Beware prolonged QT, torsades; should be used only for refractory nausea/vomiting.
      4) **Phenothiazines:** Avoid in epilepsy, head trauma. Promethazine (Phenergan) 25-50 mg q4-6h PO/IM/PR risks dystonia and seizures less than prochlorperazine (Compazine).
      5) **Metoclopramide** (Reglan): 10 mg IV/IM q2-3h or 10-30 mg PO qid before meals and qhs. A motility agent. Avoid in GI obstruction. Good for gastroparesis.
   c. **Antihistamines:** E.g., meclizine (Antivert) 25 mg PO qid. Suppresses the vestibular apparatus in vertigo.
   d. **Anticholinergics** (q. v., p. 168): E.g., scopolamine.
      1) **Indications:** Motion sickness.
      2) **Contraindications:** Outlet obstruction, DM gastroparesis, glaucoma.
   e. **Central:** E.g., ondansetron (Zofran) 4 mg IV or 8 mg PO, or granisetron (Kytril) 750 µg IV or 1 mg PO.

HEART

A. **Cardiac code calls:**
   1. **What you need:** Call code team; bag-valve ventilator, 12-lead EKG; cardiac and oxygen monitor; large-bore IV access; stat blood gas, electrolytes, and CBC; defibrillator and code cart. Arrange for an ICU bed.
   2. **Basic life support:** For all cases, two initial breaths, then compressions 80-100 per minute.
      a. **One rescuer:** 15:2 ratio of compressions to ventilations.
      b. **Two rescuers or pediatric:** 5:1 ratio of compressions to ventilations.
   3. **Advanced cardiac life support:** See Figures 31 and 32.
B. **Neurological complicaions of heart dz:** Embolic stroke, global hypoxia. MIs are RFs for stroke and vice versa. A fib, mechanical valves, and LV thrombus are all reasons for anticoagulation to prevent stroke.

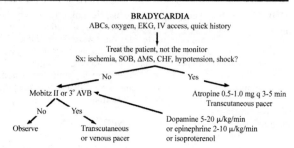

Figure 31. Bradycardia ACLS protocol.

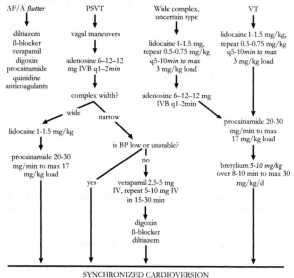

Figure 32. Tachycardia ACLS protocol.

PULSELESS ACLS PROTOCOLS

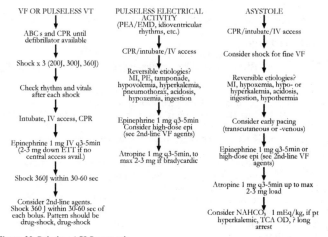

Figure 33. Pulseless ACLS protocols.

C. Arrhythmia:

1. **See also:** Electrocardiogram, p. 207.
2. **H&P:** Is pt. symptomatic during arrhythmia? What drugs is pt. on? Freq, duration, what triggers and stops rhythm.
3. **Tests:** EKG (compare with <u>old</u>), electrolytes, Ca, Mg, TSH, ABG, drug levels, CXR.
4. **Atrial fibrillation (A fib):**
   a. **Causes:** Ischemia, PE, thyroid, drugs, conduction system problem, alcohol binge, post heart surgery.
   b. **EKG:** Absent P waves. If QRS is wide, consider V tach.
   c. **Rx of new A fib:** Consider cardiology consult if unable to control rate. Unstable pts. may require immediate cardioversion.
      1) **Diltiazem:** Bolus 20 mg IV over 2 min; may repeat in 15 min. Consider verapamil or β-blockers (i.e., metoprolol 5 mg IV q5min × 3). Always give oral dose once rate controlled, as IV dosing wears off quickly.
      2) **Digoxin:** 0.5 mg IV, then 0.25 mg PO q8h × 2, then 0.125-0.25 mg qd. Takes time for effect—not always the first-line agent. See Digoxin, p. 168.
      3) **Contraindications to A fib drugs:**
         a) **Wide QRS complex:** May actually be V tach, in which Ca channel blockers may be lethal. Consider adenosine. Treat like V tach: 75 mg lidocaine, cardiovert.
         b) **Hypotension.**
         c) **Plan for DC cardioversion:** Digoxin may make cardioversion dangerous.

    4) DC cardioversion: <u>Emergent</u> if there is angina, low BP, CHF.

    5) Anticoagulation: See Anticoagulants, p. 160.

5. AV block:

  a. 1st degree = Long PR. Do not treat unless bradycardic. Consider digoxin toxicity as cause.

  b. 2nd degree:

    1) Mobitz I (Wenckebach): Above bundle of His.

      a) EKG: Gradual PR lengthening, narrow QRS, RR gradually shorter.

      b) Rx: Usually benign. If pt. is symptomatic or if there is bundle branch block, give atropine or pace.

    2) Mobitz II: The lesion is usually below the bundle of His. May go to complete heart block.

      a) EKG: PR constant; usually wide QRS; occasional nonconducted P wave.

      b) Rx: Cardiology consult. Needs pacer even if pt. is asymptomatic. In the mean time, if symptomatic, use atropine, isoproterenol, or external pacing.

  c. 3rd degree: Complete heart block. Treat as Mobitz II, but more urgently.

6. Bradycardia: See Cardiac code calls, p. 203.

7. Junctional rhythm:

  a. EKG: Narrow QRS but no P waves.

  b. Rx: Treat underlying condition (ischemia, dig toxicity). Treat paroxysmal junctional tach like SVT, but carotid massage does not work as well.

8. Premature beats: (PACs, PVCs). Usually treat only if pt. is symptomatic, but check with cardiology—some PVCs are "malignant."

9. Supraventricular tachycardia (SVT, AKA PSVT):

  a. DDx: V tach; rapid A fib, sinus tach.

  b. EKG: Narrow-complex tachycardia always preceded by P waves. Tachycardia can cause ST depression and T wave inversion, without ischemia, even after tachycardia has resolved.

  c. Rx: See Cardiac code calls, p. 203. Consult cardiology.

    1) Adenosine if narrow-complex tachycardia.

      a) Dosing: Run rhythm strip; give 6-12-12 mg rapid bolus through peripheral IV (3-6-6 if central line) q1-2min.

      b) Complications: Watch for bronchospasm and low BP. If pt. is on theophylline, adenosine may not work.

      c) Specific conditions: Okay to use in Wolff-Parkinson-White (WPW). In A fib/flutter, adenosine will uncover a string of nonconducted Ps.

    2) Cardioversion if pt. has angina, hypotension, or CHF.

    3) Carotid sinus massage ± Valsalva maneuver. Need IV access and EKG monitoring. Rule out bruits first. Massage carotids only one side at a time: 10 sec on R; if no response, then 10 sec on L. This may convert A flutter to A fib.

    4) Nodal blockers:

      a) Contraindications: Avoid in wide-complex tachycardia, hypotension.

        b) Verapamil: 5-10 mg IV over 2-3 min.

        c) Beta-block: Propranolol 0.15 mg/kg at 1 mg/min, or esmolol if h/o asthma.

        d) Digoxin: 0.5-0.75 mg IV/PO, then 0.25 mg q2h as needed.

10. Torsades de pointes:

  a. Causes: Things that lengthen QT interval, e.g., bradycardia, antiarrhythmics; phenothiazines; low K, Mg, or Ca; cerebral hemorrhage, ischemia, cardiomyopathy, congenital long QT, erythromycin + Seldane.

  b. EKG: QRS height varies sinusoidally, HR 160-180. Long QTc.

  c. Rx: Consult cardiology. Stop offending drugs. Give magnesium. Treat drug or metabolic imbalance. Consider lidocaine, phenytoin, isoproterenol (cautious if CAD), overdrive pacing.

11. Ventricular fibrillation (V fib): Call a code. See p. 203.

12. Ventricular tachycardia (V tach):

  a. DDx: Aberrantly conducted SVT (15%, usually with RBB), tachycardic A fib. When in doubt, treat as V tach.

  b. Causes: Ischemia, MI recovery (especially with post-MI aneurysm), cardiomyopathy, prolonged QT, mitral valve prolapse, drug toxicity, metabolic disturbance.

  c. EKG: >6 wide QRSs at 100-200 bpm. ST and T changes in direction opposite to major QRS deflection. LAD (compared with axis in sinus). AV dissociation. Monophasic or biphasic RBBB QRSs with LAD and R/S <1 in V6.

  d. Rx:

    1) Sustained V tach: Call a code. See p. 203.

    2) Nonsustained V tach: Consult cardiology immediately. Treat V tach if pt. is symptomatic during V tach or if runs are increasing in frequency or length (this has high risk of V fib).

13. Varying rhythm:

  a. Identical Ps: Suggests sinus arrhythmia; observe.

  b. Changing Ps: Suggests wandering atrial pacemaker or multifocal atrial tachycardia.

    1) Causes: COPD, hypoxia, digoxin toxicity, mitral regurgitation, myocard. scar.

    2) Rx: Correct hypoxia, electrolytes; try verapamil or diltiazem, beta-block (<u>not</u> if COPD), consider Ia antiarrhythmics, amiodarone. <u>Avoid</u> digoxin.

  c. No P waves: Suggests A fib.

D. Electrocardiogram:

  1. <u>Compare all EKGs to old ones.</u>

  2. Heart rate: Normally 60-100. One box = 0.04 sec.

  3. Rhythm: Look at both Ps and QRSs. If there is arrhythmia (see Arrhythmia, p. 205), ask:

    a. What is relation between P and QRS? Ps best seen in leads II and V1. Should be upright there.

    b. Wide or narrow QRS?

    c. QRS regular or irregular?

  4. Intervals:

    a. PR: 3-5 boxes. <0.12 sec suggests WPW; >0.2 sec = AV block.

    b. QRS: >3 boxes (0.12) suggests ventricular arrhythmia or bundle branch block (BBB). Look in widest QRS, usually V1, V5.

    c. QT: 7-10 boxes (0.28-0.40 sec) for normal rate.

       1) QTc = $QT/(RR\ interval)^{1/2}$. Less than 0.42 for men, 0.43 women.

       2) DDx: Drugs (quinidine, procainamide, TCAs, phenothiazines), hypothermia, electrolyte abnormality, pentamidine, idiopathic.

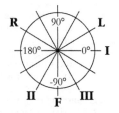

Figure 34. EKG axes.

5. Axis: Normal if upright in I, F (or, more liberally, if −30 to +90).

6. P waves: Best seen in II and VI.

    a. Absent Ps: Atrial fibrillation (q.v. p. 205).

    b. Inverted Ps in II, III, or F: Low atrial or junctional pacemaker.

7. QRS waves:

    a. Q wave = significant when more than 1 box wide or deep, or more than 1/3 of the following R wave. Normal in III, or small isolated Q in I, L, F, V4-V6. Q in III can also suggest PE.

    b. Poor R-wave progression (PRWP): DDx = anterior MI, LBBB.

    c. Too-good RWP (R in V1-V2 larger than in V3): Posterior MI, RV infarct, lateral MI, RBBB, RV hypertrophy, WPW.

    d. LV hypertrophy: S in V1 + R in V5 >35 mm. LAD, wide QRS, and T slants down slowly and returns rapidly.

8. ST segments: Compare voltages to TP segment, not PR.

    a. ST elevation: Nl <1 mm limb leads; <2 mm chest.

       1) DDx: Acute MI, LBBB, J point elevation (concave, upsloping ST in young people).

       2) Persistent ST elevations: DDx: persistent ischemia, LV aneurysm, pericarditis (concave, widespread, or anterior).

    b. ST depression: DDx: ischemia, digoxin (upsloping), exercise, strain, PE (especially lead II).

9. T waves: Can be down in III, L, F, V1-V2. Brain injury can cause nonspecific T wave changes, but this is a diagnosis of exclusion.

    a. Peaked (hyperacute) T waves: Ischemia, high K. Ts should be <5 mm in limb leads; <10 mm in chest leads.

    b. T wave flattening: Ischemia, post MI, low K.

    c. T wave inversion (TWI): Ischemia, post MI, BBB (should be in opposite direction), strain (biphasic and asymmetric in V5-V6), sometimes just from tachycardia. Normally inverted in R.

    d. Pseudonormalized Ts: I.e., formerly inverted, now flat or upright. Suggests ischemia.

    e. T wave axis: Should be <50 from QRS axis.

10. U waves: Low K, low Mg.

E. Miscellaneous EKG syndromes:

    1. Beta-blockers: Bradycardia, AV block.

    2. Bundle branch block (BBB): If QRS >0.12. Left BBBs can have fixed ST elevations not associated with MI, but always worry if the elevations change.

3. **Calcium:**
    a. **Calcium channel blockers:** Sinus arrest, AV block.
    b. **High Ca:** Short QT, tachycardia.
    c. **Low Ca:** Long QTc.
4. **Digoxin toxicity:** Upsloping ST depressions, tachycardia, AV block, junctional rhythms, bradycardic junctional escape, V tach, V fib.
5. **Potassium:**
    a. **High K:** In sequence as K rises, see peaked T (esp. V2-V4), ST depression, decreased R waves, PR lengthening, flat P, wide QRS, long QT, torsades.
    b. **Low K:** Flat T and U wave, ST depression, SVT, A fib, long QT.
6. **Pulmonary embolus:** Often nonspecific sinus tachycardia, sometimes SI-QIII-TIII (big S in I, Q, and TWI in III), right axis deviation and right BBB.

F. **Coronary artery dz:**
    1. **Acute MI:**
        a. **DDx of chest pain:** Aortic dissection, peri- or myocarditis, PE, PTX, perforated ulcer, cholecystitis, pancreatitis, rupture of the esophagus, musculoskeletal pain.
        b. **Tests:** See Rule Out MI Protocol, p. 209.
        c. **Rx:** Emergency cardiology or medicine consult.
            1) **Reduce cardiac work:**
                a) **But beware low BP** if carotid dz, renovascular dz, aortic stenosis, RV infarct, big anterior MI, tamponade.
                b) **Nitroglycerine:** SL and IV to increase coronary perfusion.
                c) **Beta-blocker:** IV metoprolol.
                    i. **Loading metoprolol:** 5 mg IVP over 2 min × 3 doses to lower heart rate, while SBP >100, HR >50, PR <0.24. Then 50 bid, and titrate up, with hold parameters.
                    ii. **Beware of PO BP drugs** that cannot reverse fast.
                    iii. **Use cautiously** in COPD, CHF, inferoposterior or big anterior MI.
                d) **Morphine:** 2-5 mg IV. Reduces pain, preload. Watch BP.
            2) **Treat clot:** Have pt. chew aspirin, IV heparin; consider lysis, angioplasty, bypass.
                a) **Heparin:** For unstable angina, ST depressions, or chest pain with a baseline BBB.
                b) **Consider thrombolysis:** For ST elevations. <u>Absolute contraindications</u> = recent surgery, stroke, GI or brain bleed.
    2. **Complications of MI:**
        a. **Arrhythmias:** Cardiac monitor.
        b. **Hypotension:** Suspect right ventricle infarct in anyone with hypotension during an inferoposterior MI.
        c. **Congestive heart failure:** See p. 210.
    3. **Rule Out MI Protocol:**
        a. **Cardiology consult.**
        b. **Drugs:** Aspirin, heparin SC or IV (for unstable angina, needs several days of heparin to cool off), O_2, IV access, colace, sucralfate,

nitropaste q4h (see Admission Orders, p. 13, for doses; adjust if carotid dz or longstanding HTN).

c. Labs: CPK/troponin q8min × 3, profile 7, PTT (bid if IV hep), Ca/Mg/phos, CBC, LFTs, lipids, drug levels, EKG qAM × 3; consider echocardiogram, ETT with thallium (make pt. NPO after midnight) or Persantine- or adenosine-thallium scan (no caffeine or theophylline before scan).

d. Orders: Bed rest, check orthostatic BP, guaiac stools, I/Os, daily wts, low-salt and low-cholesterol diet, cardiac monitor (pt. may travel without), old chart to floor quickly.

4. Chest pain orders: Check vitals, EKG during pain, nitroglycerine SL q5min × 3 if SBP >90, O_2 2 L/min, call resident, post-pain EKG. Consider Mylanta, morphine.

G. Preoperative cardiac evaluation: If pt. has any of the following CAD markers, consider pre-op cardiology consult: Age >70, prior angina or MI, prior CHF or ventricular arrhythmia, DM, positive stress test.

H. Congestive heart failure (CHF):
  1. Systolic failure:
   a. H&P: Ask about SOB, check rales, JVP, edema.
   b. DDx: Lung dz, noncardiac edema.
   c. Rx: Goal = decreased preload.
     1) Acute: Sit pt. up with legs dangling. Oxygen, morphine 2-5 mg IV, nitroglycerine SL or IV, furosemide 40 mg IV.
     2) Severe: Consider digoxin, CPAP (helps LV pump, but bad if preload is low), dobutamine, intubation.
     3) Orders: R/O MI orders, fluid restrict, low salt, daily weights.
     4) Labs: Digoxin level, repeat K and CXR after diuretics, consider echocardiogram.
     5) Drugs: Digoxin, furosemide, captopril (or isosorbide dinitrate + hydralazine).
   d. Diastolic dysfunction: Goal is maintained preload, decreased afterload, and decreased contractility. Nitrates and diuretics are okay acutely, but try verapamil long term.

I. Blood pressure:
  1. Hypertension:
   a. Causes: MI, stroke, cerebral bleed, drug withdrawal or overdose, renal, endocrine, anxiety, aortic dissection or coarct, eclampsia.
   b. Hypertensive crisis: Usually DBP >130 or SBP >250, with evidence of end-organ damage: heart, brain, renal, fundi.
     1) Rx: Arterial line + IV nitroprusside or labetalol. See p. 172.
       a) Contraindications to Nipride: Cerebral edema or coronary ischemia.
       b) Avoid: SL nifedipine, which can drop BP too fast.
     2) Time course: Decrease BP gradually, by 25% in the following intervals:
       a) If cerebral hemorrhage, in 6-12 h.
       b) If papilledema, in 3-6 h.
       c) If CHF, LV failure, dissection, in 15 min.

   c. **Antihypertensive drugs:** Consider nifedipine 10 mg SL (danger
      of hypotension), or metoprolol 50 mg PO. For IV blood pressure
      control, see p. 172.
      1) **Aortic aneurysm:** <u>Use</u> labetolol (lowers HR as well as BP)
         unless there is CHF.
      2) **CHF:** <u>Use</u> ACE-I, diuretics, α_1-blockers. <u>Avoid</u> β-blockers,
         diltiazem, verapamil.
      3) **CAD:** <u>Use</u> β-blockers, Ca channel blockers, ACE-I. <u>Avoid</u>
         diuretics, hydralazine.
      4) **Cerebral bleed or stroke:** <u>Use</u> β-blockers, then α-blockers,
         then ACE-I.
      5) **COPD:** <u>Use</u> Ca blockers, ACE-I, diuretics. <u>Avoid</u> β-blockers.
      6) **DM:** <u>Use</u> ACE-I, α_1-blockers, Ca blockers. <u>Avoid</u> β-blockers,
         diuretics.
      7) **Diastolic dysfunction:** <u>Use</u> β-blockers or Ca blockers.
      8) **Heart block/bradycardia:** <u>Avoid</u> β-blockers, verapamil.
      9) **Hyperlipidemia:** <u>Use</u> α_1-blockers, Ca blockers. <u>Avoid</u>
         β-blockers, diuretics except indapamide.
      10) **Peripheral vascular dz:** <u>Use</u> Ca blockers, ACE-I, diuretics.
         <u>Avoid</u> β-blockers.
      11) **Renal failure:** <u>Use</u> loop diuretics, Ca blockers, ACE-I (espe-
         cially for DM or nephrotic syndrome, but use very cautiously).
         <u>Avoid</u> β-blockers, K-sparing diuretics.
      12) **Sexual dysfunction:** <u>Use</u> ACE-I, Ca blockers. <u>Avoid</u> β-blockers,
         central α-blockers, diuretics.
2. **Hypotension:**
   a. **Causes:** Heart rate, pump, or volume problem: drug effect, blood loss,
      dehydration, sepsis, third-spacing, adrenal insufficiency, tension PTX.
   b. **Tests:** EKG, ABG, orthostatics, chem. 20, cultures, CXR.
   c. **Rx:**
      1) **Trendelenburg position:** Head of bed down 10 degrees. Of
         short-term benefit only; increases risk of aspiration.
      2) **If bradycardic:** Correct rate before giving fluid or pressor.
      3) **Normal saline IV:** Be careful if CHF.
      4) **Hold offending drugs.**
      5) **Blood:** For volume (be careful if CHF).
      6) **Oxygen:** Especially if anemic (be careful if COPD, because of
         risk of CO_2 retention).
      7) **Take cultures:** If febrile.
      8) **Pressors:** Oral rx: fludrocortisone 0.1 mg qd or midodrine
         10 mg tid. For IV pressors, see p. 172.
J. **Cholesterol emboli syndrome:**
   1. **Causes:** Often after arterial catheterization, vascular surgery.
   2. **Sx:** Necrotic foot lesions, conjunctival petechiae, renal failure, depres-
      sion and dementia, nausea and anorexia.
   3. **Rx:** Symptomatic.
K. **Pulmonary artery catheter** (Swann-Ganz catheter):
   1. **Alternatives:** Green dye cardiac output (requires arterial line and cen-
      tral line); noninvasive cardiac output (NICO) monitor, echocardiogra-
      phy, a better physical exam. . . .

2. **Indications:** Note there is no evidence that Swanns improve outcome. They may worsen it. They are useful for telling cause of shock (e.g., septic vs. cardiogenic); cause of pulmonary edema (e.g., cardiogenic vs. increased permeability); monitoring the effects of fluids, inotropes, pressors, afterload agents, and vasodilators; and optimizing oxygen transport.

3. **Relative contraindications:** Coagulopathy, thrombocytopenia, endocardial pacemaker, severe pulmonary hypertension, ventricular arrhythmias, left bundle branch block (have external pacer ready in case of complete heart block), prosthetic right heart valve.

4. **Complications:** Include these risks on the consent form.
   a. **During puncture:** Arterial puncture, pneumo- or hemothorax, air embolism, nerve injury, thrombosis.
   b. **During advancement of catheter:** Arrhythmias, cardiac perforation and tamponade, bundle branch block.
   c. **During maintenance of catheter:** <u>Pulmonary artery rupture</u>, mural thrombus, infection, valve damage, pulmonary infarction.

5. **Normal values:**
   a. **CVP:** Central venous pressure, 5-8 mm Hg.
   b. **RA:** Right atrial pressure, 0-8 mm Hg.
   c. **RV:** Right ventricular pressure, (15-30)/(0-4) mm Hg.
   d. **PA:** Pulmonary artery pressure, (15-30)/(6-12) mm Hg.
   e. **PCWP:** Pulmonary capillary wedge pressure, 1-10 mm Hg.
   f. **LVP:** Left ventricular pressure, (100-140)/(3-12) mm Hg.
   g. **CO:** Cardiac output, 4-8 L/min ($=$ HR $\times$ stroke volume).
   h. **CI:** Cardiac index, 2.5-4.2 $L/min/m^2$.
   i. **SVR:** Systemic vascular resistance, 770-1500 $dynes/sec/cm^5$.
   j. **PVR:** Pulmonary vascular resistance, 20-120 $dynes/sec/cm^5$.
   k. **MAP:** Mean art. pressure, 70-105 mm Hg $= 1/3$ (SBP $-$ DBP) $+$ DBP.

INFECTION

A. **See also:** CNS Infections, p. 54.

B. **Fever workup:**
   1. **H&P:** Pain, cough, shortness of breath, dysuria, diarrhea, new drugs. Vital signs; lung, cardiac, abdomen, mouth, skin, fundi.
   2. **Tests:** CBC, UA, urine culture, CXR; consider sputum culture, stool culture for *C. difficile*, wound culture, line tip culture throat swab, LP, shunt tap, ascites tap, induced sputum for TB, HIV test, echocardiogram. . . . Drug fever and tumor fever $=$ dx of exclusion.
      a. **Blood cultures:** If T $>101.5°F$. If pt. has a central line, draw one off each port and one peripherally.
      b. **LP:** If neurological signs, encephalopathy, severe HA, meningismus, recent brain trauma, or surgery. See Lumbar Puncture, p. 224; Cerebrospinal Fluid, p. 19.

C. **Infection precautions:** Refer to institutional policies for specifics. These lists are not complete.
   1. **Contact:** For pts. with certain skin and enteric infections.

      a. **Use:** Hand hygiene, glove, gown, dedicated equipment, private room or coinfected roommate.

      b. **Agents:** Methicillin-resistant *S. aureus* (MRSA), vancomycin-resistant *Enterococcus* (VRE), chickenpox or disseminated VZV, *C. difficile*, others.

  2. **Droplet:** Spread by large respiratory droplets when the pt. coughs, sneezes, talks.

      a. **Use:** Hand hygiene, disposable surgical mask when within 3 feet of pt., private room.

      b. **Agents:** Meningococcal infection, *H. influenzae* meningitis or respiratory infection, *Mycoplasma* pneumonia, rubella.

  3. **Airborne:** Spread by small droplets when the pt. breathes.

      a. **Use:** Hand hygiene, fitted respirator, isolation room with negative pressure. Nonimmune personnel should avoid exposure to patient if possible.

      b. **Agents:** Tuberculosis, chickenpox or disseminated VZV, measles, SARS, avian flu.

  4. **Neutropenic precautions:** If absolute neutrophil count <500 (where ANC = WBC × %PMNs).

      a. **Inpts need:** Positive pressure rooms to avoid infection, contact and droplet precautions, bleeding precautions if platelets <20, nystatin swish and swallow 10 cc qid.

      b. **Agents:** HIV, bone marrow transplants, chemotherapy. . . .

      c. **Infection and neutropenia:** Does an HIV pt. with TB get a positive pressure room inside a negative pressure room?

D. Human immunodeficiency virus (HIV): See also neurological consequences of HIV, p. 227.

  1. **Protease inhibitors:** Agenerase = amprenavir, Crixivan = indinavir, Invirase = saquinavir, Kaletra = lopinavir/ritonavir, Norvir = ritonavir, Viracept = nelfinavir.

  2. **NRTIs:** Nucleoside reverse transcriptase inhibitors. They may cause distal symmetric peripheral polyneuropathy. Hivid = ddC (zalcitabine), Videx = DDI (didanosine), Zerit = D4T (stavudine).

  3. **NNRTIs:** Nonnucleoside reverse transcriptase inhibitors. Epivir = 3TC (lamivudine), Rescriptor = delavirdine, Retrovir = AZT (zidovudine), Sustiva = efavirenz, Viramune = nevirapine.

  4. **Secondary infections:** Bacterial, pneumocystis, toxoplasmosis, fungal, mycobacterial, viral (PML, CMV, HSV, VZV), syphilis. . . .

      a. **Prophylactic Abx:** Pts. should get azithromycin for *Mycobacterium avium* when CD4 <50, Bactrim for pneumocystis and toxoplasmosis when <200 and toxoplasmosis when <100, itraconazole for histoplasmosis in endemic areas when <100.

  5. **Secondary neoplasms:** Kaposi's sarcoma; lymphoma.

E. Antibiotic recommendations for adults: See also Abx resistance tables, p. 215. These are rough guidelines only. Revise Abx when culture data become available. Except when you must give Abx immediately, make sure all cultures have been taken before starting Abx. Not all febrile pts. need Abx.

Suspected Cause	First Choice
Community-Acquired Pneumonia	
H. flu, M. catarr. or unclear	Ceftriaxone IV ± macrolide
Aspiration/oral flora	Penicillin IV ± metronidazole
Strep. pneumoniae	Penicillin IV
Staph. aureus	Nafcillin
GNR, or recent hospital stay	Ceftriaxone or cefepime ± metronidazole
Sepsis Syndrome	
Intra-abdominal/pelvic source	Ampicillin + metronidazole + levofloxacin
Urosepsis	Ampicillin + gentamicin
Unknown source	Vancomycin + ceftriaxone + metronidazole
Neutropenic host with fever	Cefepime
Acute Bacterial Meningitis	
Immunocompetent host	Ceftriaxone + vancomycin
Immunocompromised host	Ceftriaxone + ampicillin + vancomycin
IVDA, head trauma/surgery	Nafcillin + [ceftriaxone or ceftazidime]
Skin and Soft Tissue Infection	
No underlying dz	Nafcillin or cefazolin
Underlying dz (DM, IVDA...)	Ampicillin-sulbactam or piperacillin-tazobactam
Urinary Tract Infection	
Patients who need IV Abx	Ampicillin + gentamicin
Acute Septic Arthritis	
No underlying disease	Nafcillin or cefazolin
Prosthetic joint	Vancomycin + gentamicin
Likely gonorrhea	Ceftriaxone

Table 56. Empiric antibiotic recommendations. (MGH data, 2005. These guidelines are not useful outside the USA. Courtesy of David Hooper, MD.)

F. Remove foreign bodies: Change central lines, consider removal of bladder catheter, ventricular shunt. . . .
G. Control fever: E.g., with acetaminophen; consider cooling blanket. Fever can worsen infarct size, strain the heart, and cause dehydration.
H. Fever and neutropenia: See Neutropenic precautions, p. 213.

KIDNEYS

A. H&P: Fluid intake, drugs (include NSAIDs), urine output, pain. Cardiac exam, kidney tenderness, palpable bladder, edema.
B. Neurological complications of kidney failure:
   1. Uremic encephalopathy:
      a. H&P: Renal dz ± precipitating illness, with obtundation or agitation, myoclonus, asterixis, generalized seizures in 30%.
      b. DDx: Malignant HTN, dialysis disequilibrium syndrome, stroke.

	Ampicillin	Piper–tazo	Cefazolin	Cefriaxone	Cefepime	Aztreonam	Meropenem	Gentamicin	Amikacin	Ciprofloxacin	TMP–SMX	Chloramphen	Tetracycline	Nitrofurant
Acinetobacter	0	66	0	0	39	-	74	46	81	43	58	-	45	0
Aeromonas	0	90	0	93	100	100	100	100	100	97	97	-	-	-
Citro. freundii	0	85	0	83	99	84	99	93	99	86	85	-	79	99
Citro. keseri	0	99	91	97	100	95	100	99	100	96	98	-	100	95
Ent. aerogenes	0	84	0	93	100	91	100	98	100	91	98	-	88	38
Ent. cloacae	0	72	0	75	97	74	100	91	99	83	84	-	73	51
E. coli	59	97	92	99	99	99	100	93	100	88	76	-	73	99
H. influenzae	72	-	-	100	-	-	-	-	-	-	77	97	-	-
Klebs. pneumo.	0	85	81	84	84	84	100	87	94	80	79	-	78	54
Klebs. oxytoca	0	90	67	93	93	92	100	93	98	92	94	-	89	93
Mo. morganii	0	97	0	97	100	91	100	92	100	91	87	-	57	11
Pr. mirabilis	81	96	97	100	100	99	100	95	100	84	87	-	0	0
Pr. vulgaris	0	97	0	84	100	92	100	100	100	100	97	-	36	5
Ps. aeruginosa	-	91	-	-	86	70	86	72	77	66	-	-	-	-
Salmonella	90	97	-	98	100	98	100	-	-	100	98	-	91	-
Se. marcescens	0	94	0	94	98	94	100	95	99	93	94	-	15	-
Shigella	62	96	-	96	100	100	100	-	-	96	46	-	24	-

Table 57. Gram-negative susceptibilities (%). (MGH data 2005; courtesy of D. Hooper, MD.)

	Penicillin	Oxacillin	Cephalothin c	Vancomycin	Clindamycin	Erythromycin	Tetracycline	Chloramphen	TMP–SMX	Levofloxacin	Rifampin	Linezolid	Nitrofurant.	Gentamicin
Staph. aureus	11	54	54	100	66	37	93	-	96	57	98	100	100	97
Coag-neg. Staph.	14	39	39	100	63	35	86	-	58	49	96	99	100	81
S. saprophyticus	-	-	-	100	89	48	86	-	97	99	100	100	100	100
S. lugdunensis	70	100	-	100	91	87	94	-	100	100	100	100	100	100
Strep. pneumo.	68	-	-	100	86	70	79	97	79	100	-	-	-	-
a-hemol. Strep.	62	-	-	100	85	56	62	-	-	93	-	-	-	-
Grp A b- Strep.	100	-	100	100	95	87	69	-	-	100	-	-	-	-
Grp B b- Strep.	100	-	100	100	86	73	13	-	-	100	-	-	-	-
Grp C, G b- Strep	100	-	100	100	94	76	44	-	-	100	-	-	-	-
S. anginosus	99	-	-	100	84	80	73	-	-	100	-	-	-	-
Enterococci	78	-	-	80	-	18	28	90	-	56	29	99	88	-
E. faecalis	100	-	-	91	-	18	27	85	-	63	41	100	100	-
E. faecium	8	-	-	13	-	2	31	97	-	4	11	94	48	-

Table 58. Gram-positive susceptibilities (%). (MGH data 2005; courtesy D. Hooper, MD.)

    c. **Rx:** Treat renal failure; seizures. DPH and levetiracetam need renal dosing (see p. 163). Although phenobarbital is excreted by kidneys, levels are unaffected by renal failure unless GFR <10.

  2. Dialysis disequilibrium syndrome: Acutely during or after dialysis, with headache, muscle cramps, confusion, seizures, or coma. Probably caused by cerebral edema.

  3. Dialysis dementia syndrome: Subacute memory loss, personality change, apraxia, dysarthria, myoclonus, seizures. EEG shows bursts of slowing and spikes.

C. Hematuria workup: Stop anticoagulants, change bladder catheter, consider irrigation, renal ultrasound, cystoscopy, antineutrophil cytoplasmic Ab (ANCA), antiglomerular basement membrane antibody.

D. Causes of acute renal failure:
  1. Prerenal: Hypovolemia or hypotension from dehydration, sepsis, bleed, or heart failure; liver failure.
  2. Renal:
    a. **Acute tubular necrosis (ATN):** From ischemia, toxins, radiocontrast agents, hemo- or myoglobinuria.
    b. **Acute tubulointerstitial nephritis:** From drug reaction, pyelonephritis, papillary necrosis.
    c. **Intrarenal precipitation:** Calcium, urates, myeloma protein.
    d. **Other:** Glomerulonephritis, DIC with cortical necrosis, arterial or venous obstruction.
  3. Postrenal: Obstruction from prostatism, tumor, or stones.

E. Tests:
  1. Blood: BUN, creatinine, electrolytes, Ca, Mg, phos, CBC, CPK.
  2. Urine: UA, sediment, culture, urine eosinophils, urine electrolytes after 6 h off diuretics (or test urine urea nitrogen if on diuretics).
  3. FENa: Fractional excretion of sodium. Not helpful in nonoliguric acute tubular necrosis.
    a. **FENa** = $100 \times (UNa \times SCr)/(SNa \times UCr)$; all in mg/dL.
    b. **Causes of low FENa:** Dehydration, Na-avid renal failure, cirrhosis, nephrotic syndrome, CHF, glomerulonephritis, oliguric contrast-induced renal failure.
    c. **Causes of high FENa:** Recent diuretics; renal failure.

	Prerenal	ATN
BUN	Up	Up
Serum Cr	~nl	Up
BUN/S Cr	>20	nl
Urine Na	<20	>40
U Cr/S Cr	>40	<20
Urine osms	>500	<350
FeNa	<1	>2
IV fluid helps?	Yes	No

Table 59. Prerenal kidney failure vs. acute tubular necrosis (ATN).

4. **24-h urine** for protein and creatinine in chronic renal failure.
   a. **Creatinine clearance** = [urine Cr (mg/dL)][vol (mL)]/{[serum Cr (mg/dL)][time (min)]}
   b. **Estimated creatinine clearance:** Inaccurate if Cr changing.
      1) **Male** = $(140 - age)(wt in kg)/(72 \times serum Cr)$
      2) **Female** = $0.85 \times male$
5. **Other tests:** Consider renal ultrasound, renal scan, glomerulonephritis workup.

F. Orders: Renal diet (<60 g protein, 2 g Na, K) unless on dialysis, when need protein supplements. Strict I/O, bladder catheter, daily wts.
1. **Stop nephrotoxins:** Gentamicin, ACE-I, NSAIDs; renally dose cimetidine and Abx.
   a. **NSAIDs** can lower Na, increase K, cause proteinuria, acute interstitial nephritis.
   b. **Gentamicin:** Pts. on dialysis can have gentamicin; redose after each dialysis.
2. **IV fluids:** If dehydrated.
3. **Diuretics:** If oliguric. Furosemide IV; consider adding chlorothiazide or mannitol. Follow I/Os q1h. Hold diuretics if pt. has no response, or furosemide level will build up and cause ototoxicity.
4. **Chronic renal failure:** Nephrocaps or equivalent vitamin supplementation 1 qd; aluminum hydroxide Amphogel 30 cc qid (avoid Mg compounds), calcium acetate (PhosLo) 1–2 tabs. Consider erythropoietin, iron, calcium, vit D, bicarb (600–1,200 mg PO bid).

LUNGS

A. Blood gases:
1. **A-a gradient:** Alveolar-to-arterial difference in oxygen tension. Lowered by diffusion defects, R-L shunts (these do not correct on 100% O_2), ventilation-perfusion (V/Q) mismatch.
   a. **Definitions:** PA O_2 = alveolar oxygen tension, PaO_2 = arterial oxygen tension, pCO_2 = arterial carbon dioxide tension, FiO_2 = fractional concentration of oxygen in inspired gas, RQ = respiratory quotient = ratio of CO_2 out to O_2 in (normally 0.8).
   b. **A-a** = $PAO_2 - PaO_2$. Normal = 3–16 mm Hg.
      1) **Age correction:** A-a should be $< 2.5 + 0.25$ (age). If pt. <30 years old, A-a should be <8 mm Hg.
   c. **PAO_2** = (FiO_2)(barom. − water vapor pressure) – pCO_2/RQ, so: $PAO_2 = (FiO_2)(713) – pCO_2/0.8$
      1) **On room air:** $(FiO_2)(713) = 143$; nl $PAO_2 = 100$ mm Hg.
      2) **On 100% ventilation:** nl $PAO_2 = 673$ mm Hg. This does not apply to 100% oxygen by face mask.
      3) **PaO_2 >70** gives full hemoglobin saturation.
   d. **FiO_2** increase of 10% adds 5 to PaO_2.
2. **Respiratory effects on pH:** See also Electrolytes, p. 194.
   a. **High pH:** Suggests hyperventilation. Rule out CHF, PTX, PE.
   b. **Normal pH + high pCO_2:** Suggests chronic CO_2 retention.
   c. **Low pH:** Suggests acute hypoxia or sepsis.

B. Acute dyspnea or hypoxia:

1. **H&P:** Check VS, temperature, alertness, respiratory rate and pattern, listen to lungs, heart; assess jugular distension, ankle swelling, ask about pleuritic pain.

2. **DDx:** Pulmonary edema (cardiac, vasogenic, neurogenic), COPD, MI, PE, PTX, effusion, upper airway obstruction, lung hemorrhage, hypoventilation from drugs or CNS problem, hyperventilation from acidosis or anxiety.

3. **Tests:**
   a. **Blood gas:** On room air if possible. See above for interpretation. Hct performed on blood gas is sometimes inaccurate.
   b. **D-dimer:** Will be high in PE, but very nonspecific.
   c. **Portable CXR.**
   d. **EKG:** Look for ischemia; signs of PE (see below).
   e. **Lung scan:** Consider PE-CT, V/Q scan (if CXR clear), or Pagram plus possible IVC filter placement.

4. **Rx:** "L-M-N-O-P": Lasix, Morphine, Nitrates, Oxygen, and Posture. Avoid low BP, especially in pts. with cerebrovascular dz.
   a. **Lasix:** For exacerbation of chronic CHF, but <u>not</u> for flash pulmonary edema.
   b. **Morphine:** For hyperventilation in pain and decreased preload in CHF. Beware of somnolence.
   c. **Nitrates:** For pulmonary edema and cardiac ischemia.
   d. **Oxygen:** Avoid causing CO_2 retention in COPD. Consider mechanical ventilation (see p. 220).
   e. **Posture:** Have pt. sit up, with legs dangling.
   f. **Benzodiazepines:** For anxiety. They can help prevent breath stacking in COPD, but beware of somnolence. If quaaludes were still used for anxiety, the mnemonic could have been L-M-N- O-P-Q.

C. COPD flare:

1. **H&P:** Baseline FEV_1 (see PFTs, p. 219), functional limitations, pack-years of smoking, home oxygen, previous intubations. Lung and heart exam.

2. **DDx:** See Acute dyspnea (see above).

3. **Tests:** ABG, CXR, EKG, K, Mg, CBC, theophylline level. Sputum for gram stain, culture. If suspect TB: PPD, sputum for AFB × 3. Consider sputum for cytology × 3.

4. **Drugs:** Write order for inhalers, not nebulizers, if pt. intubated.
   a. **Albuterol** nebulizer 0.5 cc in 2.5 cc NS q2-4h.
   b. **Ipratropium** inhaler 2 puffs qid or glycopyrrolate nebulizer 0.8 cc in 2.5 cc NS q6-8h.
   c. **Methylprednisolone:** 60 mg IV q6h, then taper (eventually switch to inhaled steroids). Ranitidine or sucralfate while on steroids.
   d. **Empiric Abx:** If signs of airway infection, e.g., increased mucus, fever, etc. See Infection, p. 212.

5. **Other orders:** Guaiac stools if on steroids. Chest physical therapy. Check peak flow.

D. Lung mass workup: Chest CT through the adrenals; consider needle biopsy or bronchoscopy.

E. Pulmonary function tests (PFTs):

	COPD	Restric-tive	Neuro-muscular
TLC (total lung capacity)	↑	↓	~
RV (residual volume)	↑	↓	~
FRC (functional residual capacity)	↑	↓	~
VC (vital capacity)	~↓	↓	↓
FEV$_1$ (forced exp. vol. in 1sec)	↓	~↑	~
MIP (mean inspiratory pressure)	~	~	↓
MEP (mean expiratory pressure)	~	~	↓

Table 60. Pulmonary function tests.

F. **Pulmonary embolus (PE):**
 1. **Risk factors:** Trauma, surgery, prior PE, bed rest, cancer, CHF, hyper-coagulable states, oral contraceptives.
 2. **Prophylaxis:** If not already anticoagulated. Heparin 5000 U SQ bid-tid or enoxaparin 40 mg SQ qd for low risk, 30 mg SQ bid for high risk, and pneumo-boots. If pt. has been in bed more than 24 h, check venous ultrasound before starting boots.
 3. **H&P:** Dyspnea, anxiety, tachycardia, pleuritic pain, cough.
 4. **DDx of PE:**
    a. **Small PE:** Pneumothorax, hyperventilation, asthma, MI, CHF, serositis.
    b. **Big PE:** RV infarct, tamponade, air embolism.
 5. **Tests:**
    a. **General labs:** ABG, D-dimer often high if recent trauma or surgery (low D-dimer is highly specific; high D-dimer is not), CXR.
    b. **EKG:** Often see only sinus tachycardia. See also Electrocardiogram, p. 207.
    c. **Venous ultrasounds (LENIs):** 97% sensitive for thrombus above the knee, 80% below. Not good for pelvic clots.
    d. **Ventilation-perfusion (V/Q) scan:** Consider going straight to pulmonary angiogram if high risk. V/Q scan may be useless if CXR is abnormal or there has been a previous PE.
    e. **Pulmonary angiogram:** Pulmonary HTN and renal failure are relative contraindications.
 6. **Rx of PE:**
    a. **Heparin:** (Unless contraindication, e.g., recent brain surgery) With bolus, for 5-7 days, then warfarin, or SQ heparin bid for at least 3 months, or longer if idiopathic or recurrent.
    b. **Thrombolyse:** If life-threatening PE.
    c. **Inferior vena cava filter:** For recurrent PE or pt. who cannot be anticoagulated.
G. **Stridor or laryngeal edema:** See Allergy, p. 191.
H. **Ventilators and oxygen delivery:**
 1. **Nonendotracheal oxygen delivery systems:**
    a. **Passive ventilation:** Nasal cannula, face mask or face tent, 100% nonrebreather.

    b. Partially assisted ventilation:
       1) Continuous positive airway pressure (CPAP): Indications: sleep apnea, or to keep alveoli open in COPD.
       2) Biphasic positive airway pressure (BIPAP): AKA intermittent positive pressure breathing. Indications: chronic neuromuscular dz; not great for COPD.
2. Endotracheal intubation: Call anesthesia, respiratory therapy.
    a. Indications: To maintain oxygenation or ventilation, protect airway or manage secretions, or to allow adequate sedation.
    Remember that intubation makes it hard to follow pts. neuro exam.
    b. Anesthetics for intubation: Most wear off fast, but neurological abnormalities may linger longer. See p. 158 and 173.
    c. Stat CXR after intubation: Endotracheal (ET) tube should be below thoracic inlet and >2 cm above carina. Check CXR daily.
3. Ventilator setting orders: Specify FiO_2, TV, IMV, PEEP, PS, and type of oxygen monitoring (e.g., continuous saturation monitor).
    a. Typical ventilator settings:
       1) Oxygen (FiO_2): 40% (start at 100%).
       2) Tidal volume (TV): 600-800 cc (7-10 cc/kg). More if COPD, less if restrictive lung dz.
       3) Respiratory rate (RR): 8-12. Less if COPD, more if restrictive dz.
       4) Positive end expiratory pressure (PEEP): Start at 5.
       5) Pressure support (PS): 10-15. PS ~8 just overcomes resistance of ET tube.
4. Ventilator modes:
    a. Intermittent mandatory ventilation (IMV, SIMV): For pts. without adequate spontaneous minute ventilation. Specify RR and TV. Can be used with backup pressure support for pts. spontaneous breaths.
    b. Pressure support (PS, PSV): For pts. with adequate spontaneous respiratory drive. Specify PS only; adjust so that TV is 7-10 cc/kg. Mode has apnea alarm so pt. will get a backup IMV breath if necessary.
    c. Pressure control (PC, PCV): For severe COPD, adult respiratory distress syndrome. Set RR, insp. pressure, and insp. time. It is like PS, but maintains a minimum RR. Pt. usually needs sedation and paralysis to tolerate PC.
5. Changing ventilator settings: In some hospitals, only respiratory technicians are allowed to do this.
    a. Ventilation increases (and thus pCO_2 decreases) with increased PS, TV, RR.
    b. Oxygenation increases with increased PEEP, FiO_2, or insp. time unless there is a significant pulmonary or cardiac shunt).
       1) To follow oxygenation across different FiO_2: Use pO_2/FiO_2 as index. Normal = $100/0.2 = 500$.
    c. PEEP vs. PS: PEEP is like CPAP, PEEP + PS is like BIPAP.
6. Ventilator complications:
    a. Infection: Most pts. get colonized; do not treat presence of bacteria in sputum with Abx unless abundant PMNs in sputum, fever, high WBC, or copious secretions.

    b. Tracheal stenosis: Associated with prolonged intubation. Generally plan tracheostomy after 21 days.

    c. Oxygen toxicity: Try to keep FiO_2 below 50%.

    d. Gastric distension: From ET tube leak. Place NG tube.

    e. Blood pressure changes: High intrathoracic pressure lowers BP.

        1) Intubation: Treat with IV fluids but remember to diurese pt. at extubation to avoid fluid overload.

        2) COPD: Inadequate exhalation (breath stacking) causes auto-PEEP and may be helped by decreasing RR.

    f. Barotrauma: From high peak inspiratory pressure.

    g. Pneumothorax.

7. Extubating:

    a. Criteria: Pt. on room air, PEEP (= CPAP) 5, no IMV, should have RR <30, few secretions, PIP <40, normal blood gas.

    b. Preparation: Empty stomach. HOB 45 degrees. Tell the respiratory technician. Extubate to 100% O_2, continuous O_2 sat monitor. Watch for laryngeal edema (see p. 191).

8. Tracheostomy wean: Consult anesthesia or surgery, speech path.

    a. Indications: Pt. can tolerate breathing off the ventilator, and no need for frequent suctioning.

    b. Methylene blue test: Put dye in tube feeds to r/o aspiration.

    c. Tracheostomy types: Usually pts. first trach is an 8 Portex tube, sutured. This may later change to a 4 cuffless Shiley tube with Passy-Muir valve. Consider a fenestrated tracheostomy.

I. Button tracheostomy: If pt. tolerates the tracheostomy wean. If there is no need for suctioning, you may eventually decannulate.

PROCEDURES

PROCEDURE NOTE

A. Should contain: Indication; consent; sterile preparation; anesthesia; findings; labs sent; pts. tolerance.

ARTERIAL BLOOD GAS

A. Need: ABG kit, optional Xylocaine + TB needle, lab slips.
B. Procedure: Expel gas from syringe, extend pt's wrist, iodine prep, inject Xylocaine, have gauze within reach, feel pulse, bevel up, impale artery vertically, let syringe fill 1-2 cc. Expel air bubbles, cap it, label it, put on ice, and send immediately.
C. Results: Hct and K values vary from that done in a heparinized tube.

ARTERIAL LINE

A. Consent: Bleeding, infection, thrombosis, nerve damage.
B. Need: Mask, Xylocaine and TB needle, 20-gauge 1¼; inch angio-catheters, heparinized saline hookup or flush and plug, wire, sterile towels or small sheet, wrist board with gauze roll wrapped in chuck, thick adhesive tape, iodine, sterile 4 × 4 gauze 10-pack, sterile gloves, 3-0 suture.
C. Check for ulnar-radial anastomosis: First check ulnar pulse. Have pt. make a fist; press on radial artery, open hand. Whole hand should turn pink, not just ulnar side.
D. Setup: Tape wrist, slightly hyperextended, to board, perhaps to bed too. Prep arm, sterile drape, flush catheter tip with heparinized saline, put on gloves, anesthetize wrist, unwrap wire.
E. Stick: Impale artery bevel up, at 45 degrees, flatten angiocath somewhat. When blood spurts out, thread wire, remove needle, and advance catheter.
F. Secure: If flow looks good, remove wire, connect catheter to transducer; suture catheter, cover with clear plastic dressing.
G. Removal: Hard hand pressure for 5 min; check for continued bleeding.

BLOOD DRAWS

A. Electrolytes: Green top (heparinized) or tiger top (serum separator).
B. CBC, blood bank: Lavender top (EDTA as anticoagulant)
C. General chemistries: Red top (plain, allows clotting).
D. PT/PTT: Blue top (citrate). Test is not accurate if tube not filled.
E. Glucose: Grey top (K oxalate)
F. Hypercoagulability panel: Usually 4 blue tops and a large red top.

CALORIC TESTING

A. Check ears: TM perforation is contraindication. Wax can block test.
B. Tilt head: 30 degrees backward in supine position. This makes horizontal canal perpendicular to floor.

C. Instill water: Use angiocath (with needle removed). Temperature should be 7 degrees above and below body temperature: wait 5 min after each. In comatose pt., use ice water.

D. Interpretation:
   1. **Normal:** Normally start seeing nystagmus at end of infusion or within 1 min. <u>COWS</u> (<u>C</u>old <u>O</u>pposite, <u>W</u>arm <u>S</u>ame) describes normal direction of the fast component of nystagmus.
   2. **Brainstem damage:** Smaller or absent response on damaged side.
   3. **Inner ear dz:** Smaller or absent response on damaged side.
   4. **Cerebellar dz:** Fixation does not suppress nystagmus (normally does).

CENTRAL VENOUS LINE

A. See also: Venous Access, p. 226.
B. Indication: Pressors, Nipride, nitroglycerine >400 µg/min.
C. Check: PT, PTT before placing line.
D. Consent: Complications = bleeding, clot, infection, PTX, air embolus, nerve damage.
E. Need: Central line kit, 10 cc heparin 100 U/cc (<u>not</u> 1,000), sterile gloves, sterile sponges, Betadine, suture, dressing. Prepare replacement caps for all ports, sterile gown, sterile towels, mask.
F. IJ (internal jugular) vs. SC (subclavian) access: Internists like IJs because they are safer—a laceration can be compressed. Surgeons like SCLs because they are quicker. Neurologists like SCLs—they want to avoid a carotid stick, or possible obstruction to endovascular approach. And because the neck is sacred—it's the only thing that keeps the head attached to the body.
G. Preparation:
   1. **Positioning:** Clear space behind bed. Put pt. in Trendelenburg to keep air bubbles from brain. Towel roll between pts. shoulders. Tape open heparin flush bottle upside down to IV pole for easy sterile access.
   2. **Sterility:** Iodine prep from ear to sternal notch for IJ; consider prepping SCL region too. Open towels; use their drape to cover pts. abdomen. Open kit, extra gloves, sutures onto field. Drape pt. sterilely, leaving enough room to identify landmarks. Then put on sterile gloves and gown.
   3. **Needle prep:** Remove cap from brown port, for wire to go through. Do not let line touch any nonsterile surface. Place needles on syringes, line, suture, and extra gauze within reach. Xylocaine to skin. Then fill that syringe with heparin flush. Leave a few cc to suck air out of catheter.
H. Internal jugular: Easiest from right of pt.
   1. **Find vein:** Use small needle. Anesthetize. Stand on R side of pt., feel carotid, aim with syringe on small needle through the triangle between the bellies of the sternocleidomastoid to the ipsilateral nipple. Aspirate as you go in until you hit IJ and get blood.
   2. **Thread wire:** Slip syringe on larger needle (with catheter) next to the smaller one, while aspirating. Withdraw the smaller needle; withdraw

larger syringe leaving catheter in place, thread wire down catheter and tube down wire to SVC (about 15 cm). Always hold the wire with one hand.

3. **Insert line:** Remove needle from wire, cut down along wire with scalpel, insert and remove dilator. Thread line down over wire. At some point, you will need to start pushing wire back up into line. Go about 15 cm, to SVC. Remove wire. As wire passes brown port clamp, clamp it to avoid air embolus before you screw on cap. Use heparin syringe to suck air from each port and then flush port.

4. **Secure line:** Anesthetize and suture line, tying to inner holder only; then clip outer holder on. (This allows moving line without resuturing.) Suture far end too. Cover with iodine gel, gauze, Tegaderm.

5. **Check line:** Stat CXR with immediate read to check line placement (should be in superior vena cava) and r/o PTX.

I. **Subclavian:** Easiest from left of pt.

1. **Find vein:** Use medium needle. Find middle third (angle) of clavicle, start about 2 cm away, aim straight at lower edge with lidocaine needle; march down it, injecting and pulling back, until you are underneath. Insert the large needle, noting position of bevel (up). Hold needle with left hand, aspirate with right. Consider putting little finger in sternal notch as landmark. March the same way, aspirating with large needle, until you are under the clavicle; then rotate syringe so that you are parallel with clavicle and bevel is pointing down towards toes. Keep against clavicle, advance aspirating, until you are in vein.

2. **Thread wire, insert line, and secure line:** Follow IJ protocol above, but go 17 cm for L subclavian.

J. **Taking line out:**

1. **Need:** Suture removal kit, chuck, pt. in Trendelenburg position.

2. **Procedure:** Have pt. exhale slowly as you withdraw the line, to prevent air emboli.

LACERATIONS

A. **Need:** Saline, sterile bowl, kidney bowls to irrigate into, 60 cc luer lock, 20-gauge angiocath, gauze, towels, chuck, 1% lidocaine, syringe + needle, sterile gloves, suture (for skin, 5-0 or 4-0 prolene; for scalp, galea and muscle, Vicryl).

LUMBAR PUNCTURE

1. **Indications:** To rule out meningitis, hemorrhage; help diagnose carcinomatosis, demyelinating dz.

2. **Contraindications:**

   a. **Increased ICP from mass lesion:** Check for papilledema and retinal hemorrhages; CT for signs of mass effect (if there is high suspicion of meningitis, start Abx before CT or LP). Posterior fossa mass/edema.

   b. **Coagulopathy:** 2 units FFP usually brings INR to <1.5.

   c. **Obstruction to CSF flow:** Avoid LP if suspicion of mass lesion that might block spinal canal, especially in cervical/thoracic area.

   d. **Infection over area to be punctured:** Never do an LP in a pt. with fever and back pain until you have ruled out empyema with MRI.

3. **Consent:** Headache (in 10%; see LP headache, p. 53.), bleeding, infection, nerve damage.
4. **Need:** Kit, gloves × 2, chuck, povidone, alcohol, extra black-topped tubes, extra lidocaine. Best to have a working IV before LP, in case you need to give mannitol.
5. **Position:**
   a. **Lying:** Fetal position; make sure hips are even.
   b. **Sitting:** Easier, but cannot read opening pressure. Have pt. lean over a chair.
6. **Locate L3-L4 interspace** (parallel with superior iliac crest): Sterilize skin with iodine, don sterile gloves, drape, anesthetize skin, set up tubes and manometer.
7. **Advance needle** slowly with bevel up and stylet in, parallel to bed and towards the navel. Withdraw stylet frequently to check for CSF flow.
   a. **Paresthesias:** If pt. feels tingling in a leg, angle needle away from that leg.
   b. **Difficult punctures:** Especially when the interspace is tight, or when landmarks are hard to palpate, it often helps to anesthetize a larger area and then make repeated parallel penetrations, marching up or down the spine, rather than angling the needle around within one penetration. If unsuccessful at L3-4, try L4-5 and L2-3. Try it with the pt. seated. If all fails, you can order a fluoroscopically guided LP.
8. **When you get flow**, rotate needle so bevel points towards head, attach adaptor tube and then stopcock with manometer. Measure CSF pressure.
9. **Opening pressure (OP):** Normal is <200 mm water.
   a. **If OP measurement is important:** Get pt. to straighten legs before you read it.
   b. **If OP >400-500, give mannitol:** Put stylet back, leave needle in to prevent CSF leak. Take out only amount of CSF in manometer. Infuse 20% mannitol IV 0.25-0.5 g/kg over 20-30 min (usually aim for 500 cc + urine output). Recheck pressure at end of infusion; need to get it below 400 before withdrawing needle.
10. **Collect CSF specimens:** After measuring OP, screw first white-topped tube onto bottom of manometer. Remove manometer. Change tubes when they are full. Having pt. Valsalva may speed flow.
11. **Finish LP:** Reinsert stylet, withdraw needle, clean off iodine.
12. **Send specimens:** The following are possible tests—do not run all of them on everyone. Save extra CSF. See Cerebrospinal Fluid, p. 19.
    a. **Hematology:** Tubes 1 and 4 for cell count (0.5 cc each).
    b. **Chemistry:** Glucose, protein, xanthochromia (0.5 cc), HSV PCR.
       1) **Xanthochromia:** To spin it yourself, put 1 cc in centrifuge × 2 min; look at supernatant. (Do not bother if fluid is clear.)
    c. **Immunology:** Oligoclonal bands (>2.5 cc), IgG, IgM titers.
    d. **Microbiology:** (>3 cc). Culture (bacterial ± fungal), VDRL (only if serum positive or if high suspicion), antigens (*H. influenzae*; streptococcus, meningococcus, and cryptococcus), AFB stain (2.5 cc), Lyme titer. Cultures are useful if drawn less than 2 h after starting empiric Abx.
    e. **Cytology:** 2-3 cc.
    f. **Others:** Lactate + pyruvate to rule out mitochondrial dzs (covered, on ice), paraneoplastic antibodies, protein 14-3-3.

NASOGASTRIC TUBE

A. Indications: Feeding (small tube, e.g., Enteroflex), to rule out GI bleed or protect lungs from vomiting (large tube, e.g., Salem sump).

B. Contraindications: Esophageal varices.

C. Need: tube (NG tube or Enteroflex), large syringe with correct tip (Luer for Enteroflex, catheter tip for Salem sump), lubricating jelly, cup of water + straw, stethoscope, sterile saline if lavage, basin for aspirated contents, tape, benzoin, safety pin.

D. Insertion:
1. **Measure distance** between pts. nose and stomach to get idea of how far to advance it. Lubricate tip.
2. **Position pt.:** Have pt. sit completely upright, head bent forward. If pt. cooperative, give a straw and water.
3. **Push tube** straight back while pt. swallows water.
4. **To rule out GI bleed,** aspirate contents and guaiac them (acidity of stomach contents sometimes causes false-positive result), then lavage with ice-cold saline.

E. Checking placement:
1. **Feel back of mouth with finger:** Tube may curl. Watch for biters.
2. **Listen to belly:** Cover extra holes in tube with your fingers. Blow air into gut and listen with stethoscope for bubbles. Check aspirates.
3. **Secure the tube:** Tape tube to pts. nose and pin it to pt's. garment. Consider soft restraints in confused pts.
4. **Get a CXR:** This checks tube position and rules out PTX. If tube is an Enteroflex, check the CXR before pulling the wire.

F. Med orders: If drugs must now go down NG tube, stop extended-release drugs, since they cannot be ground. Write order to flush tube after all drugs. Sucralfate can clog tubes.

VENOUS ACCESS

A. Peripheral IVs:
1. **Need:** Gloves, chuck, gauze, iodine/alcohol prep, lidocaine, tourniquet, angiocatheter, extension set or plug, saline flushes in 3-cc syringes, Tegaderm, tape.
2. **Placement:** Try for the forearm; antecubital IVs pinch off when the pt. moves his arm. In pts. with poor arm veins, consider the feet and, occasionally, external jugular.

B. Percutaneously inserted central catheters (PICC lines):
1. **Indications:** For pt. who will need an IV more than 7 days or who needs central delivery of drug. Especially good for home IV therapy. You should not draw blood samples off them.
2. **Placement:** Often done by specially trained PICC nurse. Difficult ones may be done fluoroscopically.

C. Central venous neck lines (IJ, SC):
1. **Indication:** Urgent central delivery of drugs, e.g., pressors, Nipride, nitroglycerine >400 µg/min; or frequent blood draws. Consider PICC as nonemergent alternative.
2. **Placement:** See Central Venous Line, p. 223.

D. Quinton catheters: For dialysis, pheresis. Usually inserted by surgeons.

E. Hickman catheters: Surgically placed semi–long-term (e.g., several months) central access, e.g., for chemotherapy. External ports on chest.

F. Portacaths: Surgically placed long-term (e.g., years) central access, e.g., for chemotherapy. Has subcutaneous ports in chest.

G. Clogged catheters: Try urokinase: slowly instill 5,000 units.

INDEX

Page numbers followed by *f* indicate figures; those followed by *t* indicate tables.

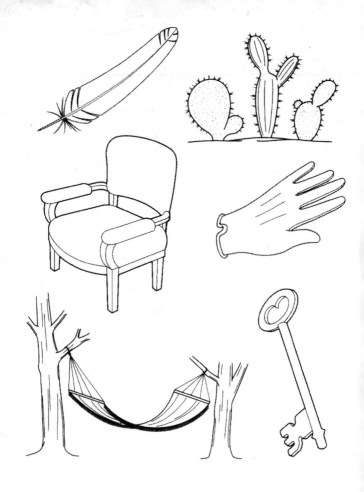

Baseball player.
I got home from work.
They heard him speak on the
radio yesterday evening.

Figure 35. Tests for anomia and alexia from the NIH Stroke Scale.